Understanding Benign Paroxysmal Positional VERTIGO

Understanding Benign Paroxysmal Positional VERTIGO

Editors
Alessandro De Stefano MD PhD
Associate Professor
Audiology and Speech Disorders Department of ASL of Lecce
Lecce, Italy

Francesco Dispenza MD PhD
Consultant of Otorhinolaryngology
UOC Otorinolaringoiatria–Azienda Universitaria
Ospedaliera Policlinico 'P Giaccone'
Palermo, Italy

Foreword
Adolfo M Bronstein

JAYPEE *The Health Sciences Publisher*
Philadelphia | New Delhi | London | Panama

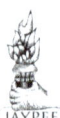 **Jaypee Brothers Medical Publishers (P) Ltd**

Headquarters
Jaypee Brothers Medical Publishers (P) Ltd.
4838/24, Ansari Road, Daryaganj
New Delhi 110 002, India
Phone: +91-11-43574357
Fax: +91-11-43574314
E-mail: jaypee@jaypeebrothers.com

Overseas Offices

J.P. Medical Ltd.
83, Victoria Street, London
SW1H 0HW (UK)
Phone: +44-20 3170 8910
Fax: +44(0)20 3008 6180
E-mail: info@jpmedpub.com

Jaypee-Highlights Medical Publishers Inc.
City of Knowledge, Bld. 235, 2nd Floor, Clayton
Panama City, Panama
Phone: +1 507-301-0496
Fax: +1 507-301-0499
E-mail: cservice@jphmedical.com

Jaypee Medical Inc.
325 Chestnut Street
Suite 412
Philadelphia, PA 19106, USA
Phone: +1 267-519-9789
E-mail: support@jpmedus.com

Jaypee Brothers Medical Publishers (P) Ltd.
17/1-B, Babar Road, Block-B, Shaymali
Mohammadpur, Dhaka-1207
Bangladesh
Mobile: +08801912003485
E-mail: jaypeedhaka@gmail.com

Jaypee Brothers Medical Publishers (P) Ltd.
Bhotahity, Kathmandu, Nepal
Phone: +977-9741283608
E-mail: kathmandu@jaypeebrothers.com

Website: www.jaypeebrothers.com
Website: www.jaypeedigital.com

© 2017, Jaypee Brothers Medical Publishers

The views and opinions expressed in this book are solely those of the original contributor(s)/author(s) and do not necessarily represent those of editor(s) of the book.

All rights reserved. No part of this publication and may be reproduced, stored or transmitted in any form or by any means, electronic, mechanical, photocopying, recording or otherwise, without the prior permission in writing of the publishers.

All brand names and product names used in this book are trade names, service marks, trademarks or registered trademarks of their respective owners. The publisher is not associated with any product or vendor mentioned in this book.

Medical knowledge and practice change constantly. This book is designed to provide accurate, authoritative information about the subject matter in question. However, readers are advised to check the most current information available on procedures included and check information from the manufacturer of each product to be administered, to verify the recommended dose, formula, method and duration of administration, adverse effects and contraindications. It is the responsibility of the practitioner to take all appropriate safety precautions. Neither the publisher nor the author(s)/editor(s) assume any liability for any injury and/or damage to persons or property arising from or related to use of material in this book.

This book is sold on the understanding that the publisher is not engaged in providing professional medical services. If such advice or services are required, the services of a competent medical professional should be sought.

Every effort has been made where necessary to contact holders of copyright to obtain permission to reproduce copyright material. If any have been inadvertently overlooked, the publisher will be pleased to make the necessary arrangements at the first opportunity.

Inquiries for bulk sales may be solicited at: jaypee@jaypeebrothers.com

Understanding Benign Paroxysmal Positional Vertigo

First Edition: 2017

ISBN: 978-93-85999-05-5

Dedication

To my wife Caterina, the greatest love of my life
To my Father and Mother for their life suggestions

Alessandro De Stefano

To my wife Vittoria and my sons Chiara and Carlo for their daily support
To my father Carlo for his teaching

Francesco Dispenza

Contributors

Mercedes FS Araújo MD MSc
Consultant
Department of Otolaryngology
University of Brasilia Medical School
Brasilia, DF, Brazil

Dimitrios G Balatsouras MD
Consultant
Department of Otolaryngology—
Head and Neck Surgery
Tzanion General Hospital
Piraeus, Greece

Ettore Bennici MD
Chief
Department of Otolaryngology
"San Giovanni di Dio" Hospital of Agrigento
Azienda Sanitaria Locale di Agrigento
Agrigento, Italy

Sebastian Bianchini MD
Consultant of Otolaryngology
"San Giovanni di Dio" Hospital of Agrigento
Azienda Sanitaria Locale di Agrigento
Agrigento, Italy

Augusto Casani MD
Associate Professor
Pisa University Medical School
Dipartimento di Patologia Chirurgica Medica, Molecolare e Area Critica
Cisanello Hospital
Pisa, Italy

Alessandro De Stefano MD PhD
Associate Professor
Audiology and Speech Disorders
Department of ASL of Lecce
Lecce, Italy

Francesco Dispenza MD PhD
Consultant of Otorhinolaryngology
UOC Otorinolaringoiatria–Azienda Universitaria
Ospedaliera Policlinico 'P Giaccone'
Palermo, Italy

Terry D Fife MD
Director
Barrow Neurological Institute
University of Arizona
College of Medicine
Phoenix, Arizona, USA

Maria Giglione MD
Consultant of Otolaryngology
"San Giovanni di Dio" Hospital of Agrigento
Azienda Sanitaria Locale di Agrigento
Agrigento, Italy

Diego Kaski MRCP PhD
Consultant of Neurology
Division of Brain Sciences
Imperial College London
London, United Kingdom

Gautham Kulamarva MS DNB DOHNS MRCS
Consultant of Otolaryngology
Kasaragod Institute of Medical Sciences (KIMS)
Kasaragod, Kerala, India

Giacinto Asprella Libonati MD
Chief
UO di Otorinolaringoiatria
Ospedale di Policoro
Matera, Italy

Salvatore Maira MD
Consultant of Otolaryngology
"San Giovanni di Dio" Hospital of Agrigento
Azienda Sanitaria Locale di Agrigento
Agrigento, Italy

Gauri Mankekar DORL MS (ENT) DNB (ENT) PhD
Consultant of Otolaryngology
Department of ENT
Hinduja Hospital
Mumbai, Maharashtra, India

Alfarghal Mohamad MD MSc AuD
Consultant of Audiology
ENT Division
National Guard Hospital
Jeddah, Saudi Arabia

Carlos A Oliveira MD PhD
Chief
Department of Otolaryngology
University of Brasilia Medical School
Brasilia, DF, Brazil

Koji Otsuka MD
Consultant
Department of Otolaryngology
Tokio Medical University
Nishi-Shinjuku, Japan

Kourosh Parham MD
Associate Professor
Director of Research
Divison of Otolaryngology—
Head and Neck Surgery
Department of Surgery
University of Connecticut Health Center
Farmington, Connecticut, USA

Akhilesh PM MD
Consultant of Otolaryngology
Kasaragod Institute of Medical Sciences (KIMS)
Kasaragod, Kerala, India

Maria Riga MD
Consultant of Otolaryngology
University Clinic of Otorhinolaryngology
Democritus University of Thrace
Alexandroupolis, Greece

Richard A Roberts MD
Director
Alabama Hearing and Balance Associates
Foley, Alabama, USA

Essam Saleh MD
Professor
Department of Otolaryngology
Faculty of Medicine
Alexandria University
Alexandria, Egypt

André LL Sampaio MD
Consultant
Department of Otolaryngology
University of Brasilia Medical School
Brasilia, DF, Brazil

Calogero Giancario Scarnà MD
Consultant of Otolaryngology
"San Giovanni di Dio" Hospital of Agrigento
Azienda Sanitaria Locale di Agrigento
Agrigento, Italy

Rosetta Stagno MD
Consultant of Otolaryngology
"San Giovanni di Dio" Hospital of Agrigento
Azienda Sanitaria Locale di Agrigento
Agrigento, Italy

Kristen Steenerson MD
Consultant of Neurology
Barrow Neurological Institute
University of Arizona
College of Medicine
Phoenix, Arizona, USA

Hamlet Suarez MD
Director
Laboratory of Otoneurology
Biomedical Engineering Program
British Hospital
Montevideo, Uruguay

Mamoru Suzuki MD
Head
Department of Otolaryngology
Tokio Medical University
Nishi-Shinjuku, Japan

Alev Uneri MD
Professor of Neurotology
Balance Center
Department of Otorhinolaryngology
Acibadem Kozyatagi Oncology and
Neurology Hospital
Istanbul, Turkey

Ayse Uneri MD
Consultant of Neurotology
Balance Center
Department of Otorhinolaryngology
Acibadem Kozyatagi Oncology and
Neurology Hospital
Istanbul, Turkey

Dario A Yacovino MD
Consultant of Otolaryngology
Neurotology Section
Neurology Research Institute
"Dr Raul Carrea" (Fleni)
Buenos Aires, Argentina

Foreword

Benign Paroxysmal Positional Vertigo (BPPV) is the most common cause of vertigo and also the most common peripheral vestibular disorder. Fortunately, the clinical developments of the last three decades have turned this condition into one of the best success stories of medicine in general. Within a few minutes, the vast majority of patients with BPPV can now be treated successfully by a doctor or paramedic in his own consulting room. No other area in medicine has seen so much of progress with so little research funding invested. The revolution in BPPV treatment is an extraordinary example of how good clinical observation and practice can still change patient outcomes.

In this book, Doctors De Stefano and Dispenza have achieved a remarkable gathering of specialists in the field. Any neurologist or ENT specialist interested in the area of vertigo can feel fully confident and backed up. He or she will now be able to proceed with even the more complicated and difficult cases of positional vertigo and be aware of the important differential diagnoses that have to be kept in mind. With so much of progress in this area, a dedicated book on BPPV was long overdue. The editors are to be congratulated on their idea and implementation of this project.

Professor Adolfo M Bronstein MD PhD FANA FRCP
Professor of Clinical Neuro-otology
Imperial College London
Consultant Neurologist and Neuro-otologist
Charing Cross Hospital (Imperial College Healthcare NHS Trust)
and National Hospital for Neurology and Neurosurgery
University College London Hospitals (UCLH)
London, United Kingdom

Preface

Vertigo is a frequent and frustrating symptom for which patients seek help from an Otolaryngologist and Benign Paroxysmal Positional Vertigo (BPPV) represents the most common cause of peripheral vertigo observed.

Typically, BPPV affects approximately 20-24% of patients suffering from vestibular diseases, but, unfortunately, it is very difficult to find a cause for this entity.

Sometimes, head trauma, vestibular neuritis and other inner ear disorders, such as Meniere's disease, labyrinthitis, herpesvirus infection, mastoid and stapes surgery, and vascular alterations (circulatory failure of anterior vestibular artery) have been associated with BPPV, but more than 50% of all the reported cases are identified as being idiopathic in nature.

Typically, in BPPV, the semicircular canals are inappropriately stimulated by loose otoconia in certain head positions, resulting in brief episodes of vertigo.

The incidence of BPPV progressively increases in the elderly population as reported by BPPV Guidelines of the American Academy of Otolaryngology-Head and Neck Surgery.

The elderly tend to have multiple comorbidities, such as hypertension, diabetes, osteoporosis, osteoarthrosis and many others, which cause major geriatric syndromes, such as falls, dementia, and limitation of mobility.

The comorbidities compromise the autonomy of elderly population, causing a quick worsening of quality of life.

Coincidentally, increasing age is directly proportional to the presence of several neurotological disorders associated with deterioration in equilibrium and hearing function, such as BPPV and other dizziness, sensorineural hearing loss, tinnitus, changes in the body balance, gait disorders, and occasional falls.

In our previously published study, we showed the relationship between recurrent BPPV attack and comorbidities in elderly population.

BPPV is a simple pathology if properly diagnosed by a physician, but it becomes formidable to reduce a patient's quality of life and increased spending for unnecessary medical imaging studies and incorrect assessments, if not recognized in time.

For these reasons, the knowledge of all the clinical signs of BPPV and its related new treatments can be a good opportunity for the work of the physicians, who meet the world of BPPV for the first time or for the expert neurotologists, who love to discover and treat these balance disorders.

Alessandro De Stefano MD PhD
Francesco Dispenza MD PhD

Contents

1. **Anatomy and Physiology of the Posterior Labyrinth**   1
   Mercedes FS Araújo, André LL Sampaio, Carlos A Oliveira
   - Anatomy *1*
   - Physiology *8*

2. **Pathophysiology of Benign Paroxysmal Positional Vertigo**   30
   Koji Otsuka, Mamoru Suzuki
   - Physiological Effects of Cupulolithiasis and Canalolithiasis in In Vivo Models *30*
   - Physiological Effects of Otoconia by Mathematical Models *32*
   - Physiological Effects of Canalolithiasis and Cupulolithiasis on SC Activity *33*
   - Functional Evaluation of the Otolithic Organ in BPPV Patients *37*

3. **Differential Diagnosis of Benign Paroxysmal Positional Vertigo**   40
   Richard A Roberts
   - Pathophysiology of BPPV *40*
   - Positioning Techniques for Eliciting BPPV *48*

4. **Central Positional Vertigo**   64
   Diego Kaski
   - Epidemiology *64*
   - Clinical Features *65*

5. **Posterior Benign Paroxysmal Positional Vertigo**   72
   Augusto Casani
   - Diagnosis and Outline of Physiopathology *76*
   - Clinical Aspects of BPPV of the PSC *76*
   - Diagnostic Maneuvers *77*
   - Physical Therapy For BPPV of the PSC *85*

6. **Horizontal Benign Paroxysmal Positional Vertigo**   94
   Giacinto Asprella Libonati
   - Pathophysiology *96*
   - Diagnosis *97*
   - Differential Diagnosis *102*
   - Therapy *103*
   - Post-treatment Complications *108*

7. Anterior Benign Paroxysmal Positional Vertigo — 122
Dario A Yacovino
- Epidemiology *122*
- History and Clinical Findings *123*
- Differential Diagnosis *126*
- Diagnostic Criteria for AC-BPPV *129*
- Treatment *130*

8. Residual Dizziness after Successful Canalith Repositioning Procedures for Benign Paroxysmal Positional Vertigo — 135
Alev Uneri, Ayse Uneri
- Diagnostic Evaluation *136*
- Theories of Pathogenesis *137*
- Management *140*

9. Complex Forms of Benign Paroxysmal Positional Vertigo — 145

9A: Cupulolithiasis — 145
Essam Saleh, Alfarghal Mohamad
- Pathogenesis *145*
- Posterior Canal Cupulolithiasis *146*
- Lateral Canal Cupulolithiasis *147*
- Diagnosis *151*

9B: Subjective Benign Paroxysmal Positional Vertigo — 157
Dimitrios G Balatsouras
- Literature Review *157*
- Reviews *162*
- Sitting-up Vertigo *163*
- Terminology and Diagnostic Criteria of Subjective BPPV *164*
- Pathogenesis *164*
- Frequency *166*
- Differential Diagnosis *166*
- Treatment *167*

9C: Canal Switch and Re-entry Phenomenon in Benign Paroxysmal Positional Vertigo — 171
Francesco Dispenza, Alessandro De Stefano, Maria Giglione, Rosetta Stagno, Sebastian Bianchini, Calogero Giancarlo Scarnà, Salvatore Maira, Ettore Bennici
- Epidemiology *176*
- Etiology *177*
- Pathophysiology *177*
- Diagnosis *178*

9D: BPPV Involving Multiple Canals — 176
Alfarghal Mohamad, Essam Saleh
- Bilateral BPPV Versus Bilaterally Symptomatizing BPPV *179*
- Anterior Canal BPPV *181*
- Apogeotropic Posterior Semicircular Canal BPPV *183*
- Bilateral Horizontal Canal BPPV *184*
- Bilateral AC-BPPV *185*
- Horizontal and Posterior Canal BPPV *186*
- Horizontal and Anterior Canal BPPV *187*
- Posterior and Anterior Canal BPPV *187*
- Treatment *188*

10. Secondary Benign Paroxysmal Positional Vertigo — 193
Maria Riga
- Definitions and Pitfalls *193*
- Incidence and Epidemiological Characteristics *194*
- Pathophysiology *198*
- Diagnostic Implications *204*
- Treatment Implications *205*
- General Considerations *208*

11. Benign Paroxysmal Positional Vertigo and Migraine-associated Vertigo — 212
Terry D Fife, Kristen Steenerson
- Vestibular Migraine *212*
- Association Between BPPV and Migraine *213*
- Possible Mechanistic Relationship Between BPPV and Migraine *214*
- Distinguishing Migraine Positional Vertigo from BPPV *215*
- Treatment of Vestibular Migraine *217*

12. Benign Paroxysmal Postural Vertigo in the Childhood — 221
Hamlet Suarez
- Clinical Presentation of BPPV in Children *221*
- Characteristic of the Positional Nystagmus *222*
- Frequent Etiology of BPPV in the Chilhood *223*
- Bppv Linked With Otologic Disease *225*
- Testing *225*

13. Medical Management of Benign Paroxysmal Positional Vertigo — 228
Kourosh Parham
- Treatment *229*
- Prevention *234*

14. Surgery for Benign Paroxysmal Positional Vertigo   240
Gauri Mankekar
- History *240*
- Indications For Surgery *240*
- Surgical Procedures *241*

15. Atlas of Diagnostic and Repositioning Techniques for BPPV   246
Gautham Kulamarva, Alessandro De Stefano, Francesco Dispenza, Akhilesh PM
- Diagnostic Test *246*
- Therapeutic Technique *250*

Index   *273*

Chapter 1

Anatomy and Physiology of the Posterior Labyrinth

Mercedes FS Araújo, André LL Sampaio, Carlos A Oliveira

ANATOMY

The membranous labyrinth arises from a vesicle that separates from the rhombencephalus in the embryo called the otocyst. This vesicle differentiates into the organs of the labyrinth: utricle, saccule, semicircular canals, and cochlea. The bony labyrinth is formed by the mesenchime surrounding the membranous labyrinth that becomes the petrous portion of the temporal bone. The bony labyrinth is therefore the hard bones that encase the membranous labyrinth and protect these structures.

Semicircular Canals

The vestibular system is the system of balance and equilibrium. It consists of five distinct sensory organs: three semicircular canals (SCCs) that are sensitive to angular accelerations (head rotations) and two otolithic organs (saccule and utricle) that are sensitive to linear accelerations (such as motion in a vehicle or an elevator). Thus, the function of the vestibular system is to sense motion of the head and to codify these movements precisely to the central nervous system (CNS).

The bony labyrinth consists of three SCCs, the cochlea, and a central chamber called the vestibule (Fig. 1.1). The bony labyrinth is filled with perilymphatic fluid that has a composition similar to that of cerebrospinal fluid (high Na:K ratio). Perilymphatic fluid communicates via the cochlear aqueduct with cerebrospinal fluid. Because of this communication, disorders that affect spinal fluid pressure (such as lumbar puncture) can also affect inner ear function (Fig. 1.2). The membranous labyrinth is suspended within the bony labyrinth by perilymphatic fluid and supportive connective tissue. It contains five sensory organs: the membranous portions of the three SCCs and the two otolithic organs, the utricle and saccule. Note that one end of each canal is widened in diameter to form an ampulla. The ampula is where the cristae of the SCCs are located. The membranous labyrinth is filled with endolymph (Fig. 1.1). In contrast to perilymph, the endolymph resembles intracellular

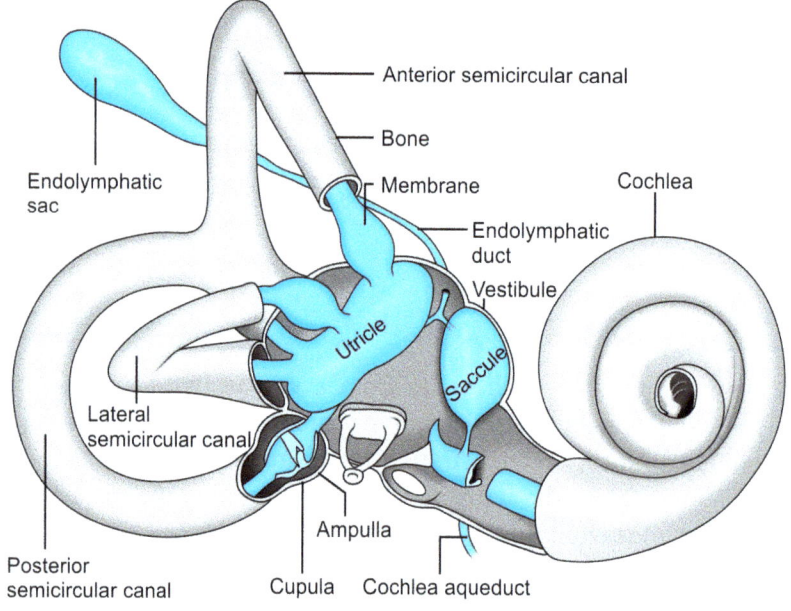

Fig. 1.1: The osseous and membranous labyrinth.

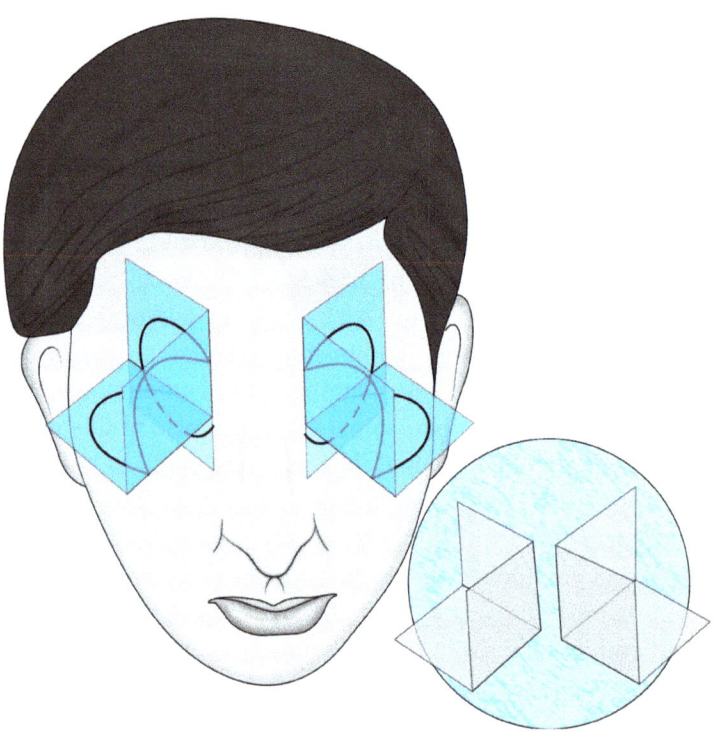

Fig. 1.2: Spatial organization of the semicircular canals.

fluid in electrolyte composition (high K:Na ratio). Under normal circumstances, there is no direct communication between the endolymph and perilymph compartments.

This section will describe the anatomic basis for the labyrinth functions. The membranous labyrinth is surrounded by the bone labyrinth of the petrous bone and is immersed in perilymph. Active transport works in order to keep differences in ions concentrations between the external perilymph and the internal endolymph.

The SCCs are membranous structures with an enlargement at the utricular end, the ampulla. A gelatinous flap completely seals one side of ampulla from the other side. The ampulla is elastic and any pressure difference across it will be detected. The membranous SCCs begin and end in the utricle. There is therefore an ampulated end and a nonampulated one. The special dispositions of these structures are fundamental for the posterior labyrinth function.

The SCCs are arranged as a set of three orthogonal sensors (*see* Fig. 1.2); that is, each canal is at approximately right angles to the other two. Furthermore, each canal is maximally sensitive to rotations that lie in the plane of that canal. The result of this arrangement is that the three canals can uniquely specify the direction and amplitude of any arbitrary head rotation. Each of the canals acts as an integrating accelerometer; thus, the necessary stimulus for the canal is an angular acceleration, but the information that is encoded by the firing of the afferent nerve fiber is more closely related to angular velocity. Finally, the canals are organized into functional pairs wherein both members of the pair lie in the same plane. Any rotation in that plane will be excitatory to one of the members of the pair and inhibitory to the other. Although in the horizontal system the two horizontal canals form a functional pair, the situation is somewhat more complex in the vertical system. Here, the anterior canal on one side is parallel and coplanar with the posterior canal on the opposite side. For example, the right anterior canal and the left posterior canal form a functional pair. Thus, when the head is turned, the membranous labyrinth moves with it but the endolymph inside has an inertial effect and that tends to oppose the turning movement.

Because the primary vestibular afferent fibers exhibit a substantial resting firing rate (60–80 spikes per second in mammals), each canal is able to report rotations in either its excitatory direction (by increasing its firing rate) or its inhibitory direction (by decreasing). This observation explains why it is possible to function reasonably well after the loss of one labyrinth.

The vestibular system forms the basis for a number of rather fundamental reflexes: the vestibulocollic reflex (VCR; head stabilization), the vestibulospinal reflex (VSR; control of upright posture), and the vestibulo-ocular reflex (VOR; retinal image stabilization). The last of these, the VOR, has been studied far more extensively than the others and is certainly the best understood; it is this reflex that forms the basis for most clinical testing (calorics, rotation tests, etc.).

This chapter describes the anatomy of the VOR in detail but without exploring every possible aspect. Many of the details that will be described have been obtained from experiments in animal species, particularly the cat and monkey; nevertheless, the information is certainly applicable to humans because the vestibular system has changed very little during the evolution of vertebrates.

Otolith Organs—the Saccule and the Utricle

The otolith organs located in the vestibule of the osseous labyrinth register forces related to linear acceleration. They respond to both linear head motion and with change of the gravitational axis. The function of the otolithic organs is illustrated by the situation of a passenger in a commercial jet. During flight at a constant velocity, the passenger has no sense that he is traveling at 300 miles/h. However, in the process of taking off and ascending to cruising altitude, he senses the change in velocity acceleration as well as the tilt of the plane on ascent. The otolithic organs respond better to changes in acceleration than in velocity.

The sensory part of the otolithic organs named secular, and utricular maculae are covered by crystals of calcium carbonate (otoliths) in gelatinous amorphous material that tops the maculae of saccule and utricle.

Like the canals, the otoliths are arranged to enable them to respond to motion in all three dimensions (Fig. 1.3). However, unlike the canals, which have one sensory organ per axis of angular motion, the otoliths have only two sensory organs for three axes of linear motion. In an upright individual, the saccule is vertical (parasagittal), whereas the utricle is horizontally oriented (near the plane of the lateral SCCs). In this posture, the saccule can sense linear acceleration in its plane, which includes the acceleration oriented along the occipitocaudal axis as well as linear motion along the anterior-posterior axis. The utricle senses acceleration in its plane, which includes lateral accelerations along the interaural axis as well as anterior-posterior motion.

The earth's gravitational field is a linear acceleration field, so in a person on the earth, the otoliths register tilt. For example, as the head is tilted laterally (which is also called roll; Fig. 1.3), shear force is exerted upon the utricle, causing excitation, but shear force is lessened upon the saccule. Similar changes occur when the head is tilted forward or backward.

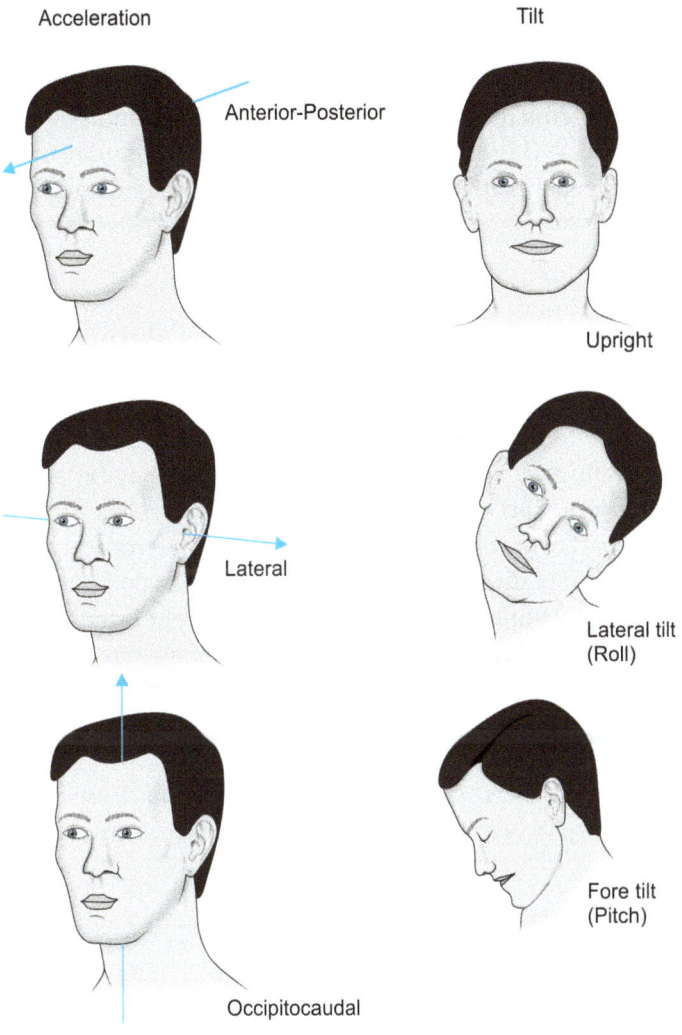

Fig. 1.3: Spatial organization of the saccule and utricle.

Because linear acceleration can come from two sources—earth's gravitational field and linear motion—there is a sensor ambiguity problem. We discuss strategies that the CNS might use to solve this problem later in the section on higher-level vestibular processing. In the otoliths, as in the canals, there is redundancy, with similar sensors on both sides of the head. Push-pull processing for the otoliths is also incorporated into the geometry of each of the otolithic membranes. Within each otolithic macula, a curving zone, the striata, separates the direction of hair-cell polarization on each side. Consequently, head increases afferent discharge from one part of a macula, while reducing the afferent discharge from another portion of the same macula. This extra level of redundancy in comparison with the SCCs probably makes the otoliths less vulnerable to unilateral vestibular lesions. Tilt increases afferent discharge from one part of a macula, while reducing the afferent discharge from another portion of the same macula. This extra level of redundancy in comparison with the SCCs probably makes the otoliths less vulnerable to unilateral vestibular lesions.

Blood Supply

The labyrinthine artery supplies the peripheral vestibular system (Fig. 1.4). The labyrinthine artery has a variable origin. Most often it is a branch of the anterior-inferior cerebellar artery (AICA), but occasionally a direct branch from the basilar artery may exist. Upon entering the inner ear, the labyrinthine artery divides into common cochlear artery and anterior vestibular artery. The anterior vestibular artery supplies the vestibular nerve, most part of the utricle, the ampulla of the anterior and lateral SCC. The cochlear artery divides into two branches, the main branch cochlear artery and the vestibulocochlear artery. The cochlear artery supplies the cochlea and the vestibulocochlear branch supplies part of the cochlea axis as well as the saccule and the ampulla of posterior SCC.

Vestibular Nerve

Vestibular nerve fibers are the afferent projections from the bipolar neurons of Scarpa's (vestibular) ganglion. The vestibular nerve transmits

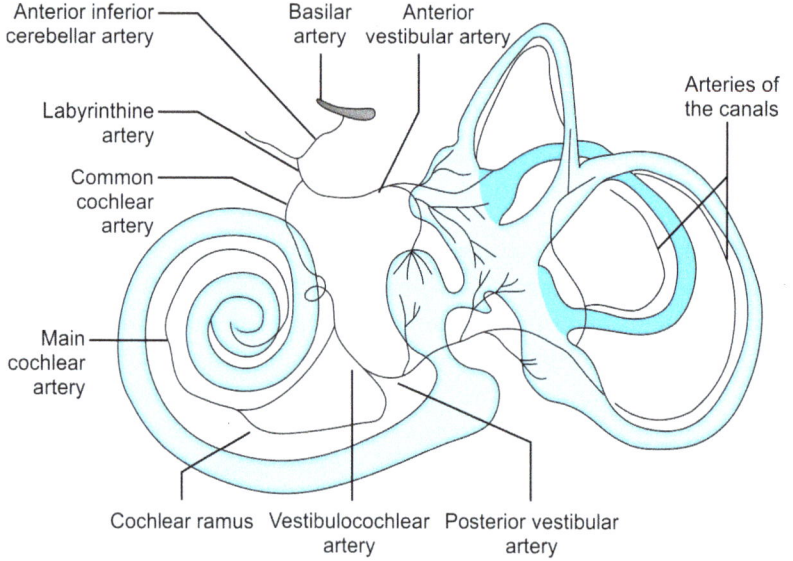

Fig. 1.4: Vascular supply of the labyrinth.

afferent signals from the labyrinths along its course through the internal auditory canal (IAC). In addition to the vestibular nerve, the IAC contains the cochlear nerve (hearing), the facial nerve, the nervus intermedius (a branch of the facial nerve which carries sensation), and the labyrinthine artery.

The IAC travels through the petrous portion of the temporal bone to open into the posterior fossa at the level of the pons. The vestibular nerve enters the brainstem at the pontomedullary junction. Because the vestibular nerve is interposed between the labyrinth and the brainstem, some authorities consider this nerve a peripheral structure, whereas others consider it a central structure. We consider it a peripheral structure.

There are two patterns of firing in vestibular afferent neurons. Regular afferents usually have a tonic rate and little variability in interspike intervals. Irregular afferents often show no firing at rest and, when stimulated by head motion, develop highly variable interspike intervals.

Regular afferents appear to be the most important type for the VOR, because in experimental animals irregular afferents can be ablated without much change in the VOR. However, irregular afferents may be important for the VSR and in coordinating responses between the otoliths and canals.

Regular afferents of the monkey have tonic firing rates of about 90 spikes per second and a sensitivity to head velocity of about 0.5 spikes per degree per second. We can speculate about what happens immediately after a sudden change in head velocity. Humans can easily move their heads at velocities exceeding 300° per second. As noted previously the SCCs are connected in a push-pull arrangement so that one side is always being inhibited while the other is being excited.

Given the sensitivity and tonic rate noted previously, the vestibular nerve, which is being inhibited, should be driven to a firing rate of 0 spikes per second, for head velocities of only 180° per second! In other words, head velocities >180° per second may be unquantifiable by half of the vestibular system. This *cutoff* behavior has been advanced as the explanation for Ewald's second law, which says that responses to rotations that excite a canal are greater than those to rotations that inhibit a canal. *Cutoff* behavior explains why a patient with unilateral vestibular loss avoids head motion toward the side of the lesion.

Vestibular Nuclei

The vestibular nuclei consist of four major nuclei, superior, descending, lateral and medial and at least more seven minor structures. The superior and medial vestibular nuclei relate to the VOR. The lateral vestibular nucleus is primary involved in the VSR. All vestibular nuclei complex is located in the medulla oblongata on the brainstem.

Endolymphatic Duct and Endolymphatic Sac

As shown in Figure 1.1, the endolymphatic duct comes out of the utricle, traverses the petrous bone toward the posterior fossa, and ends in the endolymphatic sac that lies in the posterior surface of the petrous bone in the posterior fossa. These structures have no function related to equilibrium and probably are related to endolymph absorption. In other words, there is a longitudinal flow of endolymph toward the endolymphatic sac where this fluid is resorbed. Dysfunction of the endolymphatic sac is believed to cause endolymphatic hydrops.

PHYSIOLOGY

The vestibular system's main function is to sense head movements, especially involuntary ones, and counter them with reflexive eye movements and postural adjustments that keep the visual world stable and keep us from falling. The posterior labyrinth senses head rotation and linear acceleration and sends that information to secondary vestibular neurons in the brainstem vestibular nuclei. Information above the tonic (spontaneous) firing of the type I hair cells transmitted along type I neurons is largely thought to have a stimulatory effect in contrast to a more inhibitory effect attributable to type II hair cells and type II neurons.

The reflexive nature of the vestibular system is essential for complete understanding of vestibular physiology. The brainstem interprets imbalances in vestibular input due to pathologic processes in the same way that it interprets imbalances due to physiologic stimuli. Therefore, the cardinal signs of vestibular disorders are eye movement's reflexes and postural changes. These reflexes can largely be understood as the brainstem's responses to perceived rotation around a specific axis or perceived tilting or translation of the head. Knowing the effective stimulus for each vestibular end organ allows determination of which end organ or combination of end organs must be stimulated to produce the observed motor output. Specifically, neurons encoding head movement form synapses within the ocular motor nuclei to elicit the patterns of extraocular muscle contraction and relaxation needed for the VOR (Fig. 1.5), which stabilizes gaze (eye position in space). Other secondary vestibular neurons synapse on cervical spinal motor neurons to generate the VCR or to lower spinal motor neurons to generate the VSRs. These reflexes stabilize posture and facilitate gait. Vestibular sensory input to autonomic centers, particularly information about posture with respect to gravity, is used to adjust hemodynamic reflexes to maintain cerebral perfusion. Finally, vestibular input to the cerebellum is essential for coordination and adaptation of

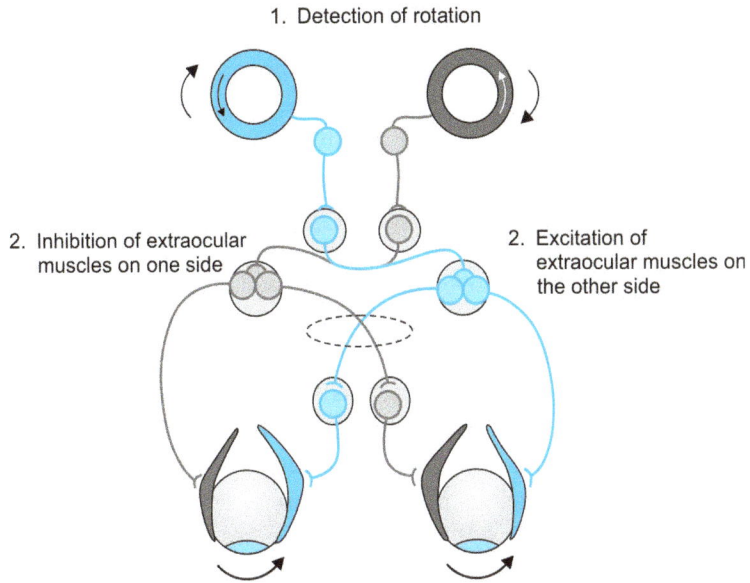

Fig. 1.5: Vestibulo-ocular reflex (VOR): when a rotational head movement is detected an inhibitory signal is triggered to extraocular muscles on one side and excitatory signal to the muscles on the other side producing compensatory eyes movement.

vestibular reflexes when changes occur such as injury to a vestibular end organ or alteration in vision (e.g. a new pair of glasses).

The sequence of events that occur during the excitation of vestibular nerve fibers is very similar to auditory system, so stereocilia deflection is the common mechanism by which vestibular hair cells transduce mechanical forces into action potentials. Movements of the head or changes in linear acceleration cause deflection of the cupula (Fig. 1.6B) or shift the gelatinous matrix of the otolithic organs with its load of otolithic crystals (Fig. 1.7B) that will result in depolarization (stimulation) or hyperpolarization (inhibition) of types I and II hair cells. When the head tilts forward the gravitational force on the otolithic membrane of the otolithic organs changes and the hair cells are subjected to a new force that displaces cilia to the side; pulls them down, away from the epithelium in the inverted position or pushes them back against the cell in the upright position. It is observed the maximal discharge of the nerve when the cilia are bent to one side and minimal when they bent to the other side. At intermediate positions there is intermediate response.

Displacement of the stereocilia either toward or away from the kinocilium influences calcium influx mechanisms at the apex of the cell that causes the release or reduction of neurotransmitters from the cell to the surrounding afferent neurons.

Semicircular Canals

The semicircular canals appear to be responsible for the equal but opposite corresponding eye-to-head movements that are commonly known as VOR, and they are primarily responsible by the sense of rotational acceleration of the head. The VOR is the most important human vestibular pathway and it is required to maintain a stable retinal image with active head movement. In order to ultimately produce conjugate versional VOR-mediated movements of the eyes, each vestibular nucleus receives electrical information from both sides that is exchanged via the vestibular commissure in the brainstem (Fig. 1.5). The organization is generally believed to be specific across the commissure. For example, neurons in the right vestibular nucleus that receive type I input from the right horizontal SCC project across commissure to the neurons found in the left vestibular nucleus that are driven by the left horizontal SCC receiving contralateral type II input and vice versa as described by Leigh and Zee.[1] The VOR is subserved by a simple three-neuron pathway: motions detected by the end organ are transduced into neural impulses that are sent via the vestibular nerve to the vestibular nuclei and rostrally through the ascending medial longitudinal fasciculus (MLF) to the oculomotor nuclei of the extraocular muscles. Secondary vestibulo-ocular connections via the reticular formation have been described, but functionally these are less important than the direct three-neuron MLF vestibulo-ocular pathway. Inhibitory-crossed connections at the levels of both vestibular and oculomotor nuclei probably also participate in the VOR. The crossed-inhibitory oculomotor connections subserve antagonistic extraocular muscles that are important in the formation of conjugate-eye movements.[2]

Sensation by SCCs works as follows. When angular acceleration in the plane of an SCC starts, inertia causes the endolymph in the canal to lag behind the motion of the membranous canal, much as coffee in a mug initially remains in place as the mug is rotated about it. Relative to the canal walls, the endolymph effectively moves in the opposite direction as the head. Inside the ampulla, a swelling at the end of the canal where it meets the utricle, pressure exerted by endolymph deflects the cupula, an elastic membrane that spans a cross section of the ampulla (Fig. 1.6A). Once the vestibular hair cells are arrayed beneath the cupula on the surface of the crista ampullaris and its stereociliary bundles are coupled to the cupula its deflection creates a shearing stress between the stereocilia and the cuticular plates at the tops of the hair cells.

Stereocilia within a bundle are linked to one another by protein strands called "tip links" that span from the side of a taller stereocilium to the tip of its shorter neighbor in the array. The tip links are believed

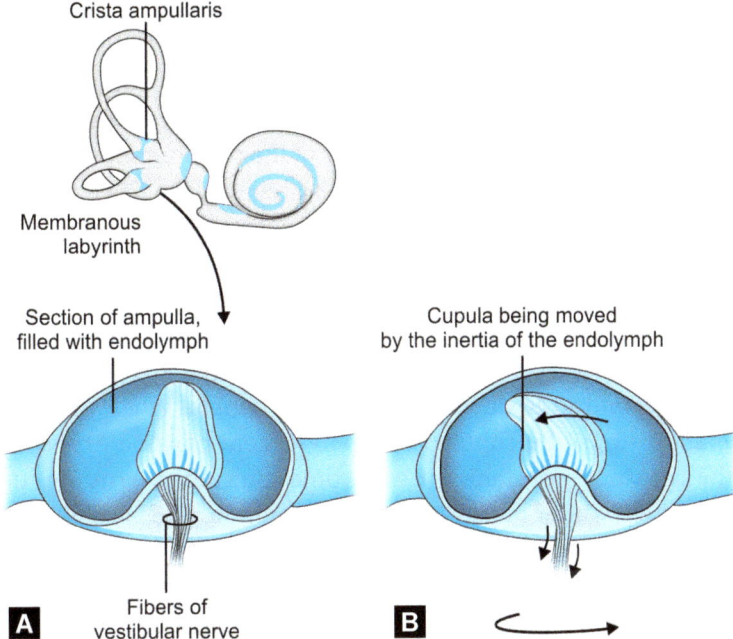

Figs. 1.6A and B: (A) The cupula spans the lumen of the ampulla from the crista to the membranous labyrinth at resting position. (B) If head moves to right, the relative flow of endolymph in the canal is therefore opposite to the direction of head acceleration. This flow produces a pressure across the elastic cupula, which suffers deflection.

to act as gating springs for mechanically sensitive ion channels, meaning that the tip links literally tug at molecular gates in the stereocilia.[3] These gates, which are cation channels, open or close (or, more precisely, spend more or less time in the open state), depending on the direction in which the stereocilia are deflected. When deflected in the open or "on" direction, which is toward the tallest stereocilium, cations, including potassium ions from the potassium-rich endolymph, rush in through the gates, and the membrane potential of the hair cell becomes more positive. This in turn activates voltage-sensitive calcium channels at the basolateral aspect of the hair cell, and an influx of calcium leads to an increase in the release of excitatory neurotransmitters, principally glutamate, from hair cell synapses onto the vestibular primary afferents. All of the hair cells on an SCC crista are oriented or "polarized" in the same direction. That is to say that their stereociliary bundles all have the tall ends pointing the same way, so that the endolymph motion that is excitatory for one hair cell will be excitatory for all of the hair cells on that crista.

Head rotation carries the membranous SCC along with it, whereas the inertia of the endolymph and cupula tend to keep these elements stationary in space (like the coffee in a mug as the mug is quickly turned).

Nevertheless, two things act to accelerate the endolymph in the same direction that the head is turning but through the smaller angle. The first is the elastic or spring-like push from the distended cupula, as it pushes against the endolymph. The second is the viscous drag exerted on the endolymph at its interface with the walls of the membranous canal.

The movement of the cupula can now be described as a function of head acceleration: during a constant, low-acceleration head rotation, cupular deflection eventually reaches a steady-state constant value. The time course of cupular displacement, in response to a constant acceleration approximates a single exponential growth, and the time constant with which cupular displacement reaches its maximum deflection is approximately 10 seconds, the time constant of the cupula. When the constant acceleration stops, the cupula returns to its zero position exponentially with the same time constant. The same time constant governs the cupular response to very brief pulses of head acceleration. Such "velocity steps" are often done as part of clinical rotary chair tests. However, the measured value of the time constant of the VOR in such testing is generally much longer than what would be anticipated by this calculated cupular response because of further processing by the brain. During sinusoidal head rotations in the range encompassing most natural head movements (~0.1–15 Hz), viscous friction dominates the cupular response, making cupular deflection proportional to head velocity.

Otolithic Organs

The otolithic organs (utricule and saccule) are primarily responsible for ocular counter-rolling with tilts of the head and for VSRs that help in the maintenance of body posture and muscle tone by sensing linear acceleration in horizontal and vertical (superoinferior) directions. These organs contain sheets of hair cells on a sensory epithelium called a macula. A gelatinous membrane sits atop the macula, and microscopic stones made of calcium carbonate, the otoliths (or otoconia), are embedded on the surface of this otolithic membrane. The sacculus (or saccule), located on the medial wall of the vestibule of the labyrinth in the spherical recess, has its macula oriented vertically. Gravity therefore tonically pulls the saccular otolithic mass inferiorly when the head is upright (Fig. 1.7A). The utriculus (or utricle) is located above the saccule in the elliptical recess of the vestibule. Its macula is oriented in roughly the same plane as the horizontal SCC, although its anterior end curves upward. When the head tilts out of the upright position (Fig. 1.7B), the component of the gravitational vector that is tangential to the macula creates a shearing force on stereocilia of utricular hair cells. The cellular transduction process is identical to that described above for the crista.

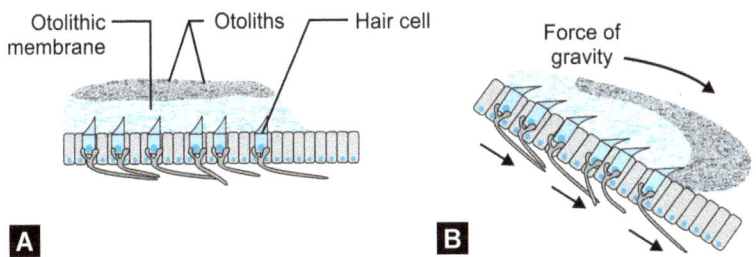

Figs. 1.7A and B: (A) Otolithic organ when head is upright. (B) Otoliths displacement when head is tilted.

However, the hair cells of the maculae, unlike those of the cristae, are not all polarized in the same direction. Instead, they are oriented relative to a curving central zone known as the striola. The utricular striola forms a C shape, with the open side pointing medially. The striola divides the utricular macula into a medial two-thirds (polarized to be excited by downward tilt of the ipsilateral ear) and a lateral one-third polarized in the opposite direction. Hair cells of the sacculus point away from its striola, which curves and hooks superiorly in its anterior portion. Each macula is essentially a linear accelerometer, with the saccular macula encoding acceleration roughly within a parasagittal plane (along the naso-occipital and superoinferior axes), and the utricular macula encoding linear acceleration roughly in an axial plane (along the naso-occipital and interaural axes). A given linear acceleration may produce a complex pattern of excitation and inhibition across the two maculas, a pattern that encodes the direction and magnitude of the linear acceleration.[4] By contrast, each of the three SCCs senses just a one-dimensional component of rotational acceleration. Modulation of neurotransmitter release from hair cells within each vestibular end organ modulates the action potential frequency, or firing rate, of vestibular nerve afferent fibers. The afferents have a baseline rate of firing, probably due to a baseline rate of release of neurotransmitter from the vestibular hair cells. Changes in vestibular nerve afferent firing are conveyed to secondary neurons in the brainstem. Baseline firing gives the system the important property of bidirectional sensitivity: firing can increase for excitatory head movements and decrease for inhibitory head movements.[5] Thus, loss of one labyrinth does not mean loss of the ability to sense one half of the head's movements.

It is common explaining movement of otoconial membrane by using the same analysis of cupular motion, but since the otoconial membrane is an inhomogeneous structure whose complexities make it very difficult to estimate the physical parameters in the model that would predict its responses under different conditions. The membrane consists of the dense otoconial layer on top, a stiff mesh layer in the middle, and an elastic gel layer on the bottom. At the macular surface, it is presumably fixed. It is unclear how tightly otoconial displacement is coupled to the motion of the stereocilia. These uncertainties lead to models that variously predict that the otoconial membrane responds to linear acceleration or velocity, but the actual behavior remains unresolved.[6]

Afferent Function

In mammals, physiologic response characteristics segregate vestibular nerve afferent fibers into two classes based on the regularity in the spacing of spontaneous action potentials.[7] Regular afferents fire at 50–100 spikes/second at rest, with very little variation in resting rate for a given fiber. In general, they respond to vestibular stimulation with tonic responses. That is, their firing modulates about the baseline, going up and down in close approximation to the stimulus (linear acceleration for the otolith organs and rotational velocity for SCCs).

Considering morphologic differences between regular and irregular vestibular afferents, they have also different action mechanisms. Irregular afferents have a wider range of spontaneous rates than do regular fibers. Irregular units show phasic responses to the stimulus acting on the end organ. That is, the response is more transient, and it approximates the rate of change of the stimulus acting on the end organ rather than simply the stimulus itself. Irregular units may have very high sensitivity to vestibular stimuli, except for a unique group of low-sensitivity calyx units in the crista, whose function is still unclear. Sensitivities to activation by efferent pathways and to galvanic stimulation also are generally greater for irregular afferents. After the peak of an action potential (caused by inward sodium currents), outward potassium currents briefly hyperpolarize the vestibular afferent membrane. The potassium conductance decays in a time-dependent manner, and the membrane potential rises again toward the threshold voltage for spike generation. Excitatory postsynaptic potentials (EPSPs) due to synaptic neurotransmitter release superimpose on this repolarization. The model assumes that variations in this potassium conductance between different afferents accounts for their regularity of discharge. In regularly discharging afferents, the model proposes that a large potassium conductance decays slowly but inexorably, so that the repolarization continues in a deterministic fashion until the membrane potential again reaches firing threshold. The model assumes that quanta of neurotransmitter released from hair cells cause relatively little variation in the trajectory of the repolarization. This deterministic nature of the repolarization means that the membrane reaches the threshold for another spike at almost the same time for each spike. Thus, the interspike intervals are all similar, and the unit's discharge is regular.

By contrast, in irregularly discharging afferents, the model assumes a potassium conductance that is high initially but decays rapidly so that it does not carry the membrane potential back up to the threshold for firing by itself. These fibers sit just below threshold voltage until driven above it by the added potential due to EPSPs. Neurotransmitter release and EPSPs are quantal and random, so that the time at which the membrane reaches firing potential is highly variable from spike to spike. Thus, the unit's discharge is irregular.

The difference about morphology and biochemistry of their membranes may be the origin of different firing characteristics between classes of afferents. They are different anatomically too: irregular units arise from the central zone of the crista or striola of the macula, and regular units arise from the peripheral zone of the crista or extrastriola of the macula. Because regular and irregular vestibular nerve afferent fibers have distinct characteristics in so many respects, it seems likely that they mediate different functions. One hypothesis holds that regular and irregular afferents may help compensate for different dynamic loads of the different vestibular reflexes.

Anatomically, regular and irregular afferents overlap extensively in their distributions to the central vestibular nuclei.[8a,b] However, physiologic evidence suggests that there is some segregation of regular and irregular inputs between central projections to the ocular motor centers and the spinal motor centers. Another role for the irregular afferents may be to initiate the vestibular reflexes with a very short latency for rapid head movements.[9] Finally, some evidence suggests that the dynamics of irregular afferents are better suited to provide the modifiable component of the VOR when gain must be changed rapidly. In addition to >10,000 afferents, each labyrinth also receives efferent innervation from ~400–600 neurons that lie on either side of the brainstem adjacent to the vestibular nuclei.[10,11] In mammals, excitation of efferents causes an increase in the background discharge of vestibular afferents, particularly irregular ones. It is hypothesized that the efferents may serve to raise baseline afferent firing rates, particularly of irregular afferents, in anticipation of rapid head movements so as to prevent inhibitory silencing. Yet Cullen and Minor[12] hypothesized that vestibular efferents may act to balance firing between the two labyrinths, a role that may be particularly important after some degree of loss of unilateral function.

The anatomic basis of SCCs physiology began with Flourens and Mach that described eye or head movements in the plane of a specific semicircular canal when it was manipulated in an isolated way in experimental animals.[13] Based on Ewald's work, who cannulated individual membranous canals in pigeons and observed the effects of endolymph motion on body, head, and eye movements.[14]

The arrangement of the canals places fluid motion sensors at the ends of relatively long, slender, fluid-filled, donut-shaped tubes. Each tube lies more or less in one plane. The most effective stimulus to move the fluid in such a planar semicircular tube is angular acceleration in that plane, about an axis perpendicular to the plane and through the center of the "donut hole." The three SCCs of the labyrinth are roughly orthogonal to each other, so that one labyrinth can sense any rotation in three-dimensional space. Canals in the two labyrinths are arranged in complementary, coplanar pairs.[15] The two horizontal canals are roughly in one plane, which is nearly horizontal when the head is in an upright position. The left anterior canal is roughly coplanar with the right posterior canal in the LARP (left anterior-right posterior) plane, which lies ~45° off the midsagittal plane with the anterior end toward the left and the posterior end toward the right. And the right anterior canal is roughly coplanar with the left posterior canal in the RALP (right anterior-left posterior) plane, again roughly 45° off the sagittal plane and orthogonal to the LARP and horizontal planes. These canal planes define the cardinal coordinate system for vestibular sensation. The power of this principle goes beyond the notion that the canal planes simply provide a coordinate system for vestibular sensation. Canal planes also provide the coordinate system for the final motor output of the VOR (and for the vestibulocolic neck reflex). The beauty of this canal-fixed (and thus head-fixed) coordinate system for eye movements is that it reduces the neural computation required for ocular motor output to exactly compensate for the head movement.

The VOR works like this: when the left horizontal canal is excited, secondary vestibular neurons that receive its afferents in the ipsilateral vestibular (medial and superior) nuclei connect to the ocular motor nuclei vestibular neurons controlling the medial and lateral rectus muscles, which also lie roughly in a horizontal plane. Secondary vestibular neurons carry excitatory signals to the ipsilateral third nucleus and contralateral sixth nucleus to excite the ipsilateral medial rectus and contralateral lateral rectus, respectively. These muscles pull the eyes toward the right as the head turns toward the left, accomplishing the goal of keeping the eyes stable in space. Other secondary vestibular neurons carry inhibitory signals to the contralateral third and ipsilateral sixth nuclei to simultaneously relax the antagonist muscles, the contralateral medial rectus and the ipsilateral lateral rectus, respectively. This reciprocal activity is typical of the extraocular muscles, which work in contraction-relaxation pairs.[16] Just as the extraocular muscles work in reciprocal pairs, so too do the coplanar SCCs.

Thanks to the nonzero baseline firing rate of vestibular afferent neurons, both of the canals in a coplanar pair can encode rotational acceleration in that plane. Like the horizontal canals and the lateral and medial recti, the vertical SCCs are linked to the vertical pairs of eye muscles, a fact that helps explain the pulling directions and insertions of the superior and inferior oblique muscles.

The alignment of canal planes and extraocular muscle planes is not exact, and the excitation of a single canal pair does not solely produce activity in a dedicated pair of extraocular muscles. Other muscles must be activated to compensate for a head rotation even when it is purely in the plane of one SCC. However, this arrangement between SCCs and extraocular muscles is remarkably constant across vertebrate species, even allowing for the shift between lateral-eyed species (e.g. rabbits) and frontal-eyed ones (e.g. humans). Robinson[17] has argued that there is an evolutionary advantage to keeping the extraocular muscles aligned with the SCCs. Such an arrangement minimizes the brainstem processing needed to activate the appropriate ensemble of eye muscles to compensate for head movement. Minimizing the number of synapses involved in the reflex preserves its remarkably short latency of ~7 ms, which in turn minimizes retinal image slip during very rapid head movements.

Because of the primacy of the canals in determining how the eyes move under vestibular stimulation, it is helpful to think about vestibular eye movements in a canal-fixed frame of reference. When we examine a patient with benign paroxysmal positional vertigo (BPPV), it is possible to observe that following Ewald's first law the eyes will move in the plane of the stimulated canal no matter where gaze is directed.

An SCC crista is excited by rotation in its plane in one direction and is inhibited by rotation in its plane in the opposite direction. So, the head's turning toward the left in the horizontal canal plane produces endolymph rotation to the left relative to space. But that endolymph rotation is less than the head rotation. Thus, relative to the canal, there is endolymph rotation to the right, and the cupula is deflected toward the utricle. The pattern of afferent activation results from the polarization of the stereocilia of the hair cells on the cristae. In the horizontal canal, the taller ends of the bundles point toward the utricle. Flow of endolymph (relative to the head) toward the ampulla—ampullopetal flow (from Latin petere, to seek), therefore excites the horizontal canal afferents, and flow of endolymph away from the ampulla—ampullofugal flow (from Latin fugere, "to flee")—inhibits these afferents. Thus, relative to the head, endolymph flow toward the ampulla occurs when the head is turning in the plane of the horizontal canal toward the same side.

The vertical canals, however, have the opposite pattern of hair cell polarization. The taller ends of the bundles point away from the utricle, so that flow away from the ampulla (ampullofugal) excites their afferents.

For the left anterior canal, whose ampulla is at its anterior end, turning the head down and rolling it to the left in the plane of the left anterior canal results in relative endolymph flow that is ampullofugal?

For the left posterior canal, whose ampulla is at its posterior end, turning the head up and rolling it to the left in the plane of the left posterior canal moves its endolymph away from the ampulla and excites its afferents. The mirror-image rotations would pertain to the right vertical canals.

What is important to know is an SCC is excited by rotation in the plane of the canal bringing the head toward the ipsilateral side instead of ampullopetal and ampullofugal flows, so the right horizontal canal is excited by turning the head rightward in the horizontal plane; the right anterior canal is excited by pitching the head nose down while rolling the head toward the right in a plane 45° off of the midsagittal plane; the right posterior canal is excited by pitching the head nose up while rolling it toward the right in a plane 45° off the midsagittal plane. It should be obvious by now that an SCC is inhibited by rotation in the plane of the canal toward the opposite side. As described previously, the arrangement of canals is such that when head rotation excites one, it inhibits its coplanar mate. As noted earlier, endolymph flows relative to the membranous canal in a direction opposite to the head rotation. Thus, the left posterior canal is excited when endolymph flows upward and toward the right in the canal—that is, ampullofugal.

Perhaps because the VOR is critical to survival of any vertebrate that needs to see and move about its environment, evolution appears to have placed a high premium on maintaining parsimonious and rapid neural connections of head rotational sensors to eye muscles and made eyes working under vestibular system demands but it will respond at same way when there is a normal stimulus or a pathologic cause. It is the same thing on concern of systems that mediate postural reflexes and perception of spatial orientation. An important point is that the brainstem (and patient) will interpret any change in firing rate from vestibular afferents as indicating head rotation, tilt, or translation that would normally produce the same change in firing rate. Secondary vestibular neurons relay the same misinformation to other reflex control centers and higher areas of conscious sensation. This leads to autonomic and postural disturbances as well as the noxious sensation of vertigo, an illusion of self-motion. A pathologic asymmetry in input from coplanar canals causes the eyes to turn in an attempt to compensate for the "perceived" head rotation. However, given the mechanical constraints imposed by the extraocular muscles, the eyes cannot continue to rotate in the same direction that the canals command for very long. Instead, rapid, resetting movements occur, taking the eyes back toward their neutral positions in the orbits. The result is nystagmus, a rhythmic; slowly forward-quickly backward movements of the eyes. The quick resetting movements (similar to saccades) are quick phases of nystagmus, and the vestibular-driven slower movements are slow phases. Nystagmus direction is described according to the direction of the quick phases, because these are more dramatic and noticeable. However, an important point is that the slow phases are the components driven by the vestibular system. By focusing on the direction of slow phases, one reduces the number of mental inversions required to identify the pathologic canal causing an observed nystagmus. This principle holds almost universally true for brief, unpredictable changes in afferent firing, but not necessarily for persistent stable changes.

By using the example of PC-BPPV, it is describe how loose otoconia and endolymph flowed in an ampullofugal direction when the affected PC was oriented vertically in the Dix-Hallpike position: the direction of endolymph flow excites the PC afferents; the eye movements resulting from excitation of the PC will be in the plane of that PC; excitation of the PC afferents will be interpreted as an excitatory rotation of the head in the plane of the PC, and the nystagmus generated would be compensatory for the perceived rotation. For the left PC, excitatory rotation consists rolling the head toward the left while bringing the nose up. To keep the eyes stable in space, the VOR generates slow phases that move the eyes down and roll them clockwise (with respect to the patient's head).

It was described by Ewald[14] that the movement of endolymph in the "on" direction for a canal produced greater nystagmus than an equal movement of endolymph in the "off" direction. It is known as Ewald's second law and it postulates an excitation-inhibition asymmetry. Excitation-inhibition asymmetries occur at multiple levels in the vestibular system. First, in the hair cells there is an asymmetry in the transduction process, which means that there is a larger receptor potential response for stereociliary deflection in the "on" direction than in the "off" direction. A second asymmetry is introduced by the vestibular nerve afferents. Recall that the afferents fire even when the head is at rest and that this firing is modulated by the hair cell responses to head acceleration after the endolymph and cupula integrate the signal to yield one representing head velocity. Vestibular afferents in mammals have baseline firing rates ranging from 50 to 100 spikes per second.[18] Although these firing rates can be driven upward to 300–400 spikes per second, they can be driven no lower than zero. This inhibitory cutoff is the most obvious and severe form of excitation-inhibition asymmetry in the vestibular system. Goldberg et al.[19] demonstrated that this asymmetry is more marked for irregular afferents.

These peripheral asymmetries may be mostly eliminated in the central vestibular connections because of the reciprocal characteristics of signals from one side compared to another. In fact, such combination of nonlinear sensors acting reciprocally on a symmetrical premotor system can increase the linear range of the vestibular reflexes when both sides are functioning appropriately.[20] However, nonlinearities in the VOR become pronounced when labyrinthine function is lost unilaterally.

Aw et al.[21] demonstrated that VOR responses may be asymmetrical in humans after unilateral labyrinthectomy. The "head thrusts" test elicit rapid passive rotatory movements and occur like this: when the head is thrust in one of the SCC planes so as to excite the canal on the intact side, the VOR that results is nearly compensatory for the head movement, but when the head is thrust in one of the SCC planes so as to excite the canal on the lesioned side, the VOR that results is markedly diminished. Although head rotation produces an excitatory contribution from the ipsilateral horizontal canal and an inhibitory contribution from the contralateral one, these contributions are markedly asymmetrical under these conditions. The inhibitory contribution from the intact canal is insufficient to drive a compensatory VOR when the head is thrust toward the lesioned side, but the excitatory contribution from the intact canal that is obtained when the head is thrust toward the intact side is almost adequate to drive a fully compensatory VOR by itself. Such a marked asymmetry may not be evident for low-frequency, low-velocity rotations, which are not dynamic enough to cut off responses in the inhibited nerve.[22] The head thrust test (HTT) has become one of the most important tools in the clinical evaluation of vestibular function. In its qualitative, "bedside" form, the examiner simply asks the subject to stare at the examiner's nose while the examiner turns the subject's head quickly along the excitatory direction for one canal. If the function of that canal is diminished, the VOR will fail to keep the eye on target, and the examiner will see the patient make a refixation saccade after the head movement is completed. When there is a loss of function well compensated, the refixation saccade may even occur while the head is completing its movement, and it may take some experience to spot the saccade while the head is still in motion. By contrast, when the head thrust is in the excitatory direction of an intact canal, the patient's gaze remains stable on the examiner's nose through-out the movement. The HTT can localize isolated hypofunction of individual SCCs.

It is not too common that natural head movements align solely with one canal plane; on the contrary, most rotations stimulate two or even all three of the pairs of canals. How much is each canal stimulated in such a rotation? The motion of the endolymph in each canal (relative to the canal) will determine the degree to which the hair cells in that canal are stimulated. The endolymph motion in each canal is proportional to the component of the head's rotational velocity acting in the plane of that canal. For example, a head rotation to the left with the head upright mostly stimulates the left horizontal canal. The component of head rotation operating on the horizontal canal is the projection onto the horizontal canal's sensitivity axis. However, note that the projections onto the sensitivity axes of the superior and posterior canals indicate excitatory stimulus acting on the ipsilateral superior canal and inhibitory stimulus acting on the ipsilateral posterior canal. The pattern of activity induced in the ampullary nerves therefore effectively decomposes a head rotation into mutually independent simultaneous components along the sensitivity axes. The actions of pairs of extraocular muscles are similarly combined. The extraocular muscles are arranged in pairs that approximately rotate the eyes around axes in the orbit that parallel the sensitivity axes of the canals. Simultaneous activation of extraocular muscle pairs in proportions similar to the proportions of canal activation will result in eye rotation around an axis parallel to that about which the head rotates, but in the opposite direction. This, of course, is the goal of the angular VOR. Given its ability to immediately sort incoming stimuli (head rotations) into spatially independent, minimally redundant channels of information, the labyrinth can be thought of as a "smart sensor" that not only measures stimuli but encodes them immediately in a maximally efficient way for downstream use in driving the angular VOR.

In this respect, it is analogous to the cochlea, which segregates sounds into separate bins of the frequency spectrum, and the retina, which spatially maps the world into a retinotopic space. Just as head rotations rarely stimulate only one pair of semicircular canals, labyrinthine disease rarely affects only one canal. The brain perceives the simultaneous activation of several canals as the head rotation that would produce the same component of activation along each canal's sensitivity axis. These components are linearly combined to produce an eye movement that would compensate for the perceived head movement. By observing the axis of the nystagmus, the examiner can deduce which combination of canals are being excited (or inhibited). This linear superposition of the canal signals for simultaneous stimulation of multiple canals was confirmed in an elegant series of experiments from Cohen and Suzuki[16,23] by using cineoculography of eye movements and electromyographic recordings from extraocular muscles in cats while electrically stimulating ampullary nerves alone and in combinations. They observed that even highly nonphysiologic combinations of ampullary nerve stimuli caused eye movements and extraocular muscle activity that could be predicted as the vector summation of responses to each stimulus alone.

Suzuki and Cohen[24] showed what occurs when all of the canals on one side become excited from their baseline firing rates. The slow phase of the observed nystagmus has a horizontal component toward the contralateral side and a torsional component that moves the superior pole of the eye toward the contralateral side. The nystagmus beats to the ipsilateral side both horizontally and torsionally. There is no vertical component to this nystagmus. This irritative nystagmus can be seen when the labyrinth is irritated, for example, early in an attack of Ménière's disease, after stapedectomy procedures, and early in the course of viral labyrinthitis.

The same static imbalance in firing rates between sides occurs with unilateral labyrinthine hypofunction. Consider the case of left unilateral labyrinthectomy, in which case all three canals on that side are ablated. Unopposed activity of the right lateral canal contributes a leftward slow phase component. Unopposed activity of the right anterior canal contributes an upward and counterclockwise slow phase component. Finally, unopposed activity of the right posterior canal contributes a downward and counterclockwise slow phase component. These components combine, with the up and down components canceling each other, and with the net result being a leftward and counterclockwise slow phase (rightward- and clockwise-beating) nystagmus.

Nystagmus due to dysfunction of SCCs has a fixed axis and direction with respect to the head and it helps to distinguish nystagmus from a peripheral vestibular disorder from nystagmus due to a central disorder. In the case of the latter, the axis or direction of nystagmus may change depending on the direction of gaze.[25] It is important to note that the magnitude of the nystagmus is not fixed depending on gaze. The reason for this is discussed in ahead.

The description of the VOR up to this point has depicted little role for brainstem and cerebellar signal processing, other than passing on the vestibular signals to the appropriate ocular motor nuclei. This "direct pathway" is the classical three-neuron reflex arc. However, the brainstem does more than serve as a conduit for the vestibular afferent signals. An "indirect pathway" through the brainstem circuits also must account for the poor performance of the vestibular end organs at low frequencies and the need for further integration of the incoming head velocity signal to generate fully compensatory eye movements. The brainstem accomplishes these tasks through processes called velocity storage and velocity-to-position integration. These two processes also lead to several important clinical phenomena, such as postrotatory nystagmus, post–head-shaking nystagmus, and Alexander's law. The last of these is another one of the cardinal signs that differentiates peripheral from central causes of nystagmus.

Velocity Storage

For head rotations at frequencies below ~0.1 Hz, the vestibular nerve afferent firing rate gives a poor representation of head velocity. In response to a constant velocity rotation, the cupula initially deflects but then returns back to its resting position, with a time constant of ~13 seconds.[26] Thus, nystagmus in response to a constant-velocity rotation would be expected to disappear after ~30 seconds. In fact, the situation would be made somewhat worse because canal afferent neural responses also tend to decay for static- or low-frequency responses. This adaptation of afferent firing is a property of the neuron itself, and it is especially pronounced for irregular afferents.

The effect of adaptation is to make afferents respond more transiently to static- and low-frequency cupular displacements. Thus, some canal afferents end up carrying a transient signal in response to low-frequency and constant-velocity rotations. This signal more closely reflects the rate of change of head velocity—that is, acceleration—than velocity itself.

Despite these tendencies for the peripheral vestibular signals to decay prematurely, experimental observations in humans have shown that the time constant of the decay of the angular VOR for constant-velocity rotation is about 20 seconds, longer than would be expected based on the performance characteristics of the canals alone.[27] Neural circuits in the brainstem seem to perseverate canal signals, stretching them out in time. The important physiologic consequence of this effect (historically called velocity storage, because it appears to "store" the head velocity information for some period of time) is that it allows the vestibular system to function better at low frequencies.

Robinson[28] proposed that velocity storage could be accomplished by a feedback loop operating in a circuit including the vestibular nuclei. Lesion studies in monkeys suggest that velocity storage arises from neurons in medial vestibular nucleus and descending vestibular nucleus whose axons cross the midline.

Velocity storage is responsible for the prolonged nystagmus that occurs after sustained constant-velocity rotation in one direction. Rotation to one side generates a positive change in afferent firing on the ipsilateral side and a negative change on the contralateral side. Because of the excitation-inhibition asymmetry inherent in the SCC signals, the net result is not zero change in the afferent firing rate sensed by the brainstem, but rather a net excitation on the ipsilateral side. The velocity storage mechanism perseverates this net excitation beyond the time that the cupula deflection has returned to zero. The brainstem thus perceives that the head continues to rotate toward the same side, and it generates an angular VOR for that perceived rotation. The slow phases of nystagmus are directed toward the contralateral side, and the fast phases are directed toward the ipsilateral side. This nystagmus decays exponentially as the velocity storage mechanism discharges with the time constant of ~20 seconds.

If the head is rotated side to side in the horizontal plane in normal subjects, the velocity storage mechanism is charged equally on both sides. There is no postrotatory nystagmus as the stored velocities decay at the same rate on either side. However, nystagmus does occur after head shaking in subjects with unilateral vestibular hypofunction. As the head is shaken from the lesioned side toward the intact side, net excitation is stored by the velocity storage mechanism. In fact, the net excitation is greater than in normal subjects because there is no inhibitory signal coming from the lesioned labyrinth. When the head is turned and rotated toward the lesioned side, there is no excitatory stimulus sent to the brainstem from that side, and only a small inhibitory stimulus from the intact labyrinth. After multiple cycles of back-and-forth rotation, a marked asymmetry develops in the velocity storage mechanism, one that signals illusory continued rotation toward the intact side. As a result, when the head stops rotating, the nystagmus is as would be expected for continued rotation toward the intact side: the slow phases go toward the lesioned side, and the fast phases toward the intact side. This pattern may even reverse after several seconds, presumably because neurons affected by velocity storage adapt to the prolonged change in firing from their baseline rates.

However, because the integrator is shared by other oculomotor systems, including the saccadic system, the ability to hold the eye in an eccentric position in the orbit is impaired when the integrator is leaky. As a result, the eyes tend to drift back to the center position in the orbits. This centripetal drift has an important effect on the observed nystagmus. When the eyes look toward the direction of the fast phase of nystagmus, the drift due to the "leakiness" of the integrator adds to the slow-phase velocity due to the vestibular imbalance, and as a result the nystagmus slow-phase velocity increases. However, when the eyes look toward the direction of the slow phase, the centripetal drift due to the leaky integrator subtracts from the slow-phase velocity due to the vestibular imbalance, and the nystagmus slow-phase decreases or may disappear. This observation has come to be known as Alexander's law.[29] Although occasionally seen in central lesions, peripheral types of nystagmus generally will obey Alexander's law, making it an important neuro-otologic examination finding in distinguishing nystagmus of central origin from that of peripheral origin.

Utricle

The utricle senses linear accelerations that are tangential to some portion of its curved surface. Most of the utricle is approximately in the plane of the horizontal canal, although its anterior end curves upward from this plane. The baseline firing of utricular afferent fibers is therefore best modulated by linear accelerations in the horizontal plane—that is, fore and aft or side to side. Hair cells in the utricle are polarized such that stereociliary deflections toward the striola excite the hair cells, and deflections away from the striola inhibit them. The organ's pattern of responses is not too simple because the orientations of the stereociliary bundles vary over its surface. Linear accelerations in different directions probably activate unique ensembles of activity in the afferents of the utricle, with some areas being excited and others inhibited. These ensemble responses may encode the direction of head acceleration. Excitation or inhibition of all regions of the utricle does not occur under normal conditions of vestibular stimulation. Thus, predicting what the brain will perceive during pathologic conditions resulting in stimulation of the whole utricle is less straightforward than was the case for the SCCs, whose hair cells are all polarized in the same direction. Thus, the brain interprets a tonic increase in firing from the utricle on one side as a net acceleration of the otoconial mass toward the ipsilateral side and a decrease or loss in firing from the utricle on one side is interpreted as a net acceleration of the otoconial mass toward the contralateral or intact side. Such acceleration could be produced by an ipsilateral tilt or by a contralateral translational movement of the head. Just how the brain distinguishes utricular signals due to tilt from those due to translation remains one of the ongoing controversies in vestibular physiology. The equivalence of tilt and translation provides the brain a seemingly irresolvable ambiguity in the utricular afferent signals. Nevertheless, the brain is somehow able to correctly resolve the source of the ambiguous stimulus under normal conditions. Low-frequency or static linear accelerations acting on the otolith organs might be interpreted as gravitational accelerations resulting from tilt, whereas transient linear accelerations might be interpreted as linear translations.[30,31] An alternative hypothesis is that the CNS integrates information from the SCCs with information from the otolith organs to distinguish tilts (which also transiently activate canals) from translations (which activate only the otolith organs).

An isolated loss of utricular nerve activity elicits a stereotypical set of static responses called the ocular tilt reaction: head tilt toward the lesioned side; disconjugate deviation of the eyes such that the pupil on the intact side is elevated and the pupil on the lesioned side is depressed (a so-called skew deviation), and a static conjugate counter-roll of the eyes rolling the superior pole of each eye away from the intact utricle. Each of these signs can be understood as the brain's compensatory response to a perceived head tilt toward the intact utricle. This perception arises from the excess of ipsilateral tilt information coming from the intact utricle.

Saccule

The saccule is almost planar and lies in a parasagittal orientation. Hair cells of the saccule, polarized so that they are excited by otoconial mass displacements away from the striola, can sense accelerations fore or aft (along the naso-occipital axis) or up and down. Most afferents from the saccule have a preferred up or down direction.[8a,b] Thus, the sacculus has a unique role of sensing upward or downward. When the head is upright in the gravitational field, the acceleration due to gravity ($9.8\,m/s^2$) constantly pulls the saccular otoconial mass toward the earth. Afferents in the inferior half of the saccule, whose hair cells are excited by this downward acceleration, have lower firing rates and lower sensitivities to linear accelerations than do those afferents in the upper half of the utricle.[8a,b] The afferents in the upper half are excited by relative upward acceleration of the otoconial mass, such as might occur when the head drops suddenly, e.g. when one is falling. Thus, sudden excitation of hair cells across the saccular macula probably would be interpreted by the brain as a sudden loss of postural tone, as in falling. The appropriate compensatory reflex would be one that activates the trunk and limb extensor muscles and relaxes the flexors to restore postural tone. Accordingly, the saccular afferents project to the lateral portions of the vestibular nuclei, which give rise to the vestibulospinal tract, in contrast to the utricular afferents, which project more rostrally to areas involved in the VORs.

As emphasized throughout this chapter, the vestibular system is efficiently designed to give stereotypical motor reflex outputs that compensate for the movements of the head. Yet a stereotypical output appropriate for one context may be inappropriate for another. For example, redirection of gaze is accomplished by turning first the eyes, then the head, toward a new visual target. During the gaze shift, there is a period during which both the eyes and head must move in the same direction. The VOR must actually be turned off during this period; otherwise, the eyes would stay fixed on the original target. This cancellation of the VOR is measurable in secondary vestibular neurons as a decrease in VOR gain when gaze is being redirected. The mechanism by which the VOR can be canceled is not clear, but secondary vestibular neurons may receive "efference copies" of the commands going to the eye muscles. These oculomotor signals may, through inhibitory connections, decrease the responses of secondary vestibular neurons participating in the VOR reflex arc. Under other circumstances, the VOR gain may need to be increased. For example, when the eyes are verged to view a target near the nose, they must rotate through a larger angle than that fore head rotation, in order to stay on target. In fact, as head rotation brings one eye closer to the target and takes the other eye farther away from it, each eye will require a different VOR gain value. Viirre et al.[32] showed that the VOR performs as needed under these demanding conditions to stabilize images on the retina, and it appears to do so within 10–20 ms of the onset of head movement—faster than could be explained by the use of any visual feedback information to correct the VOR. These investigators suggested that otolith interactions with canal signals could provide a means to constantly update an internal map of the visual target in space, allowing adjustments to the gain of the VOR for each eye.

REFERENCES

1. Leigh RJ, Zee DS. Contemporary neurology series: the neurology of the eye movements. Philadelphia, PA: FA Davies Company; 1983.
2. Highstein SM. Abducens to medical rectus pathway in the MLF: a possible cellular basis for the syndrome of internuclear ophthalmoplegia. In: Brooks BA, Bajandas FJ (Eds). Eye movements. New York: Plenum; 1976.
3. Boyle R, Goldberg JM, Highstein SM. Inputs from regularly and irregularly discharge vestibular nerve afferents to secondary neurons in the squirrel monkey vestibular nuclei. III. Correlation with vestibulospinal and vestibulo-ocular output pathways. J Neurophysiol. 1992;68:471.
4. Bronstein AM, Hood JD. The cervico-ocular reflex in normal subjects and patients with absent vestibular function. Brain Res. 1986;373:399.
5. Buchele W, Brandt T. Vestibular neuritis—a horizontal semicircular canal paresis? Adv Otorhinolaryngol. 1988;42:157.
6. Cannon SC, Robinson DA. Loss of the neural integrator of the oculomotor system from brain stem lesions in monkey. J Neurophysiol. 1987;57:1383.
7. Clendaniel RA, Lasker DM, Minor LB. Horizontal vestibuloocular reflex evoked by high-acceleration rotations in the squirrel monkey. IV. Responses after spectacle-induced adaptation. J Neurophysiol. 2001;86:1594.
8a. Fernandez C, Goldberg JM. Physiology of peripheral neurons innervating otolith organs of the squirrel monkey. III. Response dynamics. J Neurophysiol. 1976;39:996.
8b. Fernandez C, Goldberg JM. Physiology of peripheral neurons innervating otolith organs of the squirrel monkey. I. Response to static tilts and to long duration centrifugal force. J Neurophysiol. 1976;39:970.
9. Fritzsch B. Evolution of the vestibulo-ocular system. Otolaryngol Head Neck Surg. 1998;119:182.
10. Goldberg JM, Fernandez C. Conduction times and background discharge of vestibular afferents. Brain Res. 1977;122:545.

11. Goldberg JM, Fernandez C. Efferent vestibular system in the squirrel monkey: anatomical location and influence on afferent activity. J Neurophysiol. 1980;43:986.
12. Cullen KE, Minor LB. Semicircular canal afferents similarly encode active and passive head-on-body rotations: implications for the role of vestibular efference. J Neurosci. 2002;22:RC226.
13. Young LR, Henn V, Scherberger H. Grundlinien der Lehre von den Bewegungsempfindungen (Fundamentals of the Theory of Movement Perception). In: Mach E (Ed). New York: Kluwer Academic/Plenum Publishers; 2001. Young LR, Henn V, Scherberger H, translators and annotators.
14. Ewald JR. Physiologische Untersuchungen uber das Endorgan des Nervus Octavus. Wiesbaden, Germany: Bergmann; 1892.
15. Blanks RHI, Curthoys IS, Markham CH. Planar relationships of the semicircular canals in man. Acta Otolaryngol (Stockh). 1975;80:185.
16. Cohen B, Suzuki JI, Bender MB. Eye movements from semicircular canal nerve stimulation in the cat. Ann Otol Rhinol Laryngol. 1964;73:153.
17. Robinson DA. The use of matrices in analyzing the three-dimensional behavior of the vestibulo-ocular reflex. Biol Cybern. 1982;46:53.
18. Goldberg JM. Afferent diversity and the organization of central vestibular pathways. Exp Brain Res. 2000;130:277.
19. Goldberg JM, Smith CE, Fernandez C. Relation between discharge regularity and responses to externally applied galvanic currents in vestibular nerve afferents of the squirrel monkey. J Neurophysiol. 1984;51:1236.
20. Smith HLH, Galiana HL. The role of structural symmetry in linearizing ocular reflexes. Biol Cybern. 1991;65:11.
21. Aw ST, Halmagyi GM, Haslwanter T. Three-dimensional vector analysis of the human vestibulo-ocular reflex in response to high acceleration head rotations II. Responses in subjects with unilateral vestibular loss and selective semicircular canal occlusion. J Neurophysiol. 1996;76:4021.
22. Paige GD. Nonlinearity and asymmetry in the human vestibulo-ocular reflex. Acta Otolaryngol (Stockh). 1989;108:1.
23. Cohen B, Suzuki JI. Eye movements induced by ampullary nerve stimulation. Am J Physiol. 1963;204:347.
24. Suzuki JI, Cohen B. Head, eye, body and limb movements from semicircular canal nerves. Exp Neurol. 1964;10:393.
25. Leigh RJ, Zee DS. Diagnosis of central disorders of ocular motility. The Neurology of eye movements. New York: Oxford University Press; 1999.
26. Rabbitt RD, Damiano ER, Grant JW. Biomechanics of the semicircular canals and otolith organs. In: Highstein SM, Fay RR, Popper AN (Eds). The Vestibular system. New York: Springer; 2004.
27. Barr CC, Schultheis LW, Robinson DA. Voluntary, non-visual control of the human vestibulo-ocular reflex. Acta Otolaryngol (Stockh). 1976;81:365.
28. Robinson DA. Linear addition of optokinetic and vestibular signals in the vestibular nucleus. Exp Brain Res. 1977;30:447.
29. Robinson DA, Zee DS, Hain TC. Alexander's law: Its behavior and origin in the human vestibulo-ocular reflex. Ann Neurol. 1984;16:714.

30. Paige GD, Tomko DL. Eye movement responses to linear head motion in the squirrel monkey. I. Basic characteristics. J Neurophysiol. 1991;65:1170.
31. Telford L, Seidman SH, Paige GD. Dynamics of squirrel monkey linear vestibuloocular reflex and interactions with fixation distance. J Neurophysiol. 1997;78(4):1775.
32. Viirre E, Tweed D, Milner K. A reexamination of the gain of the vestibuloocular reflex. J Neurophysiol. 1986;56:439.

Chapter 2

Pathophysiology of Benign Paroxysmal Positional Vertigo

Koji Otsuka, Mamoru Suzuki

PHYSIOLOGICAL EFFECTS OF CUPULOLITHIASIS AND CANALOLITHIASIS IN IN VIVO MODELS

Benign paroxysmal positional vertigo (BPPV) has been classified into two major types based on the nature of nystagmus induced. The most common type is posterior canal canalolithiasis.[1] Nystagmus induced by posterior canal canalolithiasis is characterized by its short duration and latency. Lateral canal BPPV has been further classified into two types according to the direction of nystagmus induced. The underlying mechanism of geotropic nystagmus is thought to be canalolithiasis of the lateral canal while that of apogeotropic nystagmus is considered to be cupulolithiasis of the lateral canal.

We previously used the bullfrog labyrinth in a BPPV model study.[2] The whole membranous labyrinth was used to replicate the human vestibule. The otoconia were dislodged from the utricle by the application of mechanical vibrations to the otic capsule and were driven into the posterior canal (PC) (canalolithiasis model) (Fig. 2.1A). The cupulolithiasis model was created by placing the otoconial mass on the cupula (Fig. 2.1B). The compound action potential (CAP) of the PC nerve was recorded after placing the PC in various positions. The PC was initially placed with the cupula-to-crista axis in the horizontal plane with the utricular side upward. This was designated as the canal-down position. When the PC was placed upside down (i.e. with the canal side up), it was designated as the canal-up position.

In the canalolithiasis model, the canal-down position induced ampullofugal movement of the otoconia, resulting in an excitatory response, while the canal-up position resulted in an inhibitory response (Fig. 2.2). In the excitatory response, the average and standard deviation of the decremental time constant was 6.8 ± 1.0 seconds and the average rise time was 3.5 ± 0.4 seconds. When the otoconia moved inside the canal, neural discharges changed based on the direction of the otoconial movement. A latent period was observed before the discharge change emerged. The otoconia slowly started to move and accelerated with a positional change.

Pathophysiology of Benign Paroxysmal Positional Vertigo

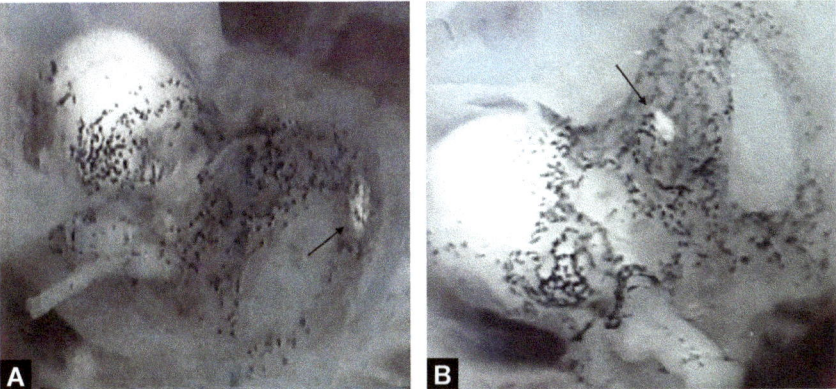

Figs. 2.1A and B: (A) An otoconial mass was detected within the posterior canal. (B) An otoconial mass was on the cupula surface.

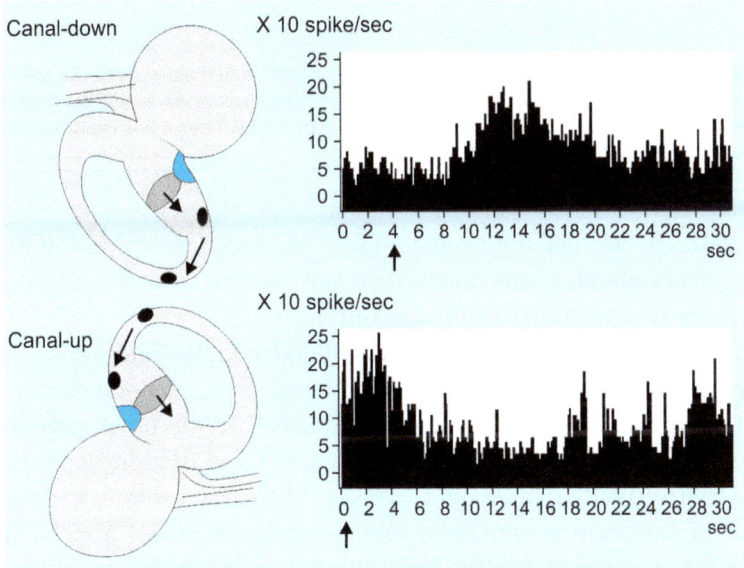

Fig. 2.2: Spike density histograms of compound action potentials in posterior semicircular canal canalolithiasis. The canal-down position induced excitatory discharges, whereas the canal-up position inhibited excitatory discharges. The arrows indicate the onset of positional changes.

The friction force between the otoconia and canal wall was responsible for this slow start of otoconial movement and latency.

On the other hand, in the cupulolithiasis model, the canal-down position induced a depression of the cupula toward the ampullofugal direction, resulting in an excitatory response, while the canal-up position similarly induced depression, resulting in an inhibitory response

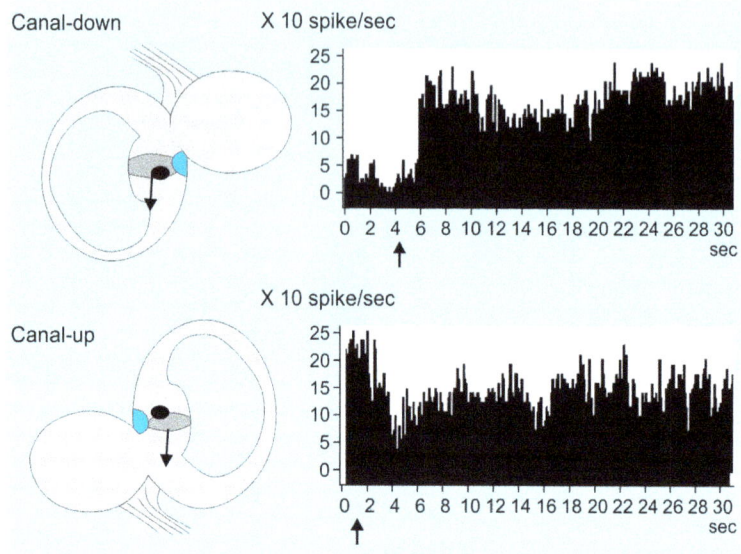

Fig. 2.3: Spike density histograms of compound action potentials in posterior semicircular canal cupulolithiasis. The canal-down position induced sustained excitatory discharges, whereas the canal-up position inhibited excitatory discharges. The arrows indicate the onset of positional changes.

(Fig. 2.3). The average time constant was >43 seconds, which was longer than that of canalolithiasis, and the average rise time was 1.8 ± 0.2 seconds, which was shorter than that of canalolithiasis.

These experiments demonstrated that both cupulolithiasis and canalolithiasis effectively stimulated the cupula and, thus, are potential mechanisms responsible for BPPV. The magnitude of CAP was previously shown to be affected by several physical factors, such as friction between the canal wall and settled otoconia as well as the weight, volume, and acceleration of the moving otoconia.[3] The findings of these model experiments are consistent with the clinical pictures of BPPV. In canalolithiasis, nystagmus has a long latency and short duration, but has a short latency and long duration in cupulolithiasis.

PHYSIOLOGICAL EFFECTS OF OTOCONIA BY MATHEMATICAL MODELS

A mathematical model has been used to analyze the mechanisms responsible for canalolithiasis and cupulolithiasis. House and Honrubia[4] investigated the biophysical fundamental properties of canalolithiasis and cupulolithiasis and reported that the pressure induced by particles moving within the semicircular canal (SC) endolymph was 0.035 dyn/cm^2. Moreover, if an individual particle had a diameter of ~10 µm, the number of particles required to develop BPPV in the cupulolithiasis model was predicted to be 490, while that required to develop BPPV in the canalolithiasis model was predicted to be 62. However, Squires et al.[5] reported that ~20 otoconia, or 0.1 µg of otoconia, was required to account for the emergence of peak nystagmus with BPPV. A mathematical model of the SCs indicated that endolymphatic pressure changed in the anterior and posterior canals when otoconia moved within the common crus in which both canals joined. The nystagmus induced may become the sum of both canals, resulting in a purely torsional effect.

PHYSIOLOGICAL EFFECTS OF CANALOLITHIASIS AND CUPULOLITHIASIS ON SC ACTIVITY

The effects of BPPV on SC function need to be determined in more detail. In BPPV, the incidence of canal paresis (CP) has been reported to be 20-50%. Canal paresis is assumed to be caused by the direct effects of the otoconia, either on the cupula or in the canal in some BPPV cases. Measurements of SC function in BPPV may enable the size of the otoconia to be evaluated and the side affected by BPPV to be identified. We previously attempted to investigate the effects of the otoconia on SC function in model experiments of BPPV.[6]

Caloric Test

Some BPPV patients have a reduced caloric response. Baloh et al.[7] reported the clinical and oculographic features of 240 cases of posterior canal BPPV (PC-BPPV). A total of 94 patients (39.2%) had CP. In 71 out of the 94 patients with CP, paresis was on the side affected by BPPV. Pagnini et al.[8] showed that 5 out of 11 patients (45.5%) with lateral canal BPPV (LC-BPPV) had caloric CP, all of which occurred on the side affected by BPPV. Baloh et al.[9] also demonstrated that 4 out of 13 patients (30.8%) with LC-BPPV had CP on the side affected by BPPV. Korres et al.[10] reported the electronystagmographic (ENG) findings of 168 BPPV patients and found that 22.1% with PC-BPPV and 21.4% with LC-BPPV had CP.

According to a histological study,[11] loose otoconia were commonly found in the lumens of all SCs. Although these loose otoconia were more commonly detected in the PC, they are also found in the LC and anterior semicircular canal (AC). The presence of the otoconia is typically asymptomatic, and this may be because a small quantity of the otoconia cannot stimulate the SC. Therefore, the presence of the otoconia in the endolymph of the LC may exert a gravitational load on the fluid and, thus, affect caloric responses in a significant number of patients with PC-BPPV.

Caloric responses in BPPV depend on the BPPV condition. Katsarkas[12] divided PC-BPPV patients into two groups according to their ENG findings; the first group was examined during the active phase of BPPV and the second group during the inactive phase. Caloric test results were frequently found to be abnormal in the first group, but within normal limits in most of the second group. Strupp et al.[13] described a patient with active LC-BPPV canalolithiasis in whom caloric weakness resolved within a few days following particle-repositioning therapy. This reversible caloric CP was attributed to functional plugging of the LC, which eliminated convective flow in the endolymph.

Rotation Test

Rotation Test for PC-BPPV

Iida et al.[14] performed a pendular rotation test with an oscillation of 360° at a frequency of 0.1 Hz in a head-tilted position (60° backward and rotated 45° to either the right or left) in PC-BPPV patients. The vestibulo-ocular reflex (VOR) response of the PC in the affected ear was smaller than that of the AC. However, the VOR improved once vertigo and nystagmus disappeared. Sekine et al.[15a] reported that VOR gains in the PC did not change in PC-BPPV canalolithiasis at any frequencies from 0.1 to 1.0 Hz, and suggested that the volume of free-floating otoconial debris associated with canalolithiasis was too small relative to the endolymph volume to change the SC dynamics.

Rotation Test for LC-BPPV

Sekine et al.[15b] performed a rotation test on LC-BPPV patients, who were rotated around the vertical axis sinusoidally at frequencies of 0.1–1.0 Hz. In canalolithiasis, no significant difference was observed in VOR gain between rotation to the affected and unaffected sides at any frequencies. Although no significant difference was noted in the VOR gain at frequencies of 0.3–1.0 Hz in cupulolithiasis, the VOR gain at 0.1 Hz was significantly smaller during rotation to the affected side than to the unaffected side. This finding suggested that the temporary impairment of LC function was induced by the mechanical restriction of cupular movements.

Head-Shaking Test

Passive high-frequency rotation of the head is commonly performed in the horizontal and sagittal planes. Lopez-Escamez et al.[16] reported the dynamics of canal responses to the horizontal and vertical head-shaking test in BPPV. Head-shaking nystagmus (HSN) was considered to be present when six consecutive beats of nystagmus with a slow-phase velocity (SPV) of at least 2° per second were detected. The main parameters were the presence of horizontal and vertical HSN, maximum SPV, and time constant of HSN. The maximum SPV of vertical HSN was significantly greater in PC-BPPV patients than in controls. Moreover, the time constant of vertical HSN was smaller for BPPV patients than for controls. These findings suggested that vestibular lithiasis had a limited contribution to the mechanism underlying the generation of HSN.

Head Impulse Test

The head impulse test(HIT) was first introduced by Halmagyi and Curthoys[17] as a clinical test of the VOR to detect lateral semicircular CP. Heidenreich et al.[18] described a patient with active LC-BPPV canalolithiasis who demonstrated robust refixation saccades on HIT, and these were most likely due to rapid mobilization of the otoconial debris. The treatment of LC-BPPV canalolithiasis immediately resolved his vertigo and the HIT results normalized in follow-up testing.

Our Experiments on SC Function in BPPV

We prepared models of canalolithiasis and cupulolithiasis using the isolated PCs of bullfrogs.[6] A glass dish filled with Ringer solution was magnetically fixed on a turntable. The specimen was placed 3 cm from the rotation center with the ampulla toward the inside and the nerve toward the outside. The crista-cupula top axis was on the line facing the rotation center. We first recorded the CAPs of normal specimens and then recorded the CAPs of the canalolithiasis and cupulolithiasis models. The turn table was sinusoidally rotated by a computer-controlled motor. Two rotation cycles, 0.1 and 0.2 Hz, were applied. The rotation cycle was initially set at 0.1 Hz, the rotation angle at 270°, and the maximum angular velocity at 84° per second (Fig. 2.4). The rotation cycle was then set at 0.2 Hz, the rotation angle at 180°, and the maximum angular velocity at 112° per second. The differences between the maximum and minimum spikes in three consecutive recordings were averaged. We designated the spike difference between the spontaneous spikes and maximum spikes as the response intensity (RI). The RIs of canalolithiasis and cupulolithiasis were expressed as a percentage, with 100% representing normal RI. We classified our experiments according to the size of the otoconial mass. An otoconial mass with a span longer than a half of the cupular height (*large otoconia*) was used. In the 0.1 Hz rotation, the RI was 54.6% in canalolithiasis and 17.7% in cupulolithiasis. Cupulolithiasis showed a larger decrease in RI than canalolithiasis. In the 0.2 Hz rotation, the RI was 72.5% in canalolithiasis and 61.8% in cupulolithiasis. The reduction in RI at 0.2 Hz was less than that in RI at 0.1 Hz in cupulolithiasis (Fig. 2.5). An otoconial mass with a span shorter than half of the cupular height

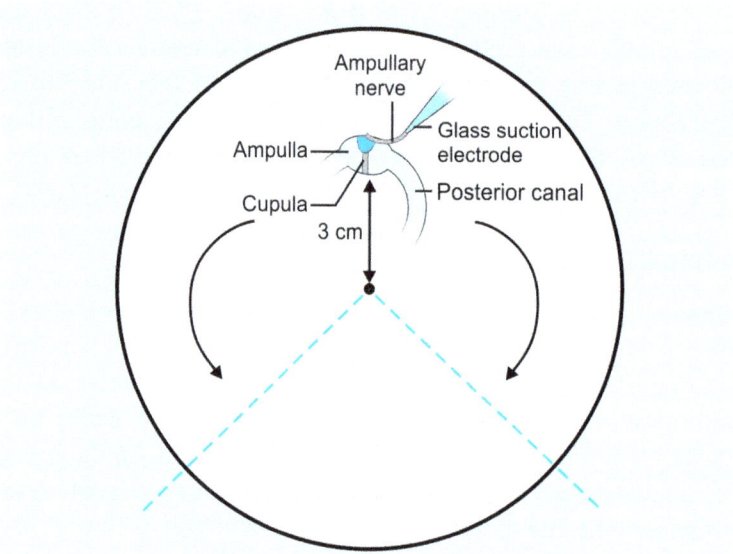

Fig. 2.4: Experimental setting on semicircular canal function in benign paroxysmal positional vertigo. The turn table was sinusoidally rotated by a computer-controlled motor. Two rotation cycles, 0.1 and 0.2 Hz, were applied.

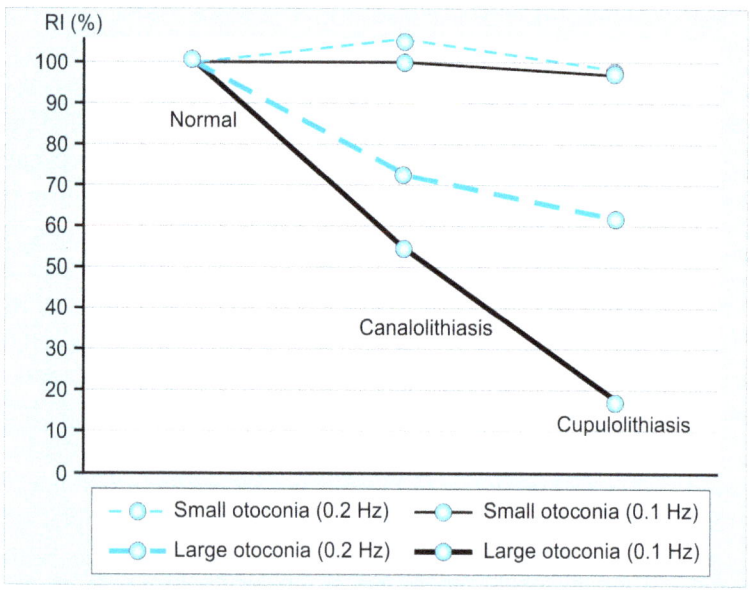

Fig. 2.5: Response intensities (RIs) in canalolithiasis and cupulolithiasis. In the case of small otoconia, the RI was not decreased in either canalolithiasis or cupulolithiasis, or at either 0.1 or 0.2 Hz. In the case of large otoconia, the RI was decreased in both canalolithiasis and cupulolithiasis models. Cupulolithiasis showed a larger decrease in RI than canalolithiasis. The RI at 0.2 Hz did not decrease as much as at 0.1 Hz in cupulolithiasis.

(*small otoconia*) was used. The RI was not decreased in canalolithiasis or cupulolithiasis at either 0.1 or 0.2 Hz (*see* Fig. 2.5).

Large Otoconia versus Small Otoconia

The CAPs markedly decreased and even disappeared in some cases of canalolithiasis involving large otoconia. The otoconia may have formed an embolus, thereby blocking endolymphatic flow. The possibility of otoconial debris forming an embolus was termed a "canalith jam" by Epley.[19] However, CAPs did not change in cases of canalolithiasis involving small otoconia. Some cases of BPPV had a decreased caloric response and VOR gain, whereas others did not. We assumed that this varied according to the size of the otoconial mass.

Canalolithiasis versus Cupulolithiasis

The RI of cupulolithiasis showed a larger decrease than that of canalolithiasis. The direct inhibition of the cupular shift was greater than the inhibition of endolymphatic flow. This suppression of CAPs may have been due to the otoconial weight, which can occur by simply blocking cupular displacement. This finding supported clinical results in which VOR gain was suppressed more in cupulolithiasis than in canalolithiasis.[15b] Our experiments suggested that reduced vestibular responses did not necessarily indicate sensory cell function damage, but rather the inhibition of cupular dynamics. This was supported by the clinical observation in which BPPV vertigo rapidly resolved with adequate physical therapy. The imbalance of cupular mobility between normal and cupulolithiasis ears may be another cause of the dizziness reported in BPPV patients.

0.1 Hz versus 0.2 Hz

The reduction in RI at 0.2 Hz was less than that in RI at 0.1 Hz in cupulolithiasis. A cupula with a large otoconial mass could be moved if the frequency was sufficiently high. This finding supported the clinical result in which VOR gain improved as angular acceleration increased in LC- BPPV.[15b]

FUNCTIONAL EVALUATION OF THE OTOLITHIC ORGAN IN BPPV PATIENTS

Utricular dysfunction has been reported in patients with BPPV. Markham et al.[20] used ocular counter-rolling as a test to reflect the utriculo-ocular reflex. In their study, abnormal ocular counter-rolling was detected in 88.9% of BPPV patients. Sugita et al.[21] examined otolith function in 23 controls and 24 BPPV patients by comparing the VOR gain of off-vertical axis rotation (OVAR) with that of earth-vertical axis rotation (EVAR). Their findings showed that VOR gain during OVAR at 0.8 Hz in BPPV patients was significantly less than that during EVAR, whereas no significant differences were observed in VOR gain between EVAR and OVAR in the controls. They analyzed their findings and suggested the existence of otolith organ dysfunction in BPPV patients.

Vestibular-evoked myogenic potential (VEMP) in cervical muscles (cVEMP) has been widely used as a clinical test of the vesibulocollic reflex, predominantly the sacculocollic reflex. Myogenic potentials around the eyes [ocular VEMP (oVEMP)] have also recently been recorded. Ocular VEMP predominantly reflects utricular functions. Nakahara et al.[22] measured oVEMP and cVEMP in 12 BPPV patients and 12 controls. More BPPV patients exhibited abnormal responses in oVEMP by stimulation on their affected side than the controls, whereas no significant differences were observed in cVEMP between BPPV patients and controls. These findings indicated that oVEMP reflected a specific abnormal condition in BPPV, i.e. utricular function was highly damaged in BPPV patients.

REFERENCES

1. Otsuka K, Ogawa Y, Inagaki T, et al. Relationship between clinical features and therapeutic approach for benign paroxysmal positional vertigo outcomes. J Laryngol Otol. 2013;127:962-7.
2. Otsuka K, Suzuki M, Furuya M. Model experiment of benign paroxysmal positional vertigo mechanism using the whole membranous labyrinth. Acta Otolaryngol. 2003;123:515-8.
3. Furuya M, Suzuki M, Sato H. Experimental study of speed-dependent positional nystagmus in benign paroxysmal positional vertigo. Acta Otolaryngol. 2003;123:709-12.
4. House MG, Honrubia V. Theoretical models for the mechanisms of benign paroxysmal positional vertigo. Audiol Neurootol. 2003;8:91-9.
5. Squires TM, Weidman MS, Hain TC, et al. A mathematical model for top-shelf vertigo: the role of sedimenting otoconia in BPPV. J Biomech. 2004;37:1137-46.
6. Inagaki T, Suzuki M, Otsuka K, et al. Model experiments of BPPV using isolated utricle and posterior semicircular canal. Auris Nasus Larynx. 2006;33:129-34.
7. Baloh RW, Honrubia V, Jacobson K. Benign positional vertigo: clinical and oculographic features in 240 cases. Neurology. 1987;37:371-8.
8. Pagnini P, Nuti D, Vannucchi P. Benign paroxysmal vertigo of the horizontal canal. ORL J Otorhinolaryngol Relat Spec. 1989;51:161-70.
9. Baloh RW, Jacobson K, Honrubia V. Horizontal semicircular canal variant of benign positional vertigo. Neurology. 1993;43:2542-9.
10. Korres SG, Balatsouras DG, Ferekidis E. Electronystagmographic findings in benign paroxysmal positional vertigo. Ann Otol Rhinol Laryngol. 2004;113:313-8.

11. Moriarty B, Rutka J, Hawke M. The incidence and distribution of copular deposits in the labyrinth. Laryngoscope. 1992;102:56-9.
12. Katsarkas A. Electronystagmographic (ENG) findings in paroxysmal positional vertigo (PPV) as a sign of vestibular dysfunction. Acta Otolaryngol. 1991;111:193-200.
13. Strupp M, Brandt T, Steddin S. Horizontal canal benign paroxysmal positional vertigo: reversible ipsilateral caloric hypoexcitability caused by canalolithiasis. Neurology. 1995;45:2072-6.
14. Iida M, Hitouji K, Takahashi M. Vertical semicircular canal function: a study in patients with benign paroxysmal positional vertigo. Acta Otolaryngol Suppl. 2001;545:35-7.
15a. Sekine K, Imai T, Morita M, et al. Vertical canal function in normal subjects and patients with benign paroxysmal positional vertigo. Acta Otolaryngol. 2004;124:1046-52.
15b. Sekine K, Imai T, Nakamae K, et al. Dynamics of the vestibulo-ocular reflex in patients with the horizontal semicircular canal variant of benign paroxysmal positional vertigo. Acta Otolaryngol. 2004;124:587-94.
16. Lopez-Escamez JA, Zapata C, Molina MI, et al. Dynamics of canal response to head-shaking test in benign paroxysmal positional vertigo. Acta Otolaryngol. 2007;127:1246-4.
17. Halmagyi GM, Curthoys IS. A clinical sign of canal paresis. Arch Neurol. 1988;45:737-9.
18. Heidenreich KD, Beaudoin K, White JA. Can active lateral canal benign paroxysmal positional vertigo mimic a false-positive head thrust test? Am J Otol. 2009;30:353-5.
19. Epley JM. Positional vertigo related to semicircular canalolithiasis. Otolaryngol Head Neck Surg. 1995;112:154-61.
20. Markham CH, Diamond SG, Ito J. Utricular dysfunction in benign paroxysmal positional vertigo. The vestibular system. In: MD Graham, J Kemink (Eds). Neurophysiologic and clinical research. New York: Raven press; 1987. pp. 255-62.
21. Sugita-Kitajima A, Azuma M, Hattori K, et al. Evaluation of the otolith function using sinusoidal off-vertical axis rotation in patients with benign paroxysmal positional vertigo. Neurosci Lett. 2007;422:81-6.
22. Nakahara H, Yoshimura E, Tsuda Y, et al. Damaged utricular function clarified by oVEMP in patients with benign paroxysmal positional vertigo. Acta Otolaryngol. 2013;133:144-9.

Chapter 3

Differential Diagnosis of Benign Paroxysmal Positional Vertigo

Richard A Roberts

INTRODUCTION

It has been found that vestibular dysfunction affects 35.4% of adults 40 years of age and older.[1] It is also well established that the most commonly diagnosed vestibular problem is benign paroxysmal positional vertigo (BPPV).[2] This finding has been reported from multiple laboratories and countries worldwide. For example, Strupp et al.[70] reported that among 17,718 patients evaluated at their respective centers, the most common diagnosis was of BPPV at 17.7% (3,036). Another investigation reported on data collected from 4,294 patients with vertigo from 13 countries over 28 months and indicated that 26.9% had BPPV.[3] Bhattacharyya et al.[59] estimate the annual costs associated with appropriate diagnosis of BPPV approach $8 billion. Further, this common problem can be quite impactful on quality of life. Using utility measures, we have shown that pretreatment health-related quality-of-life measures in patients with BPPV were comparable to measures of patients with HIV/AIDS, age-related macular degeneration, and hepatitis B.[4] The clinician must bear in mind that although BPPV impacts the life of the individual patient to this magnitude, it is highly treatable.[5,6,24] However, efficacy of treatment is dependent on accurate diagnosis of involved ear and semicircular canal. It is also important to understand that the differential for diagnosis of positional vertigo is not limited to BPPV as a sole cause, though this would be true for the majority of cases.

PATHOPHYSIOLOGY OF BPPV

The symptoms of BPPV, primarily intense vertigo with rotary nystagmus, are caused by an abnormal interaction of the semicircular canal cupula and displaced otoconia from the utricle. Clinicians often consider whether BPPV is a cupulolithiais or canalithiasis variant. Schuknecht[68] is credited with the cupulolithiasis concept based on his observation of basophilic deposits on the posterior semicircular canal cupula within the temporal bones of patients with a history of positional vertigo. The normal cupula

Table 3.1: Expectations with benign paroxysmal positional vertigo and positional vertigo with a central nervous system cause.

Characteristic	Benign paroxysmal positional vertigo (BPPV)		Central positional vertigo
	Cupulolithiasis	Canalithiasis	
Duration of response	Persistent	Transient (<1 min)	Persistent
Onset latency	None	Onset Latency	None
Fatigues on repetition	No	Yes	No
Reversal of nystagmus on supine to sitting	Yes	Yes	No
Vertigo	Yes	Yes	May or may not be present

has a specific gravity similar to the surrounding endolymph and is sensitive to angular acceleration. The presence of otoconia causes an increase in mass of the cupula, making the semicircular canal sensitive to linear acceleration. Consistent with this concept, moving the patient into a provoking position deflects the heavy cupula, causing the nystagmus and vertigo. Expectations with cupulolithiasis are shown in Table 3.1 and include an immediate onset of symptoms, as well as persistent nystagmus and vertigo as long as the patient remains in the provoking position. These specific characteristics are less commonly observed in the clinic and cupulolithiasis has been reported at an occurrence rate around 17.6% (39 of 260 patients[7]). Jackson et al.[7] reported cupulolithiasis was most common in horizontal canal BPPV (HC-BPPV; 41.9%), followed by anterior canal BPPV (AC-BPPV) with 27.3%. Only 6.3% of their patients with posterior canal BPPV (PC-BPPV) were diagnosed with cupulolithiasis. Our own clinical experience is in agreement that if cupulolithiasis exists, it is more common with HC-BPPV and AC-BPPV. However, few patients present with symptoms of BPPV consistent with expectations with cupulolithiasis which may be helpful with differential diagnosis of BPPV from other causes of positional vertigo.

More commonly, clinical observations in patients with BPPV are consistent with expectations with the canalithiasis concept of BPPV, (Table 3.1). Hall et al.[63] suggested that the displaced otoconia were mobile particles within the involved semicircular canal. The presence of otoconial debris was directly observed as an operative finding and reported by Parnes and McClure.[58] In this more common variant, the mass of otoconia moves within the semicircular canal after change in head position. This movement of the otoconia displaces the endolymphatic fluid, deflecting the cupula of the involved canal and eliciting nystagmus and vertigo (Fig. 3.1). Expected findings with canalithiasis contrast with those of cupulolithiasis in Table 3.1 and include latency from movement into provoking position until onset of symptoms, vertigo, transient

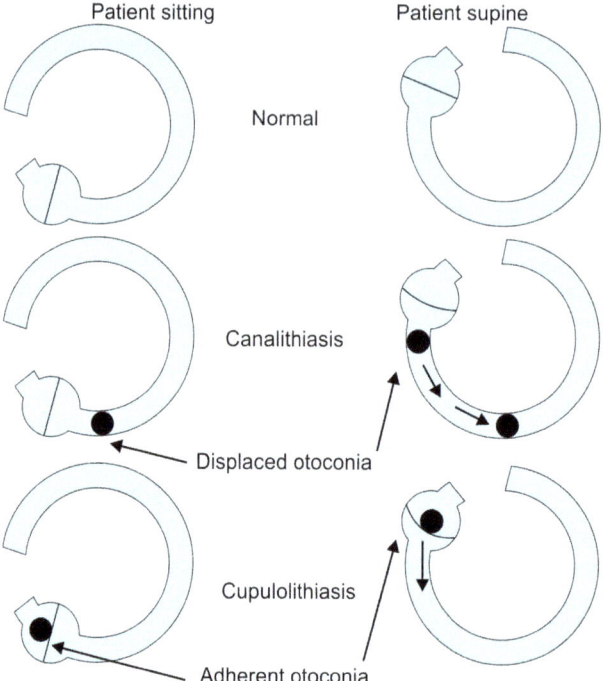

Fig. 3.1: Top panel: Posterior semicircular canal in normal patient sitting upright and then in supine position. Middle panel: Canalithiasis of the posterior semicircular canal is shown. Note the debris moving with change in position from sitting to supine and its effect on the cupula. Lower panel: Cupulolithiasis of the posterior semicircular canal is shown. Note the otoconial debris adherent to the cupula and its effect from sitting to supine. Used with permission Plural Publishing, San Diego, CA.

duration, etc. These signs and symptoms are also consistent with a model of how otoconial debris would move through canals of this size and be able to generate the force needed to deflect the cupula.[8]

The reader is referred to Table 3.2 for details on the semicircular canal and extraocular muscle connections, as well as the resulting nystagmus from BPPV. The type of nystagmus observed most often with BPPV is a rotary, upbeating nystagmus with an oblique movement toward the involved ear. This follows the fact that the posterior canal is the most often affected by BPPV and this canal is connected through the vestibulo-ocular reflex (VOR) pathway to the ipsilateral superior oblique and the contralateral inferior rectus extraocular muscles.[2,9] With HC-BPPV, a linear horizontal nystagmus is observed, which may be either geotropic or ageotropic. Geotropic refers to the nystagmus fast-phase beating toward the dependent ear, while ageotropic refers to the fast-phase beating away from the dependent ear. The horizontal canal is connected through the VOR pathway to the ipsilateral medial rectus and contralateral lateral rectus extraocular muscles.[2,9] As opposed to observations of nystagmus

Table 3.2: Semicircular canal involvement and associated nystagmus		
Canal	Paired extraocular muscles	Nystagmus fast phase
Posterior	Ipsilateral superior oblique contralateral inferior rectus	Rotary-up-beating
Horizontal (Lateral)	Ipsilateral medial rectus contralateral lateral rectus	Horizontal
Anterior (Superior)	Ipsilateral superior rectus contralateral inferior oblique	Rotary-down-beating

with PC-BPPV, a rotary downbeating nystagmus is observed with anterior canal involvement given its VOR pathway connections with the ipsilateral superior rectus and contralateral inferior oblique extraocular muscles.[2,9] An appreciation for the direction of the nystagmus is key in identification of the correct canal, which leads to selection of the appropriate management technique.

Slight modifications in the direction of nystagmus can be appreciated in patients with vertical canal BPPV by having the patient gaze in different directions. For example, the response with PC-BPPV can be made to have a more vertical aspect by having the patient gaze away from the involved ear. Gazing toward the involved ear should create a more torsional eye movement. Since potential exists for patients to unwittingly influence the nystagmus response in this way, the clinician must remain vigilant. This is especially true for downbeating nystagmus. Downbeating nystagmus has historically been interpreted as an indicator of a central nervous system (CNS) issue, but there are multiple reports in the literature that suggest purely downbeating nystagmus may also be an indicator of AC-BPPV.[10-12]

Semicircular Canal Involvement

By far, the majority of cases of BPPV involve the posterior canal. Across a number of studies, this is the involved canal in 61–97% of cases.[13-16] Most assume this is related to the inferior orientation of the posterior semicircular canal relative to the utricle. Benign paroxysmal positional vertigo can absolutely affect the other two canals. A majority of independent investigations indicate that HC-BPPV is the second most common involvement, accounting for 1–32% of cases.[13,17-19] Anterior canal BPPV, by most accounts and from clinical experience, is the least common form of BPPV and ranges from 1 to 21% of cases. Herdman et al.[65] mention the difficulty that may occur with differentiation among the vertical canals. It is possible that a better understanding of BPPV, as well as the common use of video-oculography recording of nystagmus, has made it easier to differentiate anterior canal from posterior canal involvement.

Clinicians may not have been looking for AC-BPPV so they did not see it. Any torsional nystagmus may have been attributed to posterior canal involvement.

Unilateral/Bilateral

Another interesting finding with BPPV is that it is most commonly unilateral. Bilateral BPPV is only observed in 4% to upward of 25% of cases.[20,21] Many agree bilateral involvement is more common following head trauma compared to other causes of BPPV.[22,23] Liu[23] reported significantly more bilateral BPPV (25%) in patients with post-traumatic BPPV compared to only 2% of patients with other causes of BPPV. Patients with post-traumatic BPPV were also significantly more likely (55%) to have BPPV affecting more than one canal compared to only 6.5% of other patients with BPPV. Soto-Varela et al.[69] report similar results to Liu. They also noted that in their series a history of recurrent BPPV was more common in patients with multicanal, but unilateral BPPV.

Right Ear/Left Ear

The right ear is more often affected by BPPV than the left ear.[6,24-26] von Brevern et al.[71] found only two studies, at the time, that reported more left ear than right ear involvement. From all the data, the authors estimated the right ear was involved 1.37–1.45 times more often than the left. They suggested this may be related to patient sleeping position. Lopez-Escamez et al.[67] also reported a significant association between affected ear and side during bed rest.

BPPV without Nystagmus

Benign paroxysmal positional vertigo presents in a typical manner most often. However, there are accounts of what some term subjective BPPV.[27] The only difference between typical presentation and subjective BPPV is that no nystagmus is present during vertigo provocation. Haynes et al.[64] reported on 35 patients with a presenting history and symptoms consistent with BPPV. The patients reported transient vertigo during Hallpike testing, but no nystagmus was observed by the clinician. The authors used the Semont liberatory maneuver (SLM) to treat these patients and success was achieved in 86% (i.e. 30). Huebner et al.[27] reported no difference in treatment outcome for patients with typical (with nystagmus) BPPV compared to patients with subjective BPPV. Both studies confirm that BPPV may be present in the absence of characteristic nystagmus for some patients. We would caution clinicians not to over generalize this finding to mean that numerous BPPV treatments should be imposed on all patients presenting with atypical symptoms.

Non-BPPV Causes of Positional Vertigo

It is evident that most patients with BPPV present with a history of transient, positionally provoked vertigo. That patient would be expected to have torsional and upbeating nystagmus coincident with vertigo during test positioning. The duration of the response should be for seconds. This would indicate a posterior canal involvement and slightly more often this would be the right ear. Horizontal canal BPPV is also observed as is AC-BPPV, though these are less common than PC-BPPV. Benign paroxysmal positional vertigo related to head trauma will have a greater tendency to present as bilateral and/or multicanal. There is also a group of patients who present with this history and these symptoms but do not have nystagmus during examination. Clinicians must be cautious, however, when considering identification of an "atypical variant" or a "nonclassic form" of BPPV. In those cases, the possibility increases substantially the patient may not have BPPV.

Other Peripheral Vestibular Involvement

Patients with uncompensated vestibulopathy related to some type of pathology (i.e. vestibular neuritis) may report positional dizziness during evaluation. This is usually distinguished from true vertigo during case history interview, but the patient may also report the sensation while symptoms are provoked during evaluation. This may help differentiate true vertigo from positional dizziness. Observation of nystagmus is also essential for differential diagnosis. As expected from Ewald's second law, the nystagmus from unilateral uncompensated vestibular dysfunction is direction-fixed and horizontal with the fast-phase beating toward the intact ear. This nystagmus should also suppress with a fixation target. This varies from expectations of nystagmus with BPPV as we have described. It is important for the clinician to remember that BPPV can be observed secondary to vestibular insult like vestibular neuritis, labyrinthitis, Ménière's disease, etc.[28,29] So, secondary BPPV may be present in addition to uncompensated symptoms.

Perilymphatic fistula is another peripheral vestibular issue that may cause positional vertigo. This is caused by leakage of perilymphatic fluid via an abnormal opening into the middle ear space. The associated nystagmus should be direction fixed. In addition to provocation of symptoms during positioning, changes in intracranial pressure, as well as changes in ear canal pressure may also provoke symptoms. Perilymphatic fistula and BPPV may both be associated with head trauma and could coexist.

As standard clinical practice, patients are asked to refrain from alcohol at least 48 hours prior to evaluation. Fetter et al.[62] recorded upbeating nystagmus in all 10 of their test participants. The more well-known reason for restricting alcohol consumption prior to testing is to avoid either phase of positional alcohol nystagmus (PAN I and PAN II). Aschan et al.[30,31] completed much of the work that helped explain the alcohol diffusion differential between endolymph and cupulae. This difference can result in a geotropic nystagmus 30 minutes after alcohol ingestion (PAN I). Positional alcohol nystagmus type II begins 5–10 hours after alcohol is no longer being ingested. In this second phase, a positionally provoked nystagmus can also be recorded, but with the fast-phase beating toward the upper ear (ageotropic nystagmus). Patients with either PAN I or PAN II could potentially experience vertigo along with the nystagmus, so this must be considered.

Central Nervous System Involvement

Positional vertigo related to CNS involvement may also be present. More commonly, vertical nystagmus without true vertigo may be present during positioning testing. The presence or absence of true vertigo can be helpful with differential diagnosis as vertigo should always be present with BPPV. Positional vertigo and purely vertical nystagmus can be observed with involvement of the cerebellum, Arnold-Chiari malformations, multiple sclerosis, and vertebrobasilar insufficiency (VBI).[9,32-34] Upbeating nystagmus is not too common. This type of vertical nystagmus is associated with infarct or tumor of the brain stem and/or cerebellum, multiple sclerosis, and even drug intoxication effects.[9,32,34]

Downbeating nystagmus is observed with degeneration and lesions of the cerebellum, lesions at the craniocervical junction (Arnold-Chiari malformations), multiple sclerosis, VBI, and drug intoxication.[9,32-34] Baloh and Honrubia[9] suggest the source of downbeating nystagmus is degeneration of the cerebellar flocculus and paraflocculus. This is believed to release the inhibitory pathways on the inherent upward eye movement bias from the six semicircular canals, which results in a downward nystagmus fast phase. Our own experience is that downbeating nystagmus is common in older patients with CNS changes reported on imaging studies. These changes may be interpreted as normal for the patient's age.

Downbeating nystagmus is worthy of further discussion in terms of differential diagnosis of BPPV. We mentioned previously there are several reports that indicate downbeating nystagmus can be an indicator of AC-BPPV.[10-12] In a series of 50 consecutive patients with downbeating nystagmus, Bertholon et al.[10] identified 24% (12) with no other indicators of CNS involvement except the downbeating nystagmus. These 12 patients did have symptoms and other findings consistent with BPPV. Similar to Baloh and Honrubia,[9] these authors considered an upward bias in vertical slow phase eye velocity based on calculations of angular eye velocity vectors derived from known canal geometry. Based on these calculations, Bertholon et al.[10] suggest that AC-BPPV would favor a more vertical nystagmus as opposed to the more torsional nystagmus expected and observed with PC-BPPV.

Zapala[12] stated that in the absence of other CNS symptoms and findings, patients with downbeating nystagmus should be treated for AC-BPPV. This is an interesting concept as he advocates the use of BPPV treatment to aid in differential diagnosis, a suggestion we had made for other causes of positional vertigo.[35] Ogawa et al.[11] reported findings from four patients similar to those of Bertholon et al.[10] and Zapala,[12] but are more conservative in their exclusion of CNS involvement. This caution is warranted. Considering Bertholon et al.'s series of 50 patients, 76% did actually have CNS involvement, not AC-BPPV. We remain in agreement with Zapala,[12] but for appropriate cases.

Another interesting finding is observation of ageotropic positional nystagmus in older patients, but with no vertigo or other dizziness. The lack of vertigo helps differentiate from HC-BPPV. If PAN II is also excluded, then the nystagmus is most likely caused by age-related CNS changes, which may be observed as even subtle findings on imaging studies. Alternatively, we have reported on patients with migrainous positional vertigo who also present with ageotropic nystagmus.[35] The presentation can be very similar to HC-BPPV of cupulolithiasis type, but with a persistent response and no improvement with repositioning. Others have reported similar findings. von Brevern et al.[51] reported on 10 patients with "pseudo-BPPV" who were diagnosed with migrainous vertigo. Four of the patients had positionally provoked nystagmus with concomitant vertigo during their episodes. These are most difficult to differentiate from BPPV and knowledge about history of migraine and aura symptoms is important. When diagnosis remains unclear, however, we trust to the efficacy of BPPV treatment techniques. We advocate as in studies of Roberts et al.[35] and Zapala[12] that for appropriate cases, treatment should be considered during evaluation to help differentiate BPPV from other causes of positional vertigo. If the patient is experiencing BPPV, the symptoms should be eliminated or improved with treatment.

Cervicogenic Dizziness

There are known connections between the cervical dorsal roots and vestibular nuclei. It is believed that the neck proprioceptors and joint receptors serve a role in eye-hand coordination, perception of balance, and postural adjustments.[36,37] Zuo et al.[72] suggest that bidirectional nerve fiber connections between cervical spinal and sympathetic ganglia provide a neuroanatomical basis for neck-related dizziness. Others suggest symptoms may be provoked by cervical changes on vertebro-basilar circulation.[38,39]

Regardless, patients with a history of neck injury, cervical pain, and limited cervical range of motion may present with positional dizziness as a primary complaint or during evaluation. True vertigo would be rare. Clendaniel and Landel[61] and Wrisley et al.[37] provide excellent reviews of both examination and treatment of cervical vertigo. Wrisley et al.[37] provide a decision tree to help guide the clinician. Cervicogenic dizziness can be differentiated from BPPV by lack of true vertigo and absence of nystagmus typical of BPPV.

POSITIONING TECHNIQUES FOR ELICITING BPPV

As modeled by Squires et al.,[8] the greatest transcupular pressure (and BPPV response) occurs if displaced otoconia move through the center of the semicircular canal duct. Greater pressure would also be expected if the largest mass of debris moves at one time. Patient movement can disperse the debris, which may cause a lesser amount to move at once, or debris movement may be along the semicircular canal duct wall. This could lead to no BPPV response or a less robust response, potentially impacting diagnosis. Clinicians are advised to test for BPPV prior to placing the patient in other positions.

The clinician must also consider the potential for patient issues related to the cervical spine, VBI, lower back, etc. This must be considered because the most widely taught and used technique for assessment of BPPV is the Dix-Hallpike maneuver.[2,40,41] The patient is seated on the examination table and briskly moved to a supine position with the head turned toward the test ear. The head is off the examination table, so there is extension of the neck and the test ear is in a dependent position. The clinician is to the side of the patient and holds either the shoulders or head of the patient. This extension of the neck may place the patient at risk for posterior circulation ischemia in patients with VBI.[42-45] Although less serious, patients with cervical spine issues may be very uncomfortable with this type of rotation and extension of the neck. Muscle spasm could also occur. Patients with lower back problems may have difficulty lying supine for the duration of testing. For these reasons, some have suggested that this testing (Dix-Hallpike) should never be completed in older patients. This is unsatisfactory in view of the prevalence, the financial burden, and the major impact on health-related quality of life for patients with BPPV. We are in agreement with others who suggest safer and more comfortable adaptations of the traditional Dix-Hallpike maneuver that have similar sensitivity for BPPV.[43,46,47]

Humphriss et al.[43] advocated the use of a Vertebral Artery Screening Test (VAST) to determine which patients may be at risk for possible vertebrobasilar ischemia. The sensitivity of this screening ranges from 0% to 57%.[48] Still, we feel this gives the clinician an idea of whether there may be a potential issue with VBI and such an issue could be the cause of patient symptoms. Additionally, this screening allows the clinician to gain an idea of cervical range of motion. We complete the VAST with the patient in a sitting position. The patient rotates the head to the right and then extends the neck to look upward. The clinician monitors for symptoms of dizziness, nausea, nystagmus, dysarthria, as well as pain/discomfort. This is repeated with rotation to the opposite side and extension of the neck. If the screening is positive, we suggest the clinician consider an alternative assessment technique (side-lying or fully supported Hallpike) in place of the methods that require extension of the neck (traditional Dix-Hallpike or modified Dix-Hallpike). This simple screening and knowledge of multiple assessment techniques should allow any patient to be assessed for BPPV.

Posterior/Anterior Semicircular Canal

Modified Hallpike

We will describe the modified Hallpike in place of the traditional Dix-Hallpike maneuver. This is shown in Figures 3.2A to C. As in the "Epley" and other canalith repositioning maneuvers for PC-BPPV, the examiner begins in a position standing behind the patient.[20,24,26,49] The patient turns the head toward the test ear (45° away from midline), while the clinician supports the patient's neck and back. The clinician sits as the patient is eased into the provoking supine position. The neck of the patient is slightly extended but always supported while the head is off the examination table. We do not recommend the modified Hallpike for patients in whom extension of the neck is contraindicated.

Posterior canal BPPV is the most common type so given the extraocular muscle connections discussed earlier (*see* Table 3.2), the most common nystagmus finding observed during positioning testing is upbeating with torsion toward the affected ear. There should be concomitant vertigo at nystagmus onset and a temporally correlated decay in both the vertigo and nystagmus. Less commonly, a downbeating rotary nystagmus may be provoked along with a vertigo response. This would indicate AC-BPPV and may not be recognized unless the clinician incorporates VOG recordings.[47] As noted earlier, purely vertical downbeating nystagmus can also be observed with AC-BPPV.[10,12]

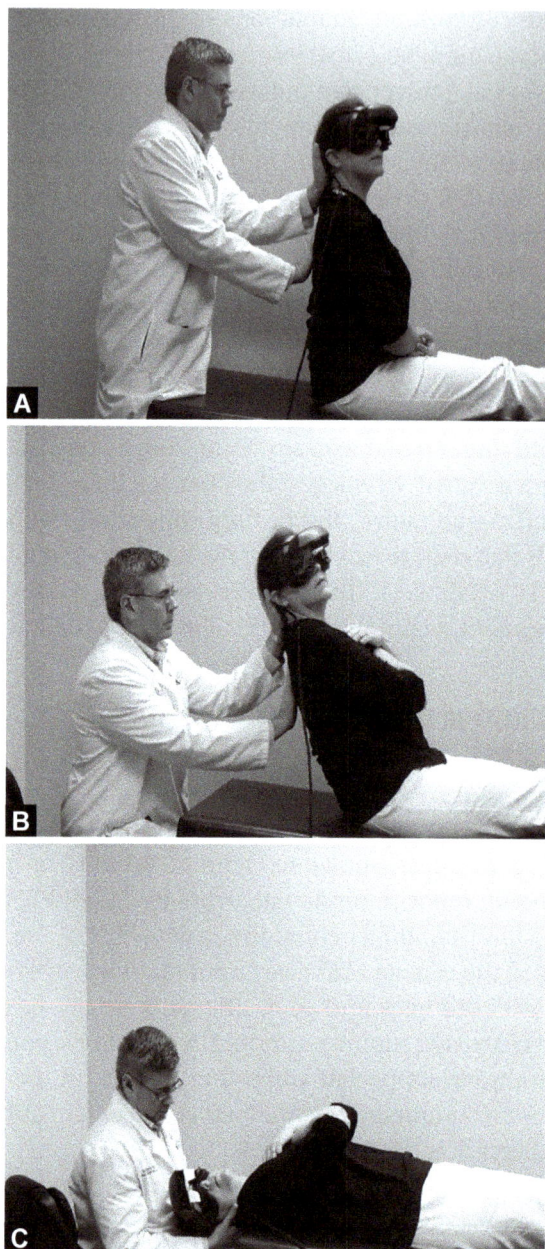

Figs. 3.2A to C: The examiner is performing a modified Hallpike to check the right posterior semicircular canal for benign paroxysmal positional vertigo (BPPV). (A) The patient is seated on the examination table with back to the examiner. The head of the patient is turned toward the ear to be tested (right ear in this example). The examiner is positioned behind the patient and provides support to the back and neck of the patient. (B) The patient is lowered to the examination table as the examiner sits. (C) The neck of the patient is hyperextended and the head is maintained 45° toward the test ear. The examiner supports the neck and head of the patient and has a clear view of the eyes of the patient. The maneuver is repeated for the left ear. Reprinted with permission from Alabama Hearing and Balance Associates, Inc., Foley, AL.

Side-Lying Maneuver

Humphriss et al.[43] suggested that the traditional Dix-Hallpike maneuver should not be performed for patients with conditions that contraindicate neck extension (i.e. VBI, cervical spondylosis, limited range of motion, etc.). They suggest side-lying maneuver as an appropriate substitute. Cohen[46] compared side-lying to traditional Dix-Hallpike testing and found no significant difference in sensitivity. This is not surprising as the side-lying maneuver is identical to the first position of the SLM[5,20,50] and the Gans repositioning maneuver[6] (Figs. 3.3A to C). While seated on the side of the examination table, the head of the patient is turned 45° away from the ear to be tested. The patient is then placed on their test side using a lateral positioning. This allows the head and neck of the patient to be fully supported on the examination table. Zapala[12] mentions this as an important reason he used side-lying to identify AC-BPPV in his case report. The side-lying maneuver is also more comfortable for patients with lower back issues or obesity who are unable to comfortably sit or bend at the waist. Side-lying is not advised for patients with significant hip problems or recent hip replacement.

Fully Supported Hallpike

There is another group of patients for whom modified Hallpike or side-lying maneuvers are contraindicated.[49] These tend to be more frail patients

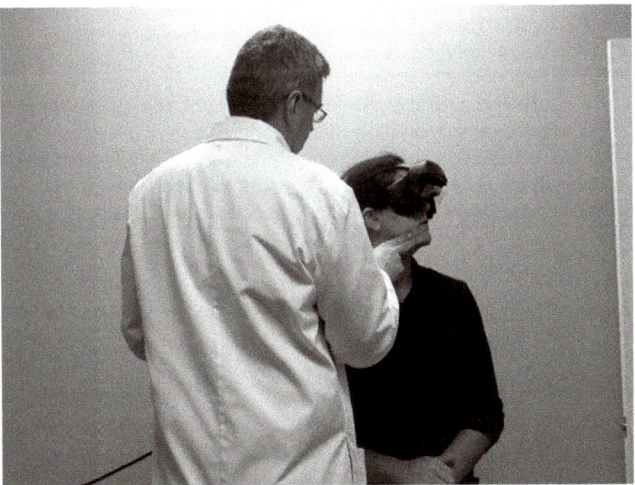

Fig. 3.3A: The examiner is performing a side-lying maneuver to check the right posterior semicircular canal for benign paroxysmal positional vertigo (BPPV). (A) The patient is seated near the center of the examination table in the side-lying position. The head of the patient is turned away from the ear to be tested.

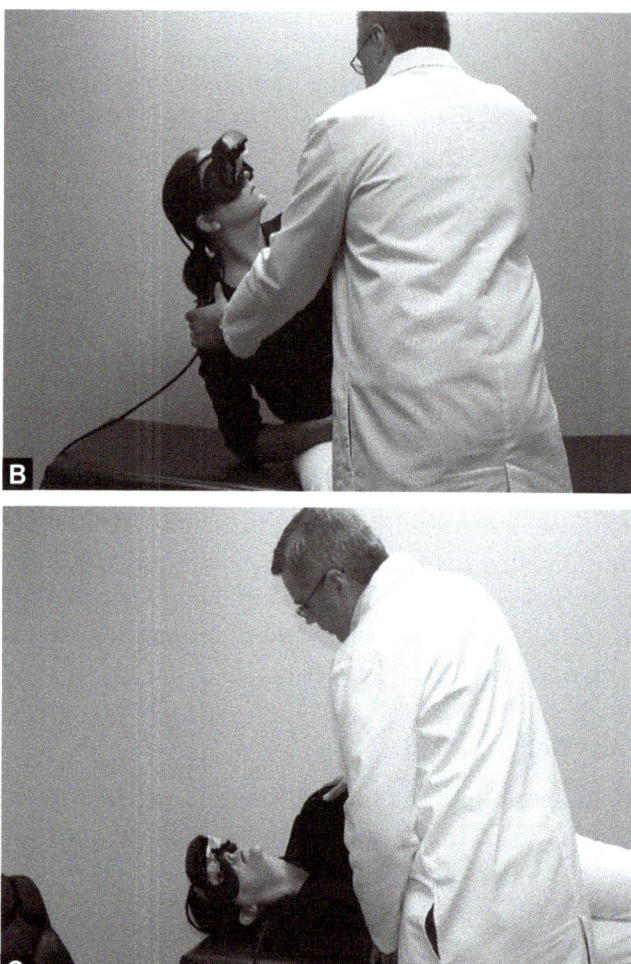

Figs. 3.3B and C: (B) The patient is positioned on the right side. (C) The legs of the patient are brought up onto the examination table. Note that the head of the patient is supported by the examination table, avoiding hyperextension of the neck. The examiner has a clear view of the eyes of the patient. The maneuver is repeated to check the left ear. Reprinted with permission from Alabama Hearing and Balance Associates, Inc., Foley, AL.

with issues that negate neck extension, recent hip replacement, rotator cuff surgery, etc. The fully supported Hallpike is performed just as the modified Hallpike except the patient is positioned so the head and neck are fully supported on the examination table. As in the traditional and modified Hallpike, the head is turned toward the test ear, (Fig. 3.4). From a logical standpoint, this maneuver should be capable of provoking symptoms of PC-BPPV as it is a position that is often reported as provoking positional vertigo in daily life, lying down in bed.

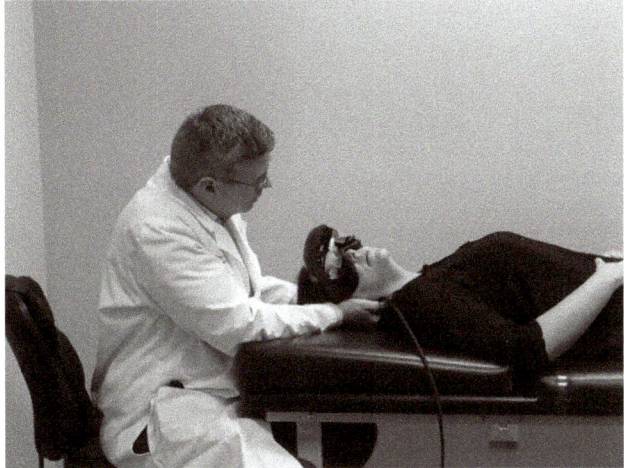

Fig. 3.4: The patient is in the fully supported Hallpike position to check for right posterior semicircular canal benign paroxysmal positional vertigo (BPPV). The head of the patient is fully supported on the examination table with the head turned 45° toward the test ear (right ear in this example). The examiner is seated behind the patient. Note that the examiner has clear view of the eyes of the patient. Maneuver is repeated to test left ear. Reprinted with permission from Alabama Hearing and Balance Associates, Inc., Foley, AL.

Supine Head-Hanging

Anterior canal BPPV is the least common type of BPPV. This type should be provoked with either modified Hallpike, side-lying maneuver, or even fully supported Hallpike. For clinicians who expect to become proficient at identification and management of all types of BPPV, there is another test position that has been advocated for the assessment of AC-BPPV, supine head-hanging, (Fig. 3.5). In the study by Bertholon et al.,[10] two of 12 patients diagnosed with AC-BPPV only experienced symptoms with this position. Ogawa et al.[11] report on four cases with possible AC-BPPV who also only provoked using this type of positioning. Bertholon et al.[10] explained that additional downward positioning of the head, with hyperextension of the neck, may be necessary to move the anterior canal ampullary segment into a vertical down pointing position needed to provoke AC-BPPV in those individuals. The reader should bear in mind that Zapala[12] was able to provoke AC-BPPV using side-lying maneuver. Even in the study by Bertholon et al.,[10] 75% (nine of 12) of their patients were identified with Dix-Hallpike positioning alone. We would reserve the supine, head-hanging position to test for AC-BPPV in individuals with a clear history consistent with BPPV, who have no contraindications to neck hyperextension, and who do not provoke with the other types of test positioning.

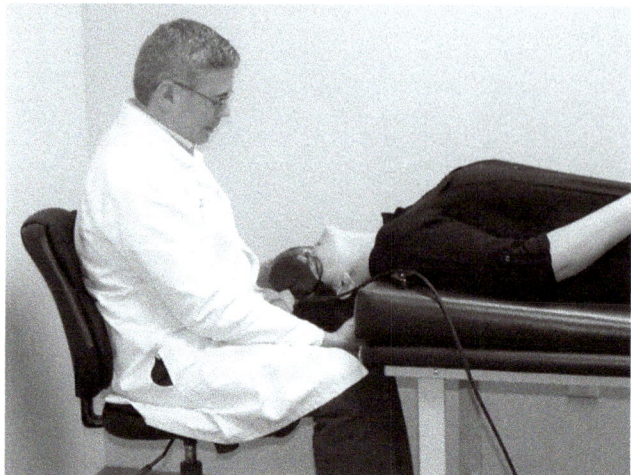

Fig. 3.5: The examiner is performing supine head-hanging technique for anterior canal benign paroxysmal positional vertigo (BPPV). Note the level of neck hyperextension. This positioning maneuver may be useful for patients who do not provoke with other techniques and in whom the hyperextension is not contraindicated. Reprinted with permission from Alabama Hearing and Balance Associates, Inc., Foley, AL.

Horizontal Canal BPPV

In some ways, HC-BPPV is potentially a more interesting type to diagnose. The impression of vertigo is often characterized by patients as more intense than with PC-BPPV. Horizontal canal BPPV presents with a horizontal nystagmus fast phase that changes direction with changes in head positioning in the plane of the horizontal semicircular canal. This may lead the inexperienced clinician to decide the patient can only have some type of CNS involvement. On the other hand, CNS involvement may certainly cause this type of vertigo response with nystagmus fast phase changing with head position.[35,51] Once the diagnosis of HC-BPPV is made, determination of involved ear can also be challenging.

Horizontal canal BPPV can be observed when assessing for vertical canal BPPV using variations of the Hallpike maneuver as discussed above, but these types of positioning will not always provoke the response. From a supine position, turning the head of the patient 90° with the ear toward the ground will provoke HC-BPPV if it is present[17,49] (Fig. 3.6). During standard vestibular evaluation, positional testing includes these positions, which are termed head right/head left. Both positions should be completed because it is important to observe the resulting nystagmus pattern with each ear dependent to help identify involved ear. This may also be helpful in determining if there could be adherent otoconia as in cupulolithiais or mobile debris in the more common canalithiasis.

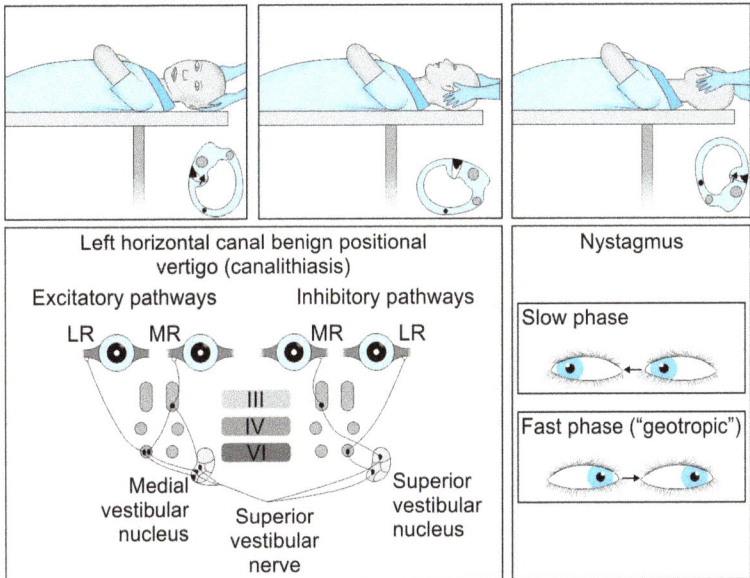

Fig. 3.6: Representation of canalithiasis variant of horizontal canal benign paroxysmal positional vertigo (HC-BPPV) with geotropic nystagmus. Upper panel shows patient during roll testing with mobile otoconial debris in the left horizontal semicircular canal. Lower panel shows the innervation and nystagmus resulting with otoconial debris moving toward the cupula with positioning on the left side. This causes an increase in neural firing. The fast phase of the nystagmus will beat toward the ground which is toward the left. Positioning on the on the right side will cause the otoconial debris in the left horizontal semicircular canal to move away from the cupula, causing decreased neural firing and a nystagmus beating toward the ground which is toward the right. Created by Jeremy Hornibrook, Christchurch, New Zealand. Courtesy of the Hindawi Publishing Corporation, New York, NY.

For many individuals, it is not possible to position the ear directly toward the ground (head right and head left). Cervical spondylosis, osteoarthritis, poor range of motion, etc. are all factors that may preclude this type of head movement. For those cases, the patient is simply moved into a lateral position to achieve the appropriate orientation of the ear to the ground, (Fig. 3.6). This is referred to as the Roll Test. For the Roll Test, the head is kept in a midline position, so there is no neck torsion.

Recall that rotary nystagmus is expected with vertical canal involvement given the connections to oblique extraocular muscles. The horizontal semicircular canals only connect with lateral and medial rectus muscles. The nystagmus pattern may be either geotropic (beating toward the dependent ear and ground regardless of position on the right or left side) or ageotropic (beating away from the dependent ear and ground regardless of position on the right or left side). Common characteristics observed with HC-BPPV are found in Table 3.3. The nystagmus may be more intense on one side, which can be helpful in determination of involved ear.

Table 3.3: Characteristics of horizontal canal benign paroxysmal positional nystagmus.

Canalithiasis	Cupulolithiasis
More common	Less common
Geotropic nystagmus	Ageotropic nystagmus
Transient duration	Transient or longer duration
Involved side has stronger response	Involved side has weaker response

The geotropic pattern of nystagmus is thought to reflect a canalithiasis variant and is reported to occur 60–83% of the time.[14,17,52,53] The nystagmus will be present when the patient is on either the right side or the left side, but the side with the more intense symptoms should be treated.[18,53,54] Figure 3.7 shows what is expected with the canalithiasis variant of HC-BPPV. Positioning of the involved ear toward the ground should move the mobile otoconia from the long arm of the lateral canal toward the ampulla. This should cause a flow of endolymph so that an utriculopetal displacement of the cupula (toward the utricle) occurs, which is excitatory for the horizontal canal. This would increase neural firing on that side. As the neural firing is greater on this side, the nystagmus beats toward the dependent ear and the ground. If the patient is positioned on the opposite side with the affected ear upward and the unaffected ear toward the ground, the otoconial debris is believed to move farther away from the ampulla, causing movement of endolymph also away from the ampulla. This creates an utriculofugal displacement of the cupula (away from the utricle) to occur, which results in an inhibitory effect on neural firing for the affected ear. As the relative difference in neural firing is greater from the dependent ear, a nystagmus with fast phase toward the unaffected ear will be present. This nystagmus would be expected to be of lower intensity compared to positioning the affected ear downward, which should be helpful in determining the involved canal.

An ageotropic nystagmus (beating away from the ground) is reported to be present 17–40% of the time.[14,52] As with HC-BPPV with geotropic nystagmus, positioning on either side is expected to elicit a nystagmus response. Most authorities agree this represents a cupulolithiasis variant and the side with the less intense response is the one that must be treated.[53,55] Figures 3.8A to D show what happens with the cupulolithiasis variant of HC-BPPV. The otoconia may be adherent to the utricle side or the canal side of the cupula.[56] Positioning of the affected ear downward toward the ground is believed to cause an utriculofugal displacement of the otoconia-weighted cupula, which results in an inhibitory effect on neural firing from the horizontal canal. An ageotropic nystagmus with fast phase toward the unaffected ear results because the neural firing from the

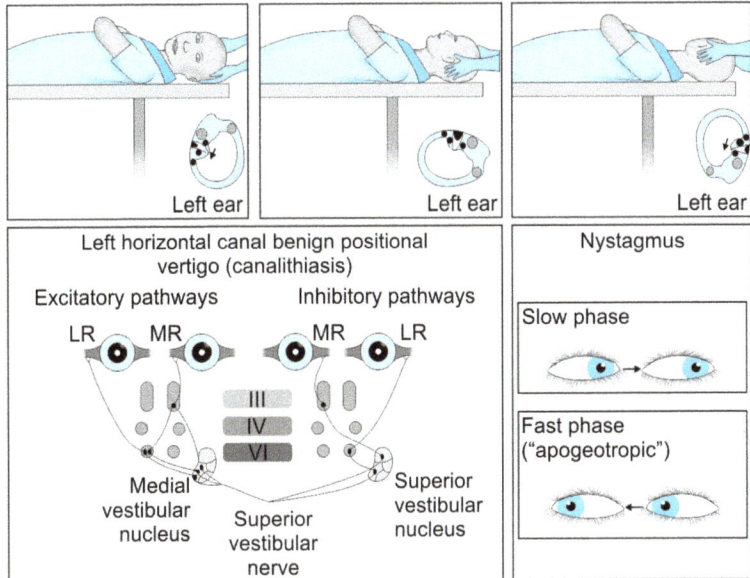

Fig. 3.7: Representation of cupulolithiasis variant of horizontal canal benign paroxysmal positional vertigo (HC-BPPV) with ageotropic nystagmus. Upper panel shows patient with otoconial debris attached to the left horizontal semicircular canal cupula. When patient is positioned onto the left side, otoconial debris pulls cupula away from the utricle, causing decreased neural firing. The fast phase of the nystagmus will beat away from the ground which is toward the right. When the patient is positioned on the right side, the otoconial debris pushes the cupula toward the utricle, causing increased neural firing and a nystagmus beating away from the ground which is toward the left. Created by Jeremy Hornibrook, Christchurch, New Zealand. Courtesy of the Hindawi Publishing Corporation, New York, NY.

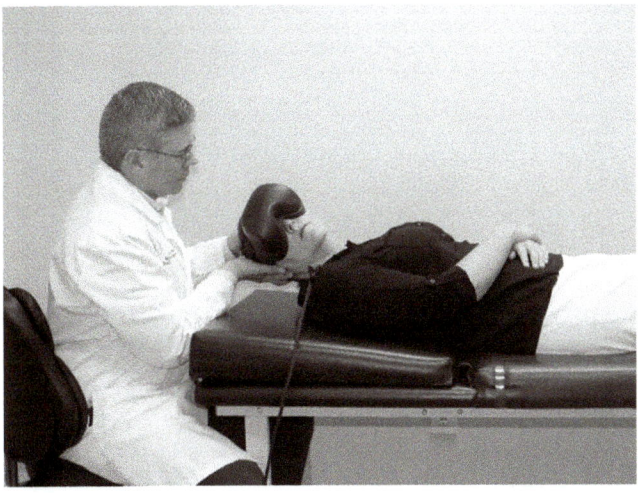

Fig. 3.8A: Test positions for horizontal canal benign paroxysmal positional vertigo are shown. Note the examiner always provides support to the head and neck of the patient. (A) Head right position with 90° rotation.

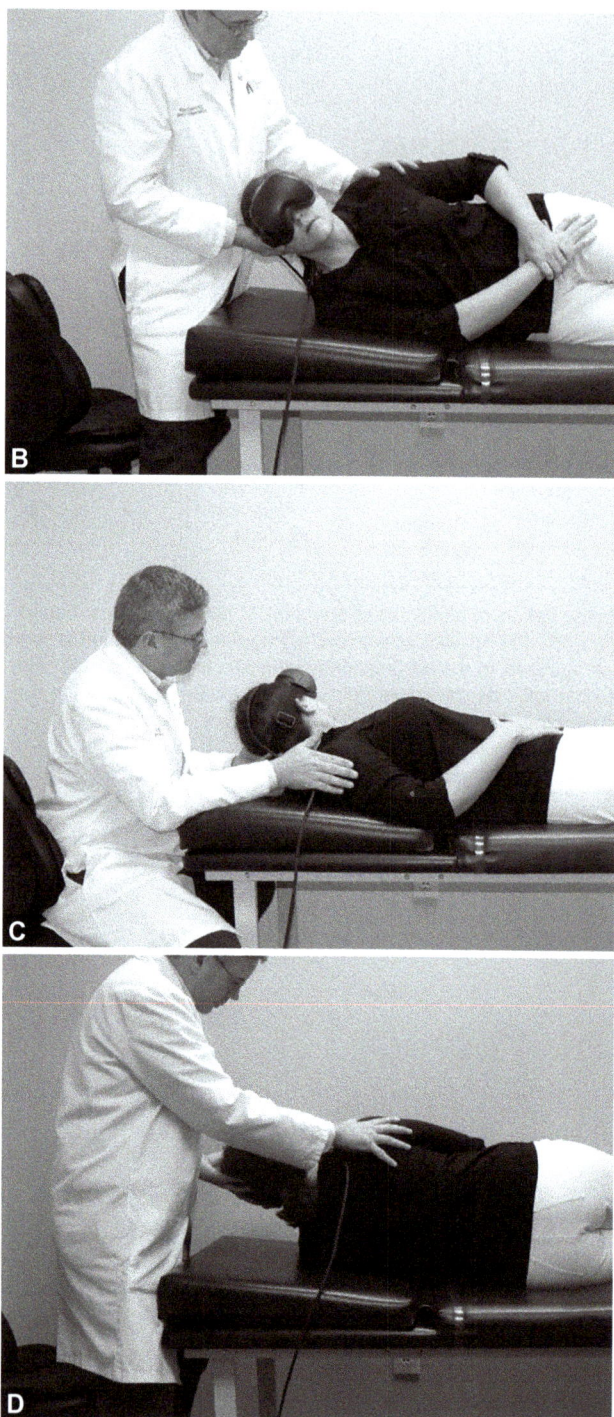

Figs. 3.8B to D: (B) Roll Test with right lateral position. (C) Head left position with 90° rotation. (D) Roll Test with left lateral position. Reprinted with permission from Alabama Hearing and Balance Associates, Inc., Foley, AL.

unaffected ear is relatively greater. When the affected ear is positioned upward (away from the ground), an utriculopetal displacement of the otoconia-weighted cupula should occur. This is excitatory and creates a stronger ageotropic nystagmus toward the uppermost ear.

The patterns described above appear often in publications and texts on HC-BPPV and seem quite clear. In clinical practice, however, the pattern may be geotropic and then switch to ageotropic on repeat testing or vice-versa. There is at least one report that describes direction-fixed nystagmus with HC-BPPV that eventually transforms to the geotropic type.[57] Some have suggested that ageotropic nystagmus may also be present when the otoconial debris is not adherent to the cupula but is located in the anterior portion of the lateral canal.[55] This makes a great deal of sense and likely provides the best explanation as to why the nystagmus pattern can (and often does) change in clinical practice with repeating the test positions. The location of the debris within the canal may dictate the nystagmus pattern (ageotropic or geotropic) as much as whether there is adherent debris. Of course, adherent debris may also become loosened on repeating positions, which could cause a change in nystagmus pattern.

Naturally, changing nystagmus patterns can make it difficult to determine the involved ear. The key factor most considered is the magnitude of the nystagmus response. The side with the more intense response with geotropic nystagmus is involved. The side with the less intense response with ageotropic nystagmus is involved. This becomes confusing if the pattern switches. In clinical practice, it may sometimes be difficult to determine which side has the greater or lesser magnitude response, further confounding identification of the involved ear. Because of this, investigators have sought other methods to aid in determination of involved ear. Koo et al.[66] investigated nystagmus patterns in patients with HC-BPPV when moved from sitting to supine. They observed that for nearly 60% of their patients, nystagmus often beat toward the involved ear for HC-BPPV with geotropic nystagmus and away from the involved ear for HC-BPPV with ageotropic nystagmus.

Another method to aid in determination of involved ear with HC-BPPV is the "bow and lean" test described by Choung et al.[60] These investigators reported that following identification of HC-BPPV, the investigators had patients bow the head forward 90° while in a seated position. Nystagmus was recorded and then patients leaned the head backward 45° and nystagmus response was also recorded. Nystagmus fast phase was toward the involved ear during the "bow" with geotropic nystagmus and toward the involved ear during the "lean" with ageotropic nystagmus.

In our own clinical experience, we adopt a somewhat practical approach to treatment of HC-BPPV. When the nystagmus pattern and magnitude are clear, we treat the expected involved ear. When the pattern changes, when it is not clear which ear has the greater or lesser response, or when initial treatment attempts are unsuccessful, we simply treat both ears.

SUMMARY

Careful consideration of history and symptoms should help narrow the differential diagnosis of positional vertigo. Identification of true vertigo and nystagmus pattern during provoking position should further differentiate BPPV from other causes, as well as isolate involved ear and canal which is essential for management. At times, CNS involvement may cause both positional vertigo and nystagmus similar to BPPV. In those cases, the response will most often persist while the patient is kept in the provoking position, while the duration is usually transient with BPPV. In the absence of other CNS indicators, BPPV treatment may be considered during evaluation given its high efficacy. Vertigo without nystagmus may also occur with BPPV and treatment may be attempted to manage subjective BPPV. For questionable cases, treatment maneuvers should reduce or eliminate symptoms with BPPV but would have no effect on other causes.

REFERENCES

1. Agrawal Y, Carey J, Della Santina C, et al. Disorders of balance and vestibular function in US adults: data from the National Health and Nutrition Examination Survey, 2001-2004. Arch Intern Med. 2009;169(10):934-44.
2. Hornibrook J. Benign paroxysmal positional vertigo (BPPV): history, pathophysiology, office treatment and future directions. Int J Otolaryngol. 2011;2011:1-13.
3. Agus S, Benecke H, Thum C, et al. Clinical and demographic features of vertigo: findings from the REVERT registry. Front Neurol. 2013;10:4-48.
4. Roberts R, Abrams H, Sembach M, et al. Utility measures of health-related quality of life in patients treated for benign paroxysmal positional vertigo. Ear Hearing. 2009;30:369-76.
5. Semont A, Freyss G, Vitte E. Curing the BPPV with a liberatory maneuver. Adv Otorhinolaryngol. 1988;42:290-3.
6. Roberts R, Gans R, Montaudo R. Efficacy of a new treatment maneuver for posterior canal benign paroxysmal positional vertigo. J Am Acad Audiol. 2006b;17:598-604.
7. Jackson L, Morgan B, Fletcher J, et al. Anterior canal benign paroxysmal positional vertigo: an underappreciated entity. Otol Neurotol. 2007;28:218-22.
8. Squires T, Weidman M, Hain T, et al. A mathematical model for top-shelf vertigo: the role of sedimenting otoconia in BPPV. J Biomechanics. 2004;37:1137-46.
9. Baloh R, Honrubia V. Clinical neurophysiology of the vestibular system, 3rd edition. New York: Oxford University Press; 2001.
10. Bertholon P, Bronstein A, Davies R, et al. Positional down beating nystagmus in 50 patients: cerebellar disorders and possible anterior semicircular canalithiasis. J Neurol Neurosurg Psychiatry. 2002;72:366-72.

11. Ogawa Y, Suzuki M, Otsuka K, et al. Positional and positioning down-beating nystagmus without central nervous system findings. Auris Nasus Larynx. 2009;36(6):698-701.
12. Zapala D. Down-beating nystagmus in anterior canal benign paroxysmal positional vertigo. J Am Acad Audiol. 2008;19(3):257-66.
13. de la Meilleure G, Dehaene I, Depondt M, et al. Benign paroxysmal positional vertigo of the horizontal canal. J Neurol Neurosurg Psychiatry. 1996;60:68-71.
14. Honrubia V, Baloh R, Harris M, et al. Paroxysmal positional vertigo syndrome. Am J Otol. 1999;20:465-70.
15. Moon S, Kim J, Kim B, et al. Clinical characteristics of benign paroxysmal positional vertigo in Korea: a multicenter study. J Korean Med Sci. 2006;21(3):539-43.
16. Ruckenstein M. Therapeutic efficacy of the Epley canalith repositioning maneuver. Laryngoscope. 2001;111:940-5.
17. Cakir B, Ercan I, Cakir Z, et al. What is the true incidence of horizontal semicircular canal benign paroxysmal positional vertigo? Otolaryngol Head Neck Surg. 2006;134:451-4.
18. Fife T. Recognition and management of horizontal canal benign positional vertigo. Am J Otol.1998;19:345-51.
19. Macias J, Lambert K, Massingale S, et al. Variables affecting treatment in benign paroxysmal positional vertigo. Laryngoscope. 2000;110:1921-4.
20. Gans R, Harrington-Gans P. Treatment efficacy of benign paroxysmal positional vertigo (BPPV) with canalith repositioning maneuver and Semont liberatory maneuver in 376 patients. Semin Hearing. 200;223:129-42.
21. Longridge N, Barber H. Bilateral paroxysmal positioning nystagmus. J Otolaryngol. 1978;7:395-400.
22. Katsarkas A. Benign paroxysmal positional vertigo (BPPV): idiopathic versus post-traumatic. Acta Otolaryngol. 1999;119:745-9.
23. Liu H. Presentation and outcome of post-traumatic benign paroxysmal positional vertigo. Acta Otolaryngol. 2012;132:803-6.
24. Epley J. The canalith repositioning procedure: for treatment of benign paroxysmal positional vertigo. Otolaryngol Head Neck Surg. 1992;119:399-404.
25. Korres S, Balatsouras D, Kaberos A, et al. Occurrence of semicircular canal involvement in benign paroxysmal positional vertigo. Otol Neurotol. 2002;23:926-32.
26. Roberts R, Gans R, DeBoodt J, et al. Treatment of benign paroxysmal positional vertigo: necessity of postmaneuver patient restrictions. J Am Acad Audiol. 2005;16:357-66.
27. Huebner A, Lytle S, Doettl S, et al. Treatment of objective and subjective benign paroxysmal positional vertigo. J Am Acad Audiol. 2013;24:600-6.
28. Balatsouras D, Ganelis P, Aspris A, et al. Benign paroxysmal positional vertigo associated with Meniere's disease: epidemiological, pathophysiologic, clinical, and therapeutic aspects. Ann Otol Rhinol Laryngol. 2012;121(10):682-8.
29. Balatsouras D, Koukoutsis G, Ganelis P, et al. Benign paroxysmal positional vertigo secondary to vestibular neuritis. Eur Arch Otorhinolaryngol. 2014;271(5):919-24.
30. Aschan G, Bergstedt M, Goldberg L, et al. Positional nystagmus in man during and after alcohol intoxication. Q J Stud Alcohol. 1956;17:381-405.
31. Aschan G. Different types of alcohol nystagmus. Acta Otolaryngol. 1958;140:69-78.
32. Brandt T. Positional and positioning vertigo and nystagmus. J Neurol Sci. 1990;95:3-28.

33. Lea J, Lechner C, Halmagyi GM, et al. Not so benign positional vertigo: paroxysmal downbeat nystagmus from a superior cerebellar peduncle neoplasm. Otol Neurotol. 2014;35(6):e204-5.
34. Leigh R, Zee D. The Neurology of eye movements, 3rd edition. New York: Oxford University Press; 2001.
35. Roberts R, Gans R, Kastner A. Differentiation of migrainous positional vertigo (MPV) from horizontal canal benign paroxysmal positional vertigo (HC-BPPV). Int J Audiol. 2006a;45:224-6.
36. Brown J. Cervical contributions to balance: cervical vertigo. In: Berthoz A, Vidal PP, Graf W (Eds). The head neck sensory motor system. New York, NY: Oxford University Press; 1992. pp. 644-7.
37. Wrisley D, Sparto P, Whitney S, et al. Cervicogenic dizziness: a review of diagnosis and treatment. J Orthop Sports Phys Ther. 2000;30(12):755-66.
38. Piñol I, Ramirez M, Saló G, et al. Symptomatic vertebral artery stenosis secondary to cervical spondylolisthesis. Spine. 2013;38(23):E1503-5.
39. Yacovino D. Cervical vertigo: myths, facts, and scientific evidence. Neurologia. 2012. S0213-4853(12)00211-3.
40. Dix R, Hallpike C. The pathology, symptomatology and diagnosis of certain common disorders of the vestibular system. Ann Otol Rhinol Laryngol. 1952;6:987-1016.
41. Lanska D, Remler B. Benign paroxysmal positioning vertigo: classic descriptions, origins of provocative positioning technique, and conceptual developments. Neurology. 1997;48:1167-77.
42. Choi K, Shin H, Kim J, et al. Rotational vertebral artery syndrome: oculo-graphic analysis of nystagmus. Neurology. 2005;65:1287-90.
43. Humphriss R, Baguley D, Sparkes V, et al. Contraindications to the Dix-Hallpike manoeuvre: a multidisciplinary review. Int J Audiol. 2003;42:166-73.
44. Nagashima C, Iwama K, Sakata E, et al. Effect of temporary occlusion of a vertebral artery on human vestibular system. J Neurosurg. 1970;33:338-94.
45. Sakata E, Ohtsu K, Sakata H. Pitfalls in which otolaryngologists often are caught in the diagnosis and treatment of vertigo. Int Tinnitus J. 2004;10:31-4.
46. Cohen H. Side-lying as an alternative to the Dix-Hallpike test of the posterior canal. Otol Neurotol. 2004;25:130-4.
47. Gans R. Overview of BPPV: pathophysiology and diagnosis. Hearing Rev. 2000;7:38-43.
48. Hutting N, Verhagen A, Vijverman V, et al. Diagnostic accuracy of premanipulative vertebrobasilar insufficiency tests: a systematic review. Manual Ther. 2013;18(3):177-82.
49. Gans R, Yellin W. Assessment of vestibular function. In: Roeser R, Valente M, Hosford-Dunn H (Eds). Audiology: diagnosis. New York: Thieme; 2007. pp. 540-66.
50. Herdman S, Tusa R, Zee D, et al. Single treatment approaches to benign paroxysmal positional vertigo. Arch Otolaryngol Head Neck Surg. 1993;119:450-4.
51. von Brevern M, Radtke A, Clarke A, et al. Migrainous vertigo presenting as episodic positional vertigo. Neurology. 2004a;62:469-72.
52. Steenerson R, Cronin G, Marbach P. Effectiveness of treatment techniques in 923 cases of benign paroxysmal positional vertigo. Laryngoscope. 2005;115:226-31.
53. White J, Coale K, Catalano P, et al. Diagnosis and management of lateral semicircular canal benign paroxysmal positional vertigo. Otolaryngol Head Neck Surg. 2005;133:278-84.

54. Appiani G, Catania G, Gagliardi M. A liberatory maneuver for the treatment of horizontal canal paroxysmal positional vertigo. Otol Neurotol. 2001;22:66-9.
55. Casani A, Vannucci G, Fattori B, et al. The treatment of horizontal canal positional vertigo: our experience in 66 cases. Laryngoscope. 2002;112:172-8.
56. Chiou W, Lee H, Tsai S, et al. A single therapy for all subtypes of horizontal canal positional vertigo. Laryngoscope. 2005;115:1432-5.
57. Califano L, Vassallo A, Melillo M, et al. Direction-fixed paroxysmal nystagmus lateral canal benign paroxysmal positioning vertigo (BPPV): another form of lateral canalolithiasis. Acta Otorhinolaryngol Ital. 2013;33(4):254-60.
58. Parnes L, McClure J. Free-floating endolymph particles: a new operative finding during posterior semicircular canal occlusion. Laryngoscope. 1992;102:988-92.
59. Bhattacharyya N, Baugh R, Orvidas L, et al. Clinical practice guideline: benign paroxysmal positional vertigo. Otolaryngol Head Neck Surg. 2008;139 (5 Suppl 4):S47-81.
60. Choung Y, Shin Y, Kahng H, et al. "Bow and lean test" to determine the affected ear of horizontal canal benign paroxysmal positional vertigo. Laryngoscope. 2006;116(10):1776-81.
61. Clendaniel R, Landel R. Cervicogenic dizziness. In: Herdman S (Ed). Vestibular rehabilitation, 3rd edition. Philadelphia, PA: F. A. Davis; 2007. pp.467-84.
62. Fetter M, Haslwanter T, Bork M, et al. New insights into positional alcohol nystagmus using three-dimensional eye-movement analysis. Ann Neurol. 1999;45:216-23.
63. Hall S, Ruby R, McClure J. The mechanics of benign paroxysmal vertigo. J Otolaryngol. 1979;8:151-8.
64. Haynes D, Resser J, Labadie R, et al. Treatment of benign positional vertigo using the semont maneuver: efficacy in patients presenting without nystagmus. Laryngoscope. 2002;112:796-801.
65. Herdman S, Tusa R, Clendanial R. Eye movement signs in vertical canal benign paroxysmal positional vertigo. In: Fuchs A, Brandt T, Buttner U, et al. (Eds). Contemporary ocular motor and vestibular research: a tribute to David A. Robinson. Stuttgart, Germany: Georg Thieme-Verlag; 1994. pp. 385-7.
66. Koo J, Moon I, Shim W, et al. Value of lying down nystagmus in the lateralization of horizontal semicircular canal benign paroxysmal positional vertigo. Otol Neurotol. 2006;27:367-71.
67. Lopez-Escamez JA, Gamiz MJ, Finana M, et al. Position in bed is associated with left or right location in benign paroxysmal positional vertigo of the posterior semicircular canal. Am J Otolaryngol. 2002;23:263-6.
68. Schuknecht H. Cupulolithiasis. Arch Otolaryngol. 1969;90:765-78.
69. Soto-Varela A, Rossi-Izquierdo M, Santos-Pérez S. Benign paroxysmal positional vertigo simultaneously affecting several canals: a 46-patient series. Eur Arch Otorhinolaryngol. 2013;270(3):817-22.
70. Strupp M, Dieterich M, Brandt T. The treatment and natural course of peripheral and central vertigo. Deutsch Ärztebl Int. 2013;110(29-30):505-16.
71. von Brevern M, Seelig T, Neuhauser H, et al. Benign paroxysmal positional vertigo predominantly affects the right labyrinth. J Neurol Neurosurg Psychiatry. 2004b;75:1487-8.
72. Zuo J, Han J, Qiu S, et al. Neural reflex pathway between cervical spinal and sympathetic ganglia in rabbit: implication for pathogenesis of cervical vertigo. Spine J. 2014;14(6):1005-9.

Chapter 4

Central Positional Vertigo

Diego Kaski

INTRODUCTION

Central positional vertigo refers to the illusion of motion caused by a change in head position with respect to gravity. In such patients, when the head is brought to an off-vertical (e.g. lateral or head-hanging) position, this induces a change in the otolithic (graviceptive) and semicircular canal inputs that precipitates nystagmus and/or vertigo. Central positional vertigo or nystagmus indicates a lesion in the posterior fossa, involving a communicating network between the vestibular nuclei and midline cerebellar structures within the vermis.

It is essential to correctly distinguish between peripheral and central vestibular dysfunction in order to instigate correct and prompt investigations and subsequent management. In most cases careful assessment of latency, direction, habituation, fatigability, and reversal of ensuing nystagmus is sufficient to distinguish the two. Such distinction may however prove difficult in individual cases, since BPPV and central positional nystagmus can share similar clinical features. It has been suggested that four main types of central positional vertigo exist:[1]

1. Positional downbeating nystagmus (with or without associated vertigo)
2. Central positional nystagmus (CPN)
3. Central paroxysmal positional/positioning vertigo (CPPV), and
4. Central positioning vomiting (CPV)

In clinical practice, there is a tendency for these terms to be used interchangeably, causing considerable confusion. Such confusion arises from a lack of systematic clinical, radiological, and oculographic evaluation of patients with positional symptoms and signs in the medical literature. In this chapter, we review the clinical features of the different types of central positional vertigo reported, the common causes, and briefly discuss possible management.

EPIDEMIOLOGY

Central positional and positioning syndromes are far less common than benign paroxysmal positional vertigo, although few studies have tried to assess its prevalence. In one study of 490 consecutive patients attending a neurootology clinic, 100 patients were found to have positional nystagmus, and of these only 12 were felt to be of central origin.[2] With an increasing awareness of this entity, an understanding of the underlying mechanism of central vertigo, and ever-improving diagnostic tools, we may see a change in the estimated prevalence of these conditions.

CLINICAL FEATURES

Positional Downbeat Nystagmus

The presence of pure downbeat nystagmus (DBN) when the patient is positioned in the head-hanging (Rose position) or lateral position (e.g. during a Dix-Hallpike maneuver) is termed positional DBN (pDBN). It is suggestive of a vestibulocerebellar nodulus lesion, as has been demonstrated following experimental ablation of the nodulus in cats[3] and in patients with focal cerebellar lesions.[4,5] The nodulus is thought to exert an inhibitory influence over the gain of the vertical vestibulo-ocular reflex, a finding that is supported abolition of lesional DBN following bilateral labyrinthectomy.[6]

Positional DBN is typically accompanied by only mild vertigo, and may be related to the DBN syndrome in which there is spontaneous DBN at rest, and in all directions of gaze (less marked on upgaze), and exacerbated by head extension. Clinical experience also suggests that DBN increases when the patient is brought into the prone position (head-forwards).[7] Positional DBN can also be seen in normal subjects, though it is typically not sustained, and usually of small amplitude, and most commonly only identified with sensitive recording methods (e.g. oculography). From a practical perspective, if it cannot be seen during fixation it is likely to be innocuous.

Positional DBN may be the only clinical sign in neurological patients, which may resolve spontaneously but more commonly persists. Recognized causes (Table 4.1) include multiple sclerosis, stroke, drug toxicity, Chiari malformations, and paraneoplastic cerebellar degeneration. Downbeat nystagmus may also be seen in patients with migrainous vertigo during an acute attack. In this setting, a structural lesion should be excluded, unless there is a clear history of previous similar episodes with normal brain imaging. In a review of 50 patients with pDBN 38 had unequivocal central nervous system (CNS) dysfunction, with multiple system atrophy ($n = 13$), cerebellar degeneration ($n = 12$), cerebrovascular disease ($n = 5$), multiple sclerosis ($n = 2$), and hydrocephalus ($n = 2$) being the commonest etiologies. Interestingly no patient in this series had an Arnold-Chiari malformation, one of the most common

Table 4.1: Causes of positional downbeat nystagmus.

Cerebellar degeneration • Multiple system atrophy • Idiopathic • Episodic ataxia type 2 • Spinocerebellar atrophy type 6
Multiple sclerosis
Developmental abnormalities • Arnold-Chiari malformation
Drug toxicity • Amiodarone • Phenytoin • Carbamazepine • Lithium
Neoplastic • Primary or secondary deposits around IVth ventricle
Paraneoplastic syndromes
Posterior circulation stroke
Migrainous vertigo

causes of spontaneous and continuous DBN.[8,9] This may indicate that the cerebellar flocculus—involved in the Arnold-Chiari malformation and shown to cause continuous DBN in animal lesion studies[10]—is not the site responsible for transient pDBN. Indeed, while floccular lesions in monkeys can produce positional nystagmus, this is horizontal-rotatory rather than downbeating.[11]

In a proportion of patients there will be no identifiable cause, although there is a suggestion that some of these patients may have migrainous vertigo, and a proportion benign paroxysmal positional vertigo with lithiasis of the anterior canal.[12] Personal experience suggests that pDBN is also seen in patients with small vessel disease (leukoaraiosis), and emerging data may help clarify this.

Central Positional Nystagmus

Positional nystagmus in the absence of vertigo points to a central pathology but the term central positional nystagmus (CPN) is often used to denote the presence of positional nystagmus with central characteristics, whether there is vertigo or not. The frequency of the nystagmus in CPN is usually lower than that of BPPV, and tends to remain constant whereas in BPPV it has a crescendo-decrescendo frequency. Nystagmus may occur in any direction (vertical, horizontal, or torsional), but when central in origin, may be direction-reversing (occurring spontaneously in two

Table 4.2: Clinical features that help distinguish between central and peripheral causes of paroxysmal positional nystagmus during a Dix-Hallpike maneuver.

	Central	Peripheral
Latency Time to onset of nystagmus from provocation maneuver	Short (<2 seconds) or absent	Present
Fatigue Diminution of nystagmus frequency and amplitude over time during provocation maneuver	Absent	Present
Habituation Diminution of nystagmus frequency and amplitude over time with repeated provocation maneuvers	Absent	Present
Nystagmus direction on Dix-Hallpike maneuver Fast-phase of eye oscillation	Pure torsional Pure upbeat Direction reversal Downbeat Not in keeping with semicircular canal activated, e.g. left-beating (ageotropic) nystagmus on right ear down Dix-Hallpike maneuver	Most commonly upbeat and geotropic (pc-BPPV) but may be pure horizontal (hc-BPPV) or rarely downbeat (ac-BPPV)

(pc-BPPV: Posterior canal benign paroxysmal positional vertigo; hc-BPPV: Horizontal canal benign paroxysmal positional vertigo; ac-BPPV: Anterior canal benign paroxysmal positional vertigo).

successive phases, without further head movements). Note that direction changing nystagmus is a feature of BPPV (usually of the horizontal canal) where the direction of the nystagmus changes when the position of the head changes. The features that help distinguish central from peripheral positional nystagmus are listed in Table 4.2.

Central positional nystagmus indicates a posterior fossa lesion, typically affecting the caudal brainstem or vestibulocerebellum.[13] Patients with CPN may also have associated cerebellar features such as gaze-evoked nystagmus, DBN, perverted head-shaking nystagmus, limb dysmetria, or gait ataxia. A prospective evaluation of 100 consecutive patients with positional nystagmus identified 12 patients in whom the nystagmus was felt to be central in origin either on the basis of the nystagmus type or identification of a CNS disorder on imaging.[2] In these patients the nystagmus was either downbeating, direction changing (vertical), apogeotropic horizontal, or geotropic horizontal. These 12 patients also suffered from a gait disturbance ($n = 7$), falls ($n = 2$), or spontaneous vertigo aggravated by head motion ($n = 5$). Isolated nodular infarctions have been reported to cause horizontal and also torsional CPN as a sole clinical feature, highlighting the importance of the sign in clinical practice.[14,15] The absence of vertigo in CPN (and possibly BPPV) is perhaps more common in the elderly and may represent abnormal cortical processing of vestibulocerebellar afferents as a result of small vessel disease (microvascular damage to the white matter tracts).

Central Paroxysmal Positional/Positioning Vertigo

Central paroxysmal positional/positioning vertigo (CPPV) is defined as paroxysmal nystagmus and vertigo that occurs immediately after position changes, does not resolve with repositioning maneuvers, and with pathology localized to the brainstem or cerebellum.[36]

There are numerous case reports and small case series describing CPPV. The change of direction is thought to represent an adaptive mechanism that acts to nullify the original pathological nystagmus.[16]

Two patients who underwent extensive investigation were found to have solitary demyelinating plaques affecting the brachium conjunctivum causes acute vertigo and DBN triggered exclusively by tonic head tilts with respect to gravity.[18] The authors argued that the brachium conjunctivum may play a pivotal role in otolithic signal processing as it carried fibers from the fastigial nucleus, that have been shown to selectively respond to otolithic stimulation in primate models.[19] A third patient with a similar solitary demyelinating left brachium conjunctivum lesion was reported 2 years later by the same authors[20] suggesting that this may be a common lesion location in patients with CPPV and may present with a paucity of accompanying cerebellar signs.

Choi et al.[36] have characterized the paroxysmal component of positional nystagmus of central origin in 17 patients. They elegantly analyzed the nystagmus characteristics and provided modeling data suggesting that the direction of the nystagmus is mostly aligned with that of the head motion during positioning, and with the sum vector of the rotational axes of the semicircular canals that are inhibited during the positioning. They report that CPPN is caused by lesions involving the nodulus and uvula. Central paroxysmal positional/positioning vertigo has also been reported in other patients with lesions of the cerebellar hemispheres,[16] cerebellar vermis,[21-23] nodulus,[14,15] around the floor of the fourth ventricle,[24-27] the cerebellopontine angle,[17,28,29] pons,[30] and nucleus prepositus hypoglossi.[31]

Central Positioning Vomiting

This syndrome refers to the presence of vomiting (often profuse) triggered by a positioning maneuver and with pathology localized to the brainstem or cerebellum. It is most commonly caused by cerebellar lesions compressing the IV ventricle. It is a misconception that patients with

BPPV often vomit during a positioning maneuver. In fact, the brevity of the nystagmus and vertigo in BPPV is usually insufficient to cause vomiting—the exception may be patients with cupulolithiasis where the nystagmus and vertigo may be prolonged. The concept of central positional vomiting with little or no nystagmus or vertigo was first described by Drachman et al. in 1977[32] and later recognized by Baloh.[33] This condition has also been termed posturally evoked vomiting, and is a poorly recognized sign of posterior fossa lesions that is often misinterpreted as a sign of peripheral vestibular disease. It may be so severe that patients will tend to hold their heads in a forced position to prevent vomiting. A case of central positional vomiting following amiodarone administration has been described, although this was also accompanied by mild vertigo, DBN, and limb ataxia.[34] It has been described as a sequelae of posterior fossa lesions[32] (usually tumors), and developmental abnormalities such as Arnold-Chiari malformation.[35] In the latter, it may be accompanied by other cerebellar signs such as broken (saccadic) pursuit and abnormal optokinetic nystagmus. The dissociation between positionally triggered vomiting and the absence of nystagmus and vertigo appears to imply a dissociation between vomiting centers in the area postrema around the periaqueductal grey and oculomotor circuitry in the dorsal cerebellar vermis.[34]

Management

Treatment of central positional vertigo will depend on the underlying cause, but symptomatic relief, particularly when nausea or vomiting are prominent, has been documented with antiemetics (e.g. prochlorperazine, hyoscine, and cyclizine) and benzodiazepines. There is no evidence to support the role of vestibular rehabilitation in central positional vertigo.

REFERENCES

1. Brandt T. Vertigo: its multisensory syndromes. Springer-Verlag; New York. 1991.
2. Bertholon P, Tringali S, Faye MB, et al. Prospective study of positional nystagmus in 100 consecutive patients. Ann Otol Rhinol Laryngol. 2006;115(8):587-94.
3. Fernandez C, Alzate R, Lindsay JR. Experimental observations on postural nystagmus. II. Lesions of the nodulus. Ann Otol Rhinol Laryngol. 1960;69:94-114.
4. Harrison MS, Ozsahinoglu C. Positional vertigo: aetiology and clinical significance. Brain. 1972;95(2):369-72.
5. Kattah JC, Kolsky MP, Luessenhop AJ. Positional vertigo and the cerebellar vermis. Neurology. 1984;34(4):527-9.
6. Allen G, Fernandez C. Experimental observations in postural nystagmus. I. Extensive lesions in posterior vermis of the cerebellum. Acta Otolaryngol. 1960;51:2-14.

7. Marti S, Palla A, Straumann D. Gravity dependence of ocular drift in patients with cerebellar downbeat nystagmus. Ann Neurol. 2002;52(6):712-21.
8. Baloh RW, Spooner JW. Downbeat nystagmus: a type of central vestibular nystagmus. Neurology. 1981;31(3):304-10.
9. Halmagyi GM, Rudge P, Gresty MA, et al. Downbeating nystagmus. A review of 62 cases. Arch Neurol. 1983;40(13):777-84.
10. Zee DS, Yamazaki A, Butler PH, et al. Effects of ablation of flocculus and paraflocculus of eye movements in primate. J Neurophysiol. 1981;46(4):878-99.
11. Takemori S, Cohen B. Loss of visual suppression of vestibular nystagmus after flocculus lesions. Brain Res. 1974;72(2):213-24.
12. Bertholon P, Bronstein AM, Davies RA, et al. Positional down beating nystagmus in 50 patients: cerebellar disorders and possible anterior semicircular canalithiasis. J Neurol Neurosurg Psychiatry. 2002;72(3):366-72.
13. Brandt T. Positional and positioning vertigo and nystagmus. J Neurol Sci. 1990;95(1):3-28.
14. Kim HA, Yi HA, Lee H. Apogeotropic central positional nystagmus as a sole sign of nodular infarction. Neurol Sci. 2012;33(5):1189-91.
15. Nam J, Kim S, Huh Y, et al. Ageotropic central positional nystagmus in nodular infarction. Neurology. 2009;73(14):1163.
16. Bassani R, Della Torre S. Positional nystagmus reversing from geotropic to apogeotropic: a new central vestibular syndrome. J Neurol. 2011;258(2):313-5.
17. Bertholon P, Antoine JC, Martin C, et al. Simultaneous occurrence of a central and a peripheral positional nystagmus during the Dix-Hallpike manoeuvre. Eur Neurol. 2003;50(4):249-50.
18. Anagnostou E, Mandellos D, Limbitaki G, et al. Positional nystagmus and vertigo due to a solitary brachium conjunctivum plaque. J Neurol Neurosurg Psychiatry. 2006;77(6):790-2.
19. Siebold C, Anagnostou E, Glasauer S, et al. Canal-otolith interaction in the fastigial nucleus of the alert monkey. Exp Brain Res. 2001;136(2):169-78.
20. Anagnostou E, Varaki K, Anastasopoulos D. A minute demyelinating lesion causing acute positional vertigo. J Neurol Sci. 2008;266(1-2):187-9.
21. Barber HO. Positional nystagmus. Otolaryngol Head Neck Surg. 1984;92(6):649-55.
22. Goto N, Hoshino T, Kaneko M, et al. Central positional vertigo—clinico-anatomic study. Neurologia Medico-Chirurgica. 1983;23(7):534-40.
23. Shoman N, Longridge N. Cerebellar vermis lesions and tumours of the fourth ventricle in patients with positional and positioning vertigo and nystagmus. J Laryngol Otol. 2007;121(2):166-9.
24. Arai M, Terakawa I. Central paroxysmal positional vertigo. Neurology. 2005;64(7):1284.
25. Katsarkas A. Vestibular and oculomotor disturbances in pathology of the fourth ventricle. Laryngoscope. 1981;91(1):71-7.
26. Maire R, Duvoisin B. Localization of static positional nystagmus with the ocular fixation test. Laryngoscope. 1999;109(4):606-12.
27. Watson P, Barber HO, Deck J, et al. Positional vertigo and nystagmus of central origin. Can J Neurol Sci. 1981;8(2):133-7.
28. Beynon GJ, Baguley DM, Moffat DA, et al. Positional vertigo as a first symptom of a cerebellopontine angle cholesteatoma: case report. Ear Nose Throat J. 2000;79(7):508-10.

29. Taylor RL, Chen L, Lechner C, et al. Vestibular schwannoma mimicking horizontal cupulolithiasis. J Clin Neurosci. 2013;20(8):1170-3.
30. Habek M, Gabelic T, Pavlisa G, et al. Central positioning upbeat nystagmus and vertigo due to pontine stroke. J Clin Neurosci. 2011;18(7):977-8.
31. Imai T, Horii A, Takeda N, et al. A case of apogeotropic nystagmus with brainstem lesion: an implication for mechanism of central apogeotropic nystagmus. Auris Nasus Larynx. 2010;37(6):742-6.
32. Drachman DA, Diamond ER, Hart CW. Posturally-evoked vomiting; association with posterior fossa lesions. Ann Otol Rhinol Laryngol. 1977;86(1 Pt 1):97-101.
33. Baloh RW. Differentiating between peripheral and central causes of vertigo. J Neurol Sci. 2004;221(1-2):3.
34. Arbusow V, Strupp M, Brandt T. Amiodarone-induced severe prolonged head-positional vertigo and vomiting. Neurology. 1998;51(3):917.
35. Pollak L, Klein C, Rabey JM, et al. Posturally evoked vomiting without nystagmus in a patient with Arnold-Chiari malformation. J Neurol Neurosurg Psychiatry. 2001;71(3):414-5.
36. Choi JY, Kim JH, Kim HJ, et al. Central paroxysmal positional nystagmus: characteristics and possible mechanisms. Neurology. 2015 Jun 2;84(22):2238-46.

Chapter 5

Posterior Benign Positional Paroxysmal Vertigo

Augusto Casani

INTRODUCTION

Benign positional paroxysmal vertigo (BPPV) represents the most frequently reported vestibular disorder in neuro-otological clinical practice and is the most frequent cause of vertigo with a prevalence in the general population of about 2.4%.[1,2]

This disorder is characterized by the recurrence of brief and violent crises of true vertigo (spinning dizziness) triggered by horizontal and vertical movements of the head. Each episode of vertigo has an abrupt and sudden onset that lasts for a short time (few seconds to 1 minute) and tends to disappear as rapidly as it appears if the patient remains still. The disorder is defined as paroxysmal on the basis of the intensity of the vertigo perceived and on the particular trend of the nystagmic findings linked to each positional crisis (positional paroxysmal nystagmus—PPNy) that tends to increase rapidly, reaching a peak that is maintained for a few seconds, and then decreasing quickly until it completely, and just as suddenly, stops. Sometimes the symptomatology appears to such an extent as to induce patients, often unconsciously, to reduce any movements of the head and of the body in order to attenuate the symptoms as much as possible. Other types of vertigo may be correlated to the choosing of certain positions but they do not reveal this particular trend.

The crises characterized by this disturbance are often repetitive and concentrated in a limited period of time (active phase), with the tendency to reoccur after a symptom-free interval of an unpredictable length (inactive phase); the percentage of recurrences is about 30–50%[3,4] and the greater part of these, about 80%, manifest during the first year after the end of the treatment. Risk factors for this include female gender, advancing of age, post-traumatic forms, the presence of an associated endolymphatic hydrops, and comorbid conditions such as osteopenia or osteoporosis. It is estimated that about 25% of recurrences occur in the contralateral ear, a finding which suggests that BPPV should not be considered a local disease but rather the expression of a more general disorder that is still not completely understood; e.g. an inherent weakness in the connecting matrix between the otoconia could be implicated that would facilitate their displacement.[5] Therefore, despite the overall benign nature of the disorder, the fact that it manifests with paroxysmal and recurring events makes it a clinical condition that is potentially capable of negatively conditioning patients' quality of life.

Although some patients experience and report a long-lasting, subcontinuous dizziness (sense of instability, etc.) sometimes associated with vertigo, in the majority of cases conducting a careful anamnesis can lead to strongly suspecting the presence of BPPV. In any case, BPPV must be distinguished from other, more serious causes of acute or episodic vertigo.

This disorder is prevalent among females according to the majority of authors, an aspect that may reflect the highest incidence of migraine in women and the fact that by now an association between this pathology and BPPV has been distinctly proved.[6] While this disorder may actually arise at any time of life, it rarely manifests in adolescents, manifesting more frequently in adults and elderly people with a peak of incidence around the 5th–7th decade of life.[7-12] In view of the lengthening of the average lifespan of the Western population, it may be hypothesized in the near future that there will be a further considerable increase in the incidence and in the prevalence of this vertigo syndrome.

The etiology of BPPV has still not been fully understood and is classified as idiopathic in >70% of cases.[7] In the remaining cases, its onset may be associated with other events that involve the labyrinth such as a viral labyrinthitis, a sudden loss of the unilateral vestibular function due to vascular causes or surgical interventions of an otological nature, all conditions that in some way could determine a direct detachment of the otoconia from the macula, or degeneration of the same, or again they could alter the endolymphatic metabolism. Benign positional paroxysmal vertigo has also been reported to be associated with osteopenia or osteoporosis and with decreased serum levels of vitamin D, associations that are not explained by age or sex.[13,14] In any event, only when a subject reports a recent trauma is it possible to identify a cause-and-effect connection and determine the disorder as secondary, or more precisely as post-traumatic. The idiopathic and post-traumatic forms of BPPV would seem to involve the posterior semicircular canal (PSC) more frequently compared to other canals that instead are more likely to be associated with a preceding episode of BPPV.[5]

The pathogenesis of BPPV is on the other hand almost certain and may be identified in the detachment of otoliths (calcium crystals that physiologically participate in the constitution of the otolithic membrane of the utricle and the saccule), and in their displacement in one of the three semicircular canals which, ordinarily sensitive only to angular

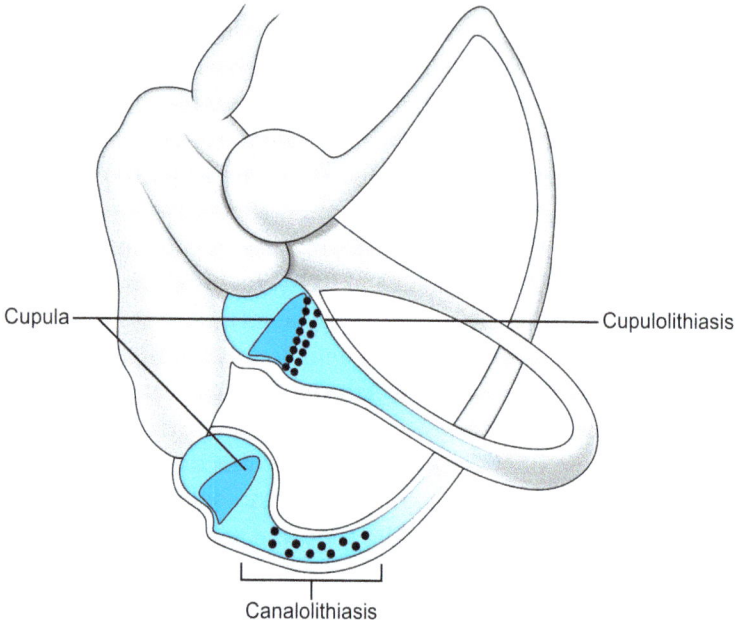

Fig. 5.1: Cupulo- and canalolithiasis.

acceleration, acquires the ability to perceive also changes of position in relation to the axis of gravity. It is also possible that particles differing from the otoconia, albeit these last equipped with a particular density (clots, white blood cells, etc.), may be responsible for the disorder. The presence of material in the lumen of the semicircular canal, that is free to move about in the endolymph, is referred to as canalithiasis. This material is described as being of such dimensions and density as to exert the effect of a pushing/sucking piston that is useful for provoking ampullopetal or ampullofugal endolymphatic currents capable of deflecting the cupola according to the movements of the head.[15] Instead the term cupololithiasis is reserved for the few cases of suspect adherence of the particles to the cupula of the canal,[16] a form that is actually less responsive to the treatment maneuvers (Fig. 5.1).

It is usually a unilateral disorder that more often involves the PSC,[17] given that it is lower down in relation to the utricle. Less frequently, in a percentage of cases that varies from 5% to 22%[18-25] but that could be underestimated since involvement at this site is more likely to remit spontaneously, there is an involvement of the lateral semicircular canal.[26] Lastly, manifestations involving the anterior semicircular canal (ASC) are rare, probably because of its uppermost position in the labyrinth, where otolithic debris is unlikely to become trapped.[27,28]

A careful anamnesis should bring forth a strong suspicion of BPPV that will be confirmed by means of a clinical examination of the patient with the use of specific diagnostic maneuvers according to which of the canals is involved. These maneuvers are performed on corresponding and specific planes in order to evidence the manifesting of typical PPNy that accompanies the vertigo in its active phase; the direction and the plane on which the PPNy is typically elicited indicate the canal that is affected and the type of stress to which the receptors are subjected. Once the diagnosis has been reached, it is important to tranquillize the patient about the essentially benign nature of the disorder in spite of the distress that it is capable of causing.[16]

A correct diagnostic approach to the disorder means avoiding a series of useless and costly instrumental tests and enables clinicians to go ahead swiftly with the treatment. In many cases, patients affected by BPPV suffer the effects of late diagnoses and the consequences of starting late with the therapy in the range of several months, a period in which they are subjected to meaningless diagnostic examinations and total inappropriate treatments.[29] The importance of timely recognition of BPPV, just as with the necessity to have effective therapies at patients' disposal, derives also from the high incidence of this pathology in the elderly population, where the presence of this disorder inevitably leads to a worsening of the capacity to carry out normal routine daily activities, determining moreover a significant increase in risk of falling, and consequent injury.[30,31] In the light of this eventuality, it is clear that a more timely identification and treatment of this disorder would have positive repercussions on the quality of life of the patient, particularly in the elderly subject, as well as containing the costs incurred by the health system and by society.[2]

As in most cases, these manifestations of vertigo can be attributed to a mechanical pathogenesis, the most effective therapy is physical. In order to obtain remission of the symptomatology, instead of opting for a direct pharmacological remedy, some maneuvers are used again, performed on the same plane of the involved canal with the aim of inducing the repositioning of the ectopic material in the vestibule. Different techniques are used that have the same aims in common, that is, to permit the force of gravity through opportune variations of the position of the patient's head, to shift the otolithic material from the canal in which it is located toward the vestibule.

In those cases that do not respond to these physical maneuvers, as also in the case of atypical nystagmus, frequently repeated recurrent episodes or where a concomitant vestibular problem is suspected, a complete reassessment of the clinical picture may be advisable and the performing of audiovestibular investigation or even imaging if thought necessary.

DIAGNOSIS AND OUTLINE OF PHYSIOPATHOLOGY

The diagnosis of BPPV, suspected after collection of strongly indicative anamnestic information, is confirmed through the finding of typical PPNy in the course of the diagnostic maneuvers. Usually the nystagmus shows an intensity to the extent that it can be opportunely assessed also without inhibiting the fixed gaze (otherwise Frenzel goggles or a video-oculography can be helpful, particularly when the nystagmus is weak or momentary). The characteristics of the eye movement express the activity of the canal involved and the connections between the semicircular canals and the extrinsic eye muscles, thus enabling clinicians often not only to confirm the diagnosis of BPPV but also to identify the canal that is responsible and the precise area of the canal hosting the particles (ampullary endings, nonampullary endings, and cupula).

The ocular movements induced by the pathological stimulation of a canal always occur on the plane of the couples of canals stimulated, analogously to what happens with physiological stimulation of the canal vestibulo-ocular reflex (VOR) (angular accelerations).

CLINICAL ASPECTS OF BPPV OF THE PSC

The form of involvement of the PSC represents the most common type of BPPV and accounts for about 80% of cases.[32] It features episodes of objective rotational vertigo (although sometimes the patient may report positional dizziness) that typically manifests in the morning or at night, when the subject sits down, goes to bed, or also when turning over in bed. Sometimes the episodes present at the moment of raising and moving the head backward or turning it abruptly or at the moment of bending down (picking something up or tying up laces). The vertigo is associated with a vagal response that is more or less intense of brief duration although patients tend to overestimate the duration when reporting symptoms. This altered perception may be attributed to the dizziness that often follows and that persists for a while after the vertigo that characterizes the single attacks. However, vertigo symptoms that last longer generally must be considered atypical and as such should require a reassessment of the diagnosis.

The natural evolution of BPPV may present with spontaneous regression of the crises over a period of time that varies from a few days to months (although actually the percentages of self-clearance are on the whole fewer compared to the forms of canalithiasis that involve the later semicircular canal); in other cases, the symptomatology does not remit even after a prolonged period of time.

In any case, since the typical vertigo crises of BPPV are often intense and hardly bearable, it is opportune to intervene with treatment.

DIAGNOSTIC MANEUVERS

The PPNy involving the PSC is triggered by a rapid movement of the head on the plane of the same canal and can be evoked by means of the positionings of Dix-Hallpike or the diagnostic positions of Semont. The presentation of PPNy that is typical elicited by the execution of these maneuvers allows formulating the diagnosis of BPPV of the PSC. Given that these diagnostic maneuvers are performed deliberately in order to trigger the typical manifestation of PPNy, it is opportune to inform the patient about the series of movements about to be executed and warn him/her about the possible onset of intense vertigo, sometimes associated with nausea that should resolve within the range of about 60 seconds.[2]

In about a quarter of subjects, above all in those observed in the late phase of the symptomatology onset, it is possible to find a mild nystagmus, while in other cases there is even a complete absence of evident ovular movements. Usually, if the patient reports vertigo with the repositioning, the typical nystagmus is more likely to emerge. Cases in which typical PPNy does not manifest, the diagnosis may only be suspected; however, if the anamnesis strongly suggests a BPPV of the PSC, a physical therapy may be anyway of potential benefit to the patient.[33] In these cases presumably the material present in the canal is effective in triggering the symptoms but not the nystagmus.[34]

The diagnosis of BPPV, or the technique adopted, must be reconsidered if the patient does not report any improvement; on the contrary, the remission of the symptomatology after the physical therapy goes to prove the diagnosis of BPPV.

Margaret Dix and Charles Hallpike were the first clinicians in 1952 to describe in detail the clinical characteristics of BPPV of the PSC and to devise a diagnostic maneuver that would reveal the typical PPNy;[35,36] still today this maneuver is considered to be the most effective in diagnosing this type of the disorder. The movements must be carried out with particular caution in patients who have previously undergone brain surgery and in subjects with cervical osteoarthrosis, given that the head must be rotated and extended during the procedure.

The maneuver begins with the patient sitting on the bed with the lower limbs extended and the upper limbs alongside the body. The examiner stands at the side of the patient[36] and rotates the patient's head for 45° toward the contralateral side, to the right or to the left, respectively (first and second Dix-Hallpike maneuver), being careful to keep the head in this position in the following phase of the maneuver. The patient (who has been instructed to keep his eyes open in a primary position in order to not modify any nystagmus) is brought to a supine position with the head hanging off the edge of the bed and slightly extended (by about 20° below

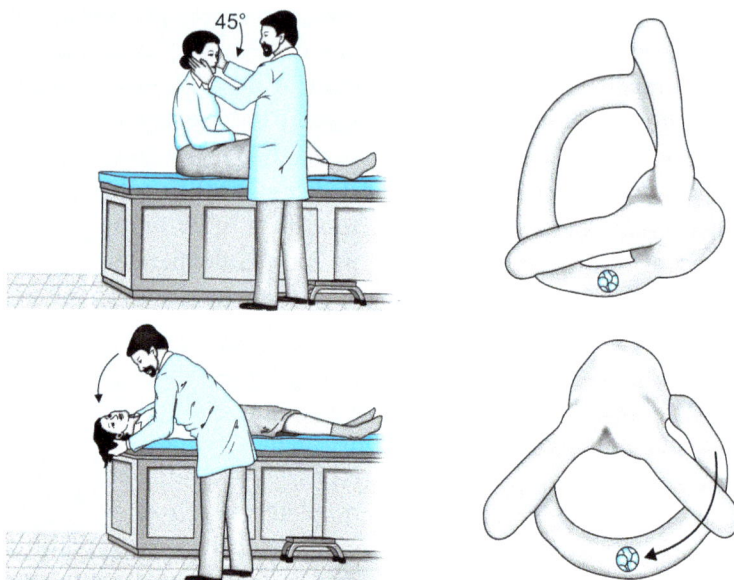

Fig. 5.2: The Dix-Hallpike maneuver to provoke positional paroxysmal nystagmus in benign positional paroxysmal vertigo involving the right posterior semicircular canal. With the patient sitting upright, the head is turned 45° to the patient's right; then he is moved from the sitting to the supine position with the head hanging below. On the right panel the movement of the debris is showed resulting in ampullofugal deviation of the cupula.

the horizontal plane) in such a way that the chin is pointing upward. In this manner, the PSC can be found on the sagittal plane in a vertical position with the ampulla higher up in relation to the nonampullary ending of the canal. In the case of a canalithiasis, the consequence is a shift of the material present inside the canal from the cupula toward the common crus; in the case of cupololithiasis, a movement of the cupula in the direction away from the utricle. In both cases the endolymphatic current flowing away from the ampulla provoked by this movement, excitatory for the posterior canals on the basis of the first law of Ewald, elicits the typical PPNy of involvement of the PSC (Fig. 5.2).

Once any dizziness and nystagmus have disappeared, the patient is slowly brought back to a sitting position. In this moment, both in the case of canalithiasis and of cupololithiasis, the material may generate an ampullopetal flow that will transform into an inhibitory discharge for the ampullary nerve, resulting in an inversion of the nystagmus. The manoeuver must be performed on both sides in order to identify which ear is involved, or perhaps to evidence involvement of both ears, a condition that manifests in a small percentage of cases, about 7.5%, and more often in the event of post-traumatic conditions.[4]

One diagnostic alternative to the Dix-Hallpike test is represented by the first step of the therapeutic maneuver devised by Alain Semont in 1988.[37]

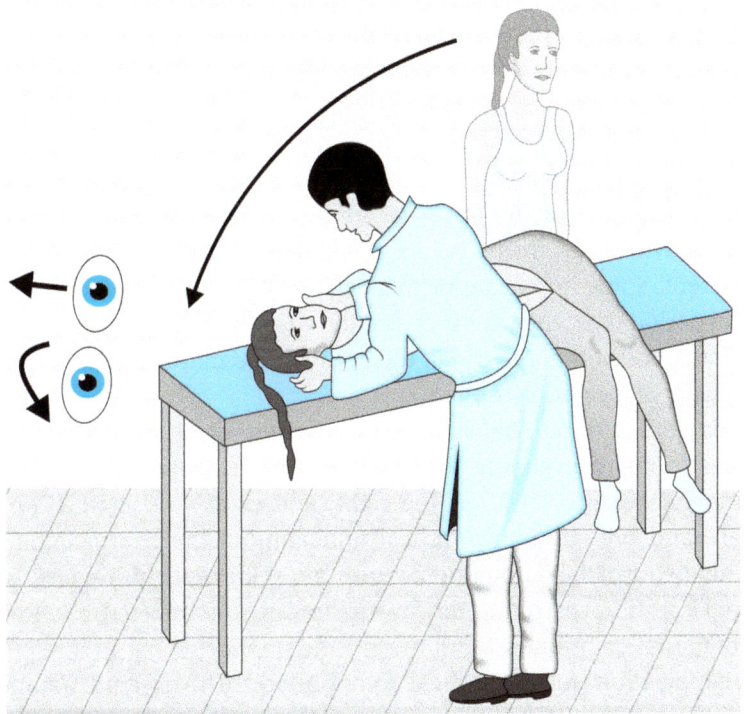

Fig. 5.3: Positional paroxysmal nystagmus caused by right benign positional paroxysmal vertigo of posterior semicircular canal elicited by a Semont diagnostic maneuver. The resulting nystagmus would be upbeat and torsional, with the top poles of the eyes beating toward the lower (right) ear.

The technique starts with the patient in a sitting position with the legs hanging down from the bed, hands on knees, and the head rotated by about 45° toward the side opposite to that on which he will be brought down. In practice the movement is performed by placing the PSC on a plane parallel to the shoulders of the patient, and in the same way as that happens during the Dix-Hallpike maneuver, determines in the cases of canalithiasis and cupulolithiasis, an excitatory ampullofugal flow that elicits the typical nystagmus indicating involvement of the PSC (Fig. 5.3). Also in this case, when the patient returns to a sitting position, nystagmus may manifest with inverse characteristics compared to the preceding one. Cawthorne, Katsarkas, and Herdman[38-40] have proposed other diagnostic maneuvers.

PPNy from Involvement of the PSC (Typical Geotropic Variant)

This form of PPNy represents the most frequent and easy to find in patients, secondary to the stimulation of the ampullary crest of the PSC. When implementing the Dix-Hallpike positioning, when the patient reaches the position with the head extended over the edge of the bed and rotated by 45° on the side being tested, the appearance of nystagmus can be observed that presents the following characteristics:

- Latency of about 3–5 seconds, probably due to the density of the endolymph—in fact, the material must overcome a certain resistance before it is able to move within the canal. This interval of time between completion of the maneuver and onset of the nystagmus represents the expression of the forces of friction that must be overcome by the gravitational thrust before manifestation of the endolymphatic current. Some important factors capable of influencing the length of the period of latency are speed of the execution of the maneuver, the spatial position of the canal, the entity of the mass of debris, and the density of the endolymph.
- It is vertical-rotational and shows aspects of dissociation in both eyes, being prevalently torsional in the ipsilateral eye (geotropic, anticlockwise for PSC on the right, and clockwise for PSC on the left) and pre-eminently vertical upbeating in the contralateral eye. The two spatial components can be evidenced more clearly by making the eyes rotate downward toward the affected ear, for the rotational component) and toward the unaffected ear in a relatively high position (for the vertical component).[41] The excitatory stimulus on the posterior ampullary nerve transforms into a contraction of the ipsilateral superior oblique and the contralateral inferior rectus muscles. This determines a slow ocular rotation that has a direct linear downbeating component that is more evident in the contralateral eye (for the contraction of the inferior rectus) and a more marked rotational component in the ipsilateral eye (for the contraction of the superior oblique), with clockwise direction for right-side PSC involvement and anticlockwise for the left-side PSC. This ocular rotation represents the slow phase of the nystagmus; the rapid phase will thus take the opposite direction both for the linear (upbeating) component and for the rotational component (anticlockwise in the event of involvement of right-side PSC and clockwise vice versa).
- It is a geotropic nystagmus since it beats in the direction of the force of gravity in the triggering positions, as the rapid phase is upbeating.
- It does not last long, from a few seconds to 1 minute, considering that by maintaining the position reached the stimulus ceases.
- It is paroxysmal: It increases rapidly in amplitude and angular velocity, reaches a plateau, and remains for a length of time before decreasing a little more slowly until it disappears.
- It may present a spontaneous inversion, in particular after an intense nystagmus. While the patient is still in the Dix-Hallpike diagnostic position, nystagmus of small amplitude may appear with the opposite direction in relation to the preceding (vertical-rotational in clockwise

direction with the head rotated to the right, vertical-rotational in an anticlockwise direction with the head rotated to the left). This spontaneous inversion of the nystagmus may be attributed to mechanisms of sensorial adjustment.[42,43]

- It inverts its direction when the patient is brought back into a sitting position. In executing this movement, both in the case that the material is free from the canal or that it is adhering to the cupula, an inhibitory ampullopetal flow is generated for the PSC with contraction of the ipsilateral inferior oblique and contralateral superior rectus muscles. The ocular movement that this triggers, still dissociated, for the slow phase is in an anticlockwise direction in the case of lithiasis of the right PSC, and in a clockwise direction for the left PSC and shows an upbeating linear component. The nystagmus from an inhibitory stimulus thus beats in a clockwise direction (right PSC) or in an anticlockwise direction (left PSC) and in both cases is downbeating. The lower intensity of the paroxysmal nystagmus that is observed after bringing the patient back to a sitting position is due to the fact that in exerting this movement an inhibitory stimulus is determined that is always weaker than the excitatory stimulus (according to the law of Ewald).

- It is fatigable, given that with repetition of the triggering positioning the nystagmus tends to reappear but becomes less and less evident showing a progressive tendency to diminish.[35] Probably this may be attributed to the fact that the material being heavier than the endolymph tends to spread, thus losing its effect of a mass (piston effect) on the endolymph and the cupula.[44]

In the presence of an anamnesis that suggests BPPV, identifying a nystagmus that presents the above-described characteristics enables clinicians to confirm the diagnosis and identify the canal involved as the PSC. In this form material that is heavier than the surrounding endolymph is free-floating in the ampullary ending of the PSC or adhering to the cupula.

When the patient is brought from a sitting position to the Dix-Hallpike position, the particles either move along the PSC, from the ampullary ending toward the common crus (pathogenetic theory of canalithiasis). According to the theory of cupololithiasis, the same movement causes compression or stretching (depending on which side—utricular or canal—they are adherent to the cupula) the ampullary receptor in the opposite direction to the utricle. In both theories, an ampullofugal stimulus is determined with consequent excitatory stimulus of the ampullary receptor of the PSC. Studies on animals have shown that a form of cupulolithiasis is more easily associated with a briefer latency and a longer-lasting nystagmus that tends to be persistent.[45] In any case to date, it is not possible to better characterize a form of BPPV of the PSC as being pertinent to the canal or to the cupula,[46] and it is likely that the aspect capable of furnishing the most indications lies in the response to the physical therapy, since it is well-known that the forms due to cupulolithiasis appear to be more resistant to maneuvers.

What we have described is the nystagmic picture that is most frequently observed and which in all its characteristics best fits with the anatomy and the physiopathology of the labyrinth. On the other hand, the nystagmic finding of posterior canalithiasis may manifest itself under a completely different aspect, without necessarily being considered atypical. It is known, in fact, that the anatomy of the semicircular canals taken singly or reciprocally, as also their caliber, can show considerable individual variations. It is possible to localize the particles in different areas along the whole canal that are potentially capable of generating nystagmic phenomena that are different from the typical manifestations. Moreover, the contemporary or sequential involvement of more than one canal in the same labyrinth has also been described, as has an involvement of both labyrinths. Different aspects of the nystagmus may also be attributed to the fact that the ocular muscles that are activated present a secondary and even tertiary action, besides that of the main action described, by virtue of which the ocular shifting may manifest in different ways.

PPNy from Involvement of the PSC (Apogeotropic Variant)

This variation described by Vannucchi involves the evoking of PPNy in the opposite direction in relation to the geotropic form, that is, a downbeating nystagmus with a clockwise torsional component (apogeotropic) in the case of right PSC and anticlockwise in the case of left PSC.[47] Any movement of the head that is executed on the vertical plane, whether coinciding with the involved PSC, with the contralateral PSC, or with the position of Rose (straight head-hanging position), can be considered a stimulus.

Unlike the typical form, this variation is associated with a less intense symptomatology of vertigo in the course of the positioning and is accompanied mostly by an irritating sensation of imbalance that is practically subcontinuous, both while standing upright and while walking.

The ocular movement observed presents the following characteristics:
- No latency
- Dissociated vertical-rotational nystagmus, prevalently rotational in the ipsilateral eye and prevalently vertical in the contralateral eye. Altogether this is a downbeating vertical nystagmus with a mild rotational component, sometimes absent, but which when present indicates the side involved. As far as the torsional component is concerned, this is in a clockwise direction when the right PSC is involved

and anticlockwise with the left PSC, while the linear component shows a rapid downbeating phase in both cases.
- Apogeotropic direction of the nystagmus, since in all three positions, when the head is outstretched, the rapid phase of the linear component is downbeating (opposite direction to that of the force of gravity).
- Variable duration but is usually long, sometimes it appears to not wear off completely during observation, despite keeping the patient for a length of time in the triggering position.
- Simil-paroxysmal trend of the nystagmus rather than purely paroxysmal, and in some cases becomes almost stationary though diminishing slowly in intensity.
- Usually there is no inversion of the nystagmus when returning the patient to a sitting position.
- Scarce fatigability (virtually none at all), given that the repetition of the triggering positions does not significantly modify the intensity of the nystagmus in comparison to that of the geotropic variation—a characteristic that perhaps is attributable to the fact that it is an inhibitory stimulus that generates it.

As is well known, a nystagmus with the characteristics described above has been thought for a long time to be caused by a lithiasis of the ASC of the opposite side to that explored by the diagnostic maneuver. Actually, this finding can be explained also with the finding of material in the nonampullary ending of the PSC, immediately before it merges with that of the ASC to form the common crus. Movements of the head on a vertical plane would appear to determine the sliding of detritus toward the ampulla and the ampullopetal stimulus, inhibitory for the PSC, would seem to be responsible for the nystagmus described, determined by the contraction of the ipsilateral oblique and the contralateral superior rectus muscles.

PPNy from Bilateral Involvement of the PSCs

The multicanal forms of paroxysmal positional vertigo, for the most part consequent to (and to be suspected in the case of recent brain traumas), include situations that may involve two different canals of the same side, the same canals of both sides or, more rarely, different canals of both sides. Clinically speaking, the PPNy of these forms can represent the epiphenomenon of a complicated interaction between ocular muscles (strengthened activation or of elision), caused by simultaneous stimulation of multiple canals.

In the case of an actual bilateral lithiasis of the PSC, performing a first Dix-Hallpike positioning maneuver, we would observe an anticlockwise vertical upbeating paroxysmal nystagmus, while during a second

Dix-Hallpike we would see a clockwise vertical upbeating paroxysmal nystagmus. In passing rapidly from the sitting position to the supine straight head hanging position (despite not acting exactly on the plane of the two posterior canal), we can obtain a bilateral ampullofugal stimulus; this will induce, bilaterally and simultaneously, a sum of nystagmi caused by the excitement of the two posterior canals. However, the nystagmus will be purely vertical (upbeating) because the two rotational components, given that they have clockwise and anticlockwise directions, tend to cancel each other out. To observe such a finding, we must necessarily hypothesize a stimulus that is equal and symmetrical in the two posterior canals; in the event of the contrary, the prevalent direction of the rotational component will indicate the PSC that is more involved or that, in supine straight head hanging position, is more stimulated.

Atypical Positional Nystagmus

If the nystagmus observed in the patient reflects the characteristics described in the typical variant of BPPV of the PSC, the diagnosis may be considered to be certain. However, not all the forms of positional vertigo and not all the forms of positional nystagmus are benign and express a peripheral problem. A positional nystagmus is generally defined atypical in reference to the loss or to the lack of clarity regarding one or more of the typically found characteristics. The most important atypical features of a positional nystagmus are the following: absence of typical latency for each canal, absence of paroxysmal trend (increase, plateau, and decrease), extreme duration, lack of exhaustibility, absence of inversion of the direction bringing the patient back to the sitting position, and absence of fatigability with repetition of the maneuvers.

The finding of these atypical forms may simply represent a variation of a typical form having the following causes: unusual collocation of the material, incorrect execution of the maneuver, unusual characteristics of the debris, alterations of the cupula, and anatomical variations of the planes of the canals. Nevertheless, an atypical positional nystagmus may also be the expression of a condition of inefficient central control of the VOR evoked by the kinematics of the various maneuvers, which is indicative of a pathology of the central nervous system (CNS). In an attempt to standardize the characteristics of the forms of atypical BPPV in order to better recognize them, Soto-Varela et al.[5] proposed the following criteria:

- Presence of symptoms or associated neurological signs
- Nystagmus in the absence of vertigo during the positioning
- Nystagmus with atypical direction (in particular downbeating or multidirectional) when placing the patient in the same position several times

- Poor response to physical therapy
- Highly frequent recurrence.

Manifestation of one of the above findings according to the authors indicates the need for further instrumental investigations.

In particular, positional downbeating nystagmus may be also attributable to a lesion of the CNS in the posterior cranial fossa (mainly cerebellar).

On that account, in the case of atypical positional nystagmus, where a not perfectly consistent anamnesis coexists with a condition of BPPV, clinicians should search for any symptoms and signs suggesting a central involvement. Also the reporting of closely repeated recurrent episodes should arouse some suspicion. In any case, in the face of an atypical form, the diagnosis cannot be certain and it may be useful to repeat the diagnostic maneuvers, speeding up the movements, and if necessary implementing ex adjuvantibus therapy. If this should prove efficacious, with the patient free from symptoms and no longer with evident nystagmus, then it is possible to confirm the diagnosis. Otherwise it is correct to exclude other causes of vertigo, in particular central vertigo, and proceed with neuroradiological investigations.[2]

PHYSICAL THERAPY FOR BPPV OF THE PSC

Over the last years, numerous techniques of physical therapy have been developed to cure BPPV of the posterior canal, which all have in common the objective of freeing the canal or the cupola from otoconial debris. Practice guidelines published in 2008 independently by the American Academy of Neurology[48] and the American Academy of Otolaryngology—Head and Neck Surgery[2] recommend only the use of Epley's maneuver for BPPV involving the posterior canal. This technique is considered safe and efficacious, and is recommended for patients of all ages. Semont's maneuver is classified as only "possibly effective" due to the lack of class I and class II studies. Nevertheless, evidence from the most recent literature recommends this maneuver as well as others.[49,50] Some of these appear to be more suitable in cases of canalithiasis, others in cases of cupololithiasis, and yet others demonstrate equal efficacy in both situations.

The most frequently used techniques, listed here below, can be essentially divided into the following categories:
- Techniques for the dispersion of debris
- Techniques for the repositioning of particles
- Techniques that propose to eliminate the debris from the canal exploiting the effect of an abrupt deceleration.

The techniques of dispersion can be associated with the exercises proposed by Brandt and Daroff in 1980 that though initially used as a

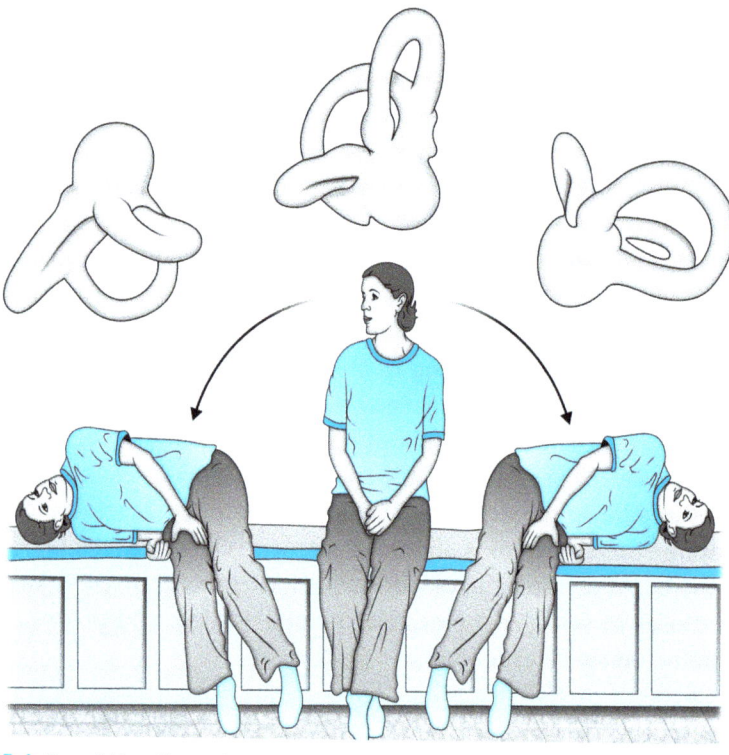

Fig. 5.4: Brandt-Daroff exercises.

proper therapeutic treatment, once classified as being of poor validity in comparison with other methods available, were then widely used as "gymnastics" exercises, to be carried out at home after the therapeutic maneuver with a view to preventing the disorder from recurring.[51] All the studies that have touched on these techniques, however, would appear to show controversial results, observing modifications neither in the number of relapses, nor in the risk of recurrence.[52] The pattern of exercises to be repeated originally consisted in sessions every 3 hours in the timespan of a day. The patient is placed sitting in the center of the bed and from here is brought rapidly to a lying-down position on his side without moving the head in any particular way, but with the aim of having the ear touch the surface of the bed. The subject is invited to remain in this position until any vertigo triggered by the movement passes away, and then maintain the position for a further 60 seconds. The subject is then required to take up the original sitting position again, in the center of the bed, which must be maintained for about 60 seconds. After this he is made to lie on the opposite side with the same method, and maintain this position again for 60 seconds after the end of any vertigo presenting, returning to the initial sitting position in the center of the bed and thus proceeding with another cycle (Fig. 5.4).

A session consists of five cycles and the therapy may be interrupted once the vertigo has disappeared for at least two consecutive days when passing from one position to another.

The techniques of repositioning are based on the maneuver described by Epley in 1980.[53] In this case, it consists of a maneuver that aims to free the area from debris in the case of canalithiasis and that can be implemented immediately after the diagnostic maneuver of Dix-Hallpike. The patient is made by the therapist to carry out a series of movements with the head so as to determine the gradual shifting of the particles from the ampullary ending of the PSC to the nonampullary ending, then on to the common crus and finally into the vestibule. Unlike the Brandt-Daroff exercises, this maneuver is conceived as a single approach and, is being performed by clinicians in a hospital setting, does not have to be repeated at home.[54]

In the original description, throughout the maneuver the patient wore a vibrator collocated on the mastoid of the affected ear, an expedient supposed to assist the movement of the particles in the canal in order that, under the effect of the vibration, they could overcome the force of attrition with the walls of the same canal. The results of the studies regarding the efficaciousness of this expedient would appear to be quite controversial.[55-59]

The maneuver starts with the patient sitting with his legs on the bed. He is brought by the therapist into the position of Dix-Hallpike that provokes the vertigo and is kept in this position for 2-3 minutes, the time necessary for the nystagmus to disappear and for the particles to collocate themselves in the sloping part of the canal that in this position is very near the nonampullary ending of the PSC.

At this point, the head of the patient is turned with a slow but continuous movement toward the unaffected side until the patient finds himself with his head facing the floor. This position is maintained for 2-3 minutes, after which the patient is slowly brought back to a sitting position (Fig. 5.5). When the patient is in the Dix-Hallpike position opposite to the affected side, or when he has been brought back to a sitting position, the nystagmus has the same direction as that evidenced with the positioning on the affected side; this indicates that the maneuver has been performed successfully, given that it evidences the movement of the detrital mass from the ampullary portion of the PSC to the common crus and then toward the utricle. Further techniques with small modifications of the one described above have been described and proposed, with the aim of simplifying the procedure; however, the results have shown to be hardly any different.[60,61]

After the maneuver, the patient is often invited to keep his head still for a few days, to sleep with the head raised, almost in a sitting position;

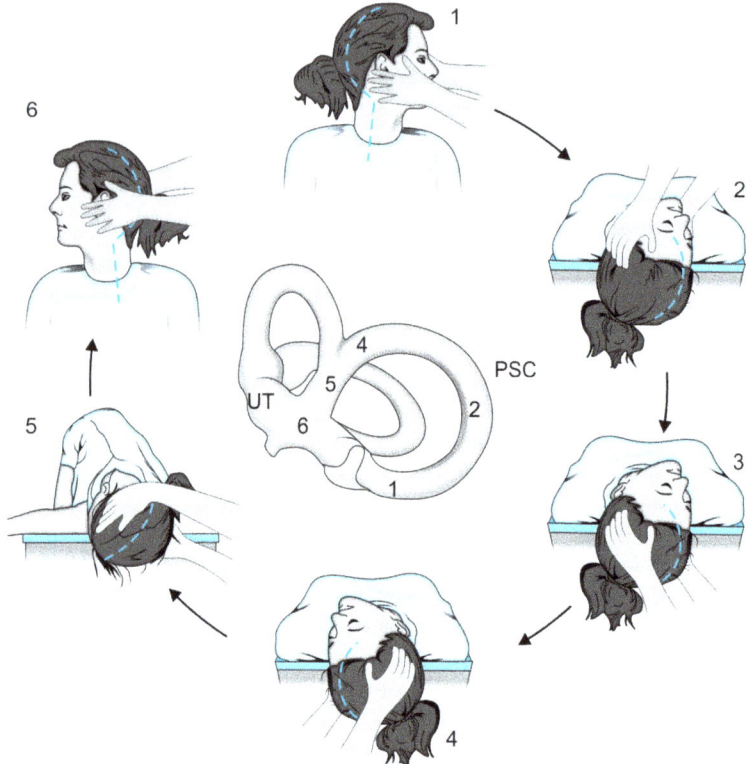

Fig. 5.5: Epley's canalith-repositioning maneuver. After resolution of positional paroxysmal nystagmus caused by a right posterior semicircular canal (PSC)-benign positional paroxysmal vertigo, after a first Dix-Hallpike maneuver (1–2), the head is turned 90° toward the unaffected (left) side (3–4): the otolithic debris move closer to the common crus. The induced nystagmus would be in the same direction as that evoked during the Dix-Hallpike maneuver. The head is turned 90° more (face-down position) (5); the trunk turned 90° in the same direction as well. The patient is then moved to the sitting position, allowing the otoliths fall into the utricule (UT), via the common crus (6).

some authors consider these precautions unnecessary insomuch as, if the therapy has been successful (and if the material has been dislodged), it is unlikely that it will go back into the canal once it has come out.[48,62,63] The success of the maneuver is assessed by the therapist after a few minutes or after a few days.

Lastly, the techniques that exploit the principle of an abrupt deceleration take the maneuver of Semont as a model.[37] The technique starts with the patient sitting on the bed with his legs hanging down and with the head rotated by 45° toward the unaffected side. The patient is then brought down onto his side corresponding to the affected side. The movement, which is a replica of the diagnostic maneuver of the same name, elicits the typical PPNy of excitement of the PSC; the position is maintained for 30 seconds to a minute. The patient is then brought to lie on the

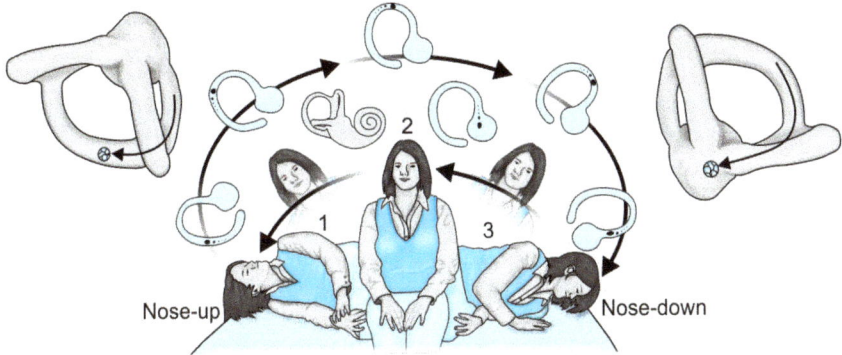

Fig. 5.6: Semont's maneuver for right benign positional paroxysmal vertigo of the posterior semicircular canal. The maneuver starts with the patient seated upright (2). Then the patient is lied on the affected side with the head turned to the left (nose up position) (1). The patient is turned to the opposite position (left) with a quick and continuous movement with the head turned to the left (nose down position) (3). Finally, the patient is seated with the head in neutral position (2).

opposite side in a single rapid movement (without stopping in the central sitting position) being careful to maintain the angle of the head. Since the new reached position is diametrically opposite, the face arrives close to the bed, facing 45° downward (Fig. 5.6). In this final position, the manifestation of a new nystagmus, still excitatory, indicates the ampullofugal migration of the otoconial mass toward the utricule; this may be considered an indication of success. Once the nystagmus has worn off and about 1 minute has passed, the patient is brought back to a sitting position while trying to maintain the head still inclined on the unaffected side. In this phase, it is important to hold the patient firmly insomuch as not infrequently he may perceive an intense sensation of pulsion forward that for a reaction will lead him to push backward. As far as the postmaneuver restrictions are concerned, the same counts here for those described for the maneuver of Epley, as also for the controls that should be carried out in the same way. The technique of Semont may be preferred in the event of the patient showing difficulty in extending the neck,[49] while on the other hand a correct execution of this maneuver may prove to be complicated in the case of elderly or obese patients.

After the maneuvers have been performed, also in the case of a successful outcome, up to two-thirds of patients may perceive a prolonged albeit mild sensation of instability, also known as "residual dizziness".[64,65] This residual symptomatology, that in part may be attributed to a state of "otolithic dysfunction", would appear to be associated with a condition of stress of the subject that in turn may be correlated in particular with the duration of the illness and therefore with age, gender, and number of recurrences.[65,66] In the light of this observation, early recognition and treatment of a clinical picture of BPPV would allow clinicians to significantly reduce the incidence of this troublesome disorder.

REFERENCES

1. Von Brevern M, Radtke A, Lezius F, et al. Epidemiology of benign paroxysmal positional vertigo: a population based study. J Neurol Neurosurg Psychiatry. 2007;78:710-5.
2. Bhattacharyya N, Baugh RF, Orvidas L, et al. Clinical practice guideline: benign paroxysmal positional vertigo. Otolaryngol Head Neck Surg. 2008;139:(Suppl 4):S47-S81.
3. Hain TC, Helminski JO, Reis IL, et al. Vibration does not improve results of the canalith repositioning procedure. Arch Otolaryngol Head Neck Surg. 2000;-126:617-22.
4. Nunez RA, Cass SP, Furman JM. Short- and long-term outcomes of canalith repositioning for benign paroxysmal positional vertigo. Otolaryngol Head Neck Surg. 2000;122:647-52.
5. Soto-Varela A, Santos-Perez S, Rossi-Izquierdo M, et al. Are the three canals equally susceptible to benign paroxysmal positional vertigo? Audiol Neurootol. 2013;18:327-34.
6. Ishiyama A, Jacobson KM, Baloh RW. Migraine and benign positional vertigo. Ann Otol Rhinol Laryngol. 2000;109:377-80.
7. Baloh RW, Honrubia V, Jacobson KM. Benign positional vertigo: clinical and oculographic features in 240 cases. Neurology. 1987;37:371-8.
8. Barber HO, Leigh RJ. Benign (and not so benign) postural vertigo: diagnoses and treatment. In: Barber HO, Sharpe JA, eds. Vestibular disorders. London: Year Book Medical; 1988. pp. 215-32.
9. Nuti D, Pagnini P. Epidemiologia della cupulolitiasi. Atti XIIa Giornata Italiana di Nistagmografia Clinica. Viterbo. 1992.
10. Katsarkas A. Dizziness in aging: a retrospective study of 1194 cases. Otolaryngol Head Neck Surg. 1994;110:296-301.
11. Gufoni M, Guidetti G, Nuti D, et al. The role of clinical history in the evaluation of balance and spatial orientation disorders in the elderly. Acta Otorhinolaryngol Ital. 2005;25:5-10.
12. Uneri A, Polat S. Vertigo, dizziness and imbalance in the elderly. J Laryngol Otol. 2008;122:466-9.
13. Jeong SH, Choi SH, Kim JY, et al. Osteopenia and osteoporosis in idiopathic benign positional vertigo. Neurology. 2009;72:1069-76.
14. Jeong SH, Kim JS, Shin JW, et al. Decreased serum vitamin D in idiopathic benign paroxysmal positional vertigo. J Neurol. 2013;260:832-8.
15. Hall SF, Ruby RF, McClure JA. The mechanics of benign paroxysmal vertigo. J Otolaryngol. 1979;8:151-8.
16. Schuknecht HF. Cupulolithiasis. Arch Otolaryngol. 1969;90:765-78.
17. Hornibrook J. Benign paroxysmal positional vertigo (BPPV): history, pathophysiology, office treatment and future directions. Int J Otolaryngol. 2011; 2011:835671.
18. De La Meilleure G, Dehaene I, Depondt M, et al. Benign paroxysmal positional vertigo of the horizontal canal. J Neurol Neurosurg Psychiatry. 1996;60:68-71.

19. Casani AP, Vannucchi G, Fattori B, et al. The treatment of horizontal canal positional vertigo: our experience in 66 cases. Laryngoscope. 2002;112:172-8.
20. Parnes LS, Agrawal SK, Atlas J. Diagnosis and management of benign paroxysmal positional vertigo (BPPV). CMAJ. 2003;169:681-93.
21. Caruso G, Nuti D. Epidemiological data from 2270 cases of PPV patients. Audiological Med. 2005;3:7-11.
22. Prokopakis EP, Chimona T, Tsagournisakis M, et al. Benign paroxysmal positional vertigo: 10-year experience in treating 592 patients with canalith repositioning procedure. Laryngoscope. 2005;115:1667-71.
23. Cakir BO, Ercan I, Cakir ZA, et al. Relationship between the affected ear in benign paroxysmal positional vertigo and habitual head-lying side during bedrest. J Laryngol Otol. 2006;120:534-6.
24. Choung YH, Shin YR, Kahng H, et al. "Bow and lean test" to determinate the affected ear of horizontal canal benign paroxysmal positional vertigo. Laryngoscope. 2006;116:1776-81.
25. Han BI, Oh HJ, Kim JS. Nystagmus while recumbent in horizontal canal benign paroxysmal positional vertigo. Neurology. 2006;66:706-10.
26. McClure JA. Horizontal canal BPV. J Otolaryngol. 1985;14:30-5.
27. Nuti D, Zee DS. Positional vertigo and benign paroxysmal positional vertigo. In: Bronstein A, ed. Oxford textbook of vertigo and imbalance. Oxford, England: Oxford University Press; 2013. pp. 217-30.
28. Casani AP, Cerchiai N, Dallan I, et al. Anterior canal lithiasis: diagnosis and treatment. Otolaryngol Head Neck Surg. 2011;144:412-8.
29. Fife TD, FitzGerald JE. Do patients with benign paroxysmal positional vertigo receive prompt treatment? Analysis of waiting times and human and financial costs associated with current practice. Int J Audiol. 2005;44:50-7.
30. Oghalai JS, Manolidis S, Barth JL, et al. Unrecognized benign paroxysmal positional vertigo in elderly patients. Otolaryngol Head Neck Surg. 2000;122:630-4.
31. Lopez-Escamez JA, Gamiz MJ, Fernandez-Perez A, et al. Long-term outcome and health-related quality of life in benign paroxysmal positional vertigo. Eur Arch Otorhinolaryngol. 2005;262:507-11.
32. Nakajama M, Epley J. BPPV and variants: improved treatment results with automated, nystagmus-based repositioning. Otolaryngol Head Neck Surg. 2005;133:107-12.
33. Balatsouras DG, Korres SG. Subjective benign paroxysmal positional vertigo. Otolaryngol Head Neck Surg. 2012;146:98-103.
34. House MG, Honrubia V. Theoretical models for the mechanisms of benign paroxysmal positional vertigo. Audiol Neurootol. 2003;8:91-9.
35. Dix MR, Hallpike CS. Pathology, symptomatology and diagnosis of certain common disorders of the vestibular system. Ann Otol Rhinol Laryngol. 1952;61:987-1016.
36. Furman JM, Cass SP. Benign paroxysmal positional vertigo. N Engl J Med. 1999;341:1590-6.
37. Semont A, Freyss G, Vitte E. Curing the BPPV with a liberatory maneuver. Adv Otorhinolaryngol. 1988;42:290-3.
38. Cawthorne T. Positional nystagmus. Ann Otol. 1954;3:481-90.

39. Katsarkas A. Nystagmus of paroxysmal vertigo: some new insights. Ann Otol Rhinol Laryngol. 1987;96:305-8.
40. Herdman SJ. Assessment and management of benign paroxysmal positional vertigo. In: Herdman SJ, ed. Vestibular rehabilitation. Philadelphia: FA Davis; 1994. pp. 331-46.
41. Harbert F. Benign paroxysmal positional nystagmus. Arch Ophthal. 1970;84:298-302.
42. Young LR, Oman CM. Model for vestibular adaptation to horizontal rotation. Aerospace Med. 1969;40:1076-80.
43. Furman JMR, Hain TC, Paige GD. Central adaptation models of the vestibulo-ocular and optokinetic systems. Biol Cybern. 1989;61:255-64.
44. Epley JM. Positional vertigo related to semicircular canalithiasis. Otolaryngol Head Neck Surg. 1995;112:154-61.
45. Otsuka K, Suzuki M, Furuya M. Model experiment of benign paroxysmal positional vertigo mechanism using the whole membranous labyrinth. Acta Otolaryngol. 2003;123:515-8.
46. Coehn HS, Sangi-Haghpeykar H. Nystagmus parameters and subtypes of benign paroxysmal positional vertigo. Acta Otolaryngol. 2010;130:1019-923.
47. Vannucchi P, Pecci R, Giannoni B. Posterior semicircular canal benign paroxysmal positional vertigo presenting with torsional downbeating nystagmus: an apogeotropic variant. Int J Otolaryngol. 2012;2012:413603.
48. Fife TD, Iverson DJ, Lempert T, et al. Practice parameter: therapies for benign paroxysmal positional vertigo (an evidence-based review): report of the Quality Standards Subcommittee of the American Academy of Neurology. Quality Standards Subcommittee, American Academy of Neurology. Neurology. 2008;70:2067-74.
49. Mandalà M, Santoro GP, Asprella Libonati G, et al. Double-blind randomized trial on short-term efficacy of the Semont maneuver for the treatment of posterior canal benign paroxysmal positional vertigo. J Neurol. 2012;259:882-5.
50. Kim JS, Zee DS. Clinical practice. Benign paroxysmal positional vertigo. N Engl J Med. 2014;370:1138-47.
51. Brandt T, Daroff RB. Physical therapy for benign paroxysmal positional vertigo. Arch Otolaryngol. 1980;106:484-5.
52. Helminski JO, Jotaspouikis D, Kovacs K, et al. Strategies to prevent recurrence of benign paroxysmal positional vertigo. Arch Otolaryngol Head Neck Surg. 2005;131:344-8.
53. Epley JM. New dimensions of benign paroxysmal positional vertigo. Otolaryngol Head Neck Surg. 1980;88:599-605.
54. Epley JM. The canalith repositioning procedure for the treatment of benign paroxysmal positional vertigo. Otolaryngol Head Neck Surg. 1992;107:399-404.
55. Li JC. Mastoid oscillation: a critical factor for success in canalith repositioning procedure. Otolaryngol Head Neck Surg. 1995;112:670-5.
56. Lopez-Escamez JA, Gonzalez-Sanchez M, Salinero J. Meta-analysis of the treatment of benign paroxysmal positional vertigo by Epley and Semont maneuvers. Acta Otorrinolaringol Esp. 1999;50:366-70.
57. Chang AK, Schoeman G, Hill M. A randomized clinical trials to assess the efficacy of the Epley maneuver in the treatment of acute benign paroxysmal vertigo. Acad Emerg Med. 2004;11:918-24.

58. Woodworth BA, Gillespie MB, Lambert PR. The canalith repositioning procedure for benign paroxysmal positional vertigo: a meta-analysis. Laryngoscope. 2004;114:1143-6.
59. Sridhar S, Panda N. Particle repositioning manoeuvre in benign paroxysmal positional vertigo: is it really safe? J Otolaryngol. 2005;34:41-5.
60. Herdman SJ, Tusa RJ, Zee DS, et al. Single treatment approaches to benign paroxysmal positional vertigo. Arch Otolaryngol Head Neck Surg. 1993;119:450-4.
61. Harvey SA, Hain TC, Adamiec LC. Modified liberatory maneuver: effective treatment for benign paroxysmal positional vertigo. Laryngoscope. 1994;104:1206-12.
62. Massoud E, Ireland DJ. Post-treatment instructions in the nonsurgical management of benign paroxysmal positional vertigo. J Otolaryngol. 1996;25:121-5.
63. Nuti D, Nati C, Passali D. Treatment of benign paroxysmal positional vertigo: non need for postmaneuver restrictions. Otolaryngol Head Neck Surg. 2000;122:440-4.
64. Di Girolamo S, Paludetti G, Briglia G, et al. Postural control in benign paroxysmal positional vertigo before and after recovery. Acta Otolaryngol. 1998;118:189-93.
65. Seok JI, Lee HM, Yoo JH, et al. Residual dizziness after successful repositioning treatment in patients with benign paroxysmal positional vertigo. J Clin Neurol. 2008;4:107-10.
66. Faralli M, Ricci G, Ibba MC, et al. Dizziness in patients with recent episodes of benign paroxysmal positional vertigo: real otolithic dysfunction or mental stress? J Otolaryngol Head Neck Surg. 2009;38:375-80.

Chapter 6

Horizontal Benign Paroxysmal Positional Vertigo

Giacinto Asprella Libonati

OVERVIEW

Benign paroxysmal positional vertigo (BPPV) is the most common cause of vertigo.

It is due to a mechanical disorder of the labyrinth that is characterized by brief and violent crises of spinning sensation showing brisk onset and rapid decrease—paroxysmal vertigo. Each crisis usually lasts from 15 to 60 seconds, and is related to head position changes with respect to gravity—positional vertigo. It usually has a favorable course and therefore is defined as "benign"; however BPPV can rarely be very disabling because of a high recurrence rate and/or a low response to the physical therapy, such that some authors prefer to omit the term benign.

Benign paroxysmal positional vertigo's peak of incidence occurs between 50 and 60 years of age but it can occur at any age, even in infants. The incidence of BPPV in children is much lower than in the adult population: in our experience only 1% of total BPPV concerns patients aged from 2 to 14 years.[1,2] Benign paroxysmal positional vertigo usually occurs spontaneously. Sometimes it can be associated with triggering mechanical events causing otoconial detachment. Such a causal relationship can be hypothesized in case of minor head trauma occurring within the last 24-72 hours (domestic injuries, sports injuries, school injuries, dental care), while only a possible or probable relationship can be assumed with viral or vascular illness. A higher BPPV incidence is reported in migrainous and Ménière population.

The labyrinthine mechanical disorder that causes BPPV is due to the presence of otoconial debris detached from the utricular macula and free floating inside the semicircular canals: canalolithiasis, or attached to the ampullary cupula: cupulolithiasis. Both of the previous conditions transform the ampullary cupula of the involved canal from a detector of angular accelerations into a detector of linear accelerations, thus becoming gravity sensitive.

According to the canalolithiasis theory, the otoconial conglomerate gravitates inside the canal because of head movements and in so doing pushes the endolymphatic column. In this way, the otoconial bolus, working like a piston,[3] provokes a hydrodynamic drag on the endolymph, which deflects the ampullary cupula, thus generating an excitatory or an inhibitory stimulus that causes the paroxysmal vertigo.

According to the cupulolithiasis theory, the otoliths are attached to the cupula that becomes heavier than the surrounding endolymph and gravity sensitive (heavy cupula). In our experience, cupulolithiasis is much more infrequent than canalolithiasis.

The most used BPPV classification in clinical practice is based on the involved canal (Table 6.1):
- Posterior semicircular canal (PSC)
- Horizontal semicircular canal (HSC) or lateral semicircular canal
- Anterior semicircular canal (ASC)
- Multicanal BPPV
    - Simultaneous involvement: Post-traumatic BPPV
    - No simultaneous involvement: canal switch.

The BPPV diagnosis shall be always based on the evoked nystagmus and not on the kind of maneuver that provokes positional vertigo. In fact, both excitatory and inhibitory stimuli of each semicircular canal are linked to a typical nystagmus, as every vestibular stimulus triggered by

Table 6.1: BPPV classification.

Involved canal	BPPV side	Variants
• Posterior semicircular canal (PSC)	• PSC-BPPV: – Left – Right – Bilateral	• Geotropic (typical) • Apogeotropic
• Horizontal semicircular canal (HSC)	• HSC-BPPV: – Left – Right – Bilateral	• Geotropic • Apogeotropic
• Anterior semicircular canal (ASC)	• ASC-BPPV: – Left – Right – Bilateral	

• Multicanal involvement	• Multicanal BPPV:
	– Simultaneous involvement
	– Post-traumatic BPPV
	   ▪ Unilateral
	   ▪ Bilateral
	– No-simultaneous involvement
	– Postmaneuver canal conversion
	   ▪ Unilateral	

(BPPV: Benign paroxysmal positional vertigo).

each ampullary cupula deflection provokes the contraction of a couple of extrinsic ocular muscles, thus generating a specific and characteristic eye movement in response to each ampullary nerve input. Therefore, there are maneuvers suggested to diagnose every single type of BPPV, but the pathognomonic nystagmus for a specific subtype of BPPV is sometimes evoked performing the maneuver recommended to diagnose a different BPPV subtype. Thus it is the evoked nystagmus and not the kind of the performed maneuver that allows us to properly diagnose which one is the involved semicircular canal.

INTRODUCTION

The second most common type of BPPV is HSC BPPV, accounting for 15–25% of all BPPV cases.

The patient usually experiences his/her first HSC BPPV attack turning sideways while sleeping. The violent vertigo abruptly wakes the patient up and is generally associated with very intense neurovegetative symptoms. Each attack lasts from 30 to 60 seconds, sometimes longer. Vertigo recurs moving the head in the horizontal plane. It is more intense when the head is rotated from side to side while supine, but the patient can suffer from mid vertigo every time the otoliths inside the affected horizontal canal begin to gravitate because of head movements, e.g. by rotating the head to the upright position, by lying straight down or on one side. Crisis associated neurovegetative symptoms and dizziness while walking are usually more intense in course of HSC BPPV, rather than in PSC BPPV.

PATHOPHYSIOLOGY

The HSC BPPV pathophysiology is most frequently ascribed to free floating debris inside the HSC modifying the cupula's sensitivity to accelerations, according to the canalolithiasis theory. Therefore, the HSC cupula becomes sensitive to linear accelerations, i.e. gravity and accelerations provoked by brisk head movements on the same plane of the involved HSC. Two HSC canalolithiasis variants are known:
1. Geotropic HSC BPPV, about 75% of all HSC BPPV, is due to debris floating along the HSC nonampullary posterior arm.
2. Apogeotropic HSC BPPV, about 25% of all HSC BPPV, is due to debris floating close to the HSC ampulla.
   - *Pathophysiology of the geotropic variant:* Shortly after rotating the patient's head to the impaired side while supine, the otoliths gravitate toward the ampulla along the HSC posterior arm, generating an ampullopetal excitatory endolymphatic current, and a geotropic nystagmus beating toward the impaired ear. When the

patient's head is turned to the healthy side, the otoliths float along the HSC posterior arm toward its utricular orifice, generating an ampullofugal inhibitory endolymphatic current. As a result, the nystagmus will be geotropic once again beating to the healthy side (Fig. 6.1A).
- *Pathophysiology of the apogeotropic variant:* When the patient lies on the impaired side the debris in the ampullary segment of the HSC will move away from the cupula, resulting in an inhibitory ampullofugal endolymphatic current, which causes an apogeotropic nystagmus beating toward the healthy ear. When the head is turned to the opposite side, the otoliths will drop toward the ampulla with an excitatory discharge and an apogeotropic nystagmus beating toward the affected side will be observed (Fig. 6.1B).

DIAGNOSIS

The diagnosis is performed identifying the HSC BPPV canalolithiasis nystagmus whose typical features are reported in Table 6.2.

The typical paroxysmal nystagmus is sometimes evoked only after repeating the diagnostic HSC BPPV maneuver again and again.[4] This could happen in patients with a delayed diagnosis, because the otoliths are initially spread out inside the HSC. In fact, the movement of otoliths is effective in deflecting the cupula only if they are conglomerated, thus acting like a piston. The repeated head rotations move debris by gathering them due to the forces of superficial adhesion.

The diagnostic maneuver for HSC BPPV is the "supine head roll test" or "McClure-Pagnini test".[5,6] This maneuver is performed by turning the head 180° to either side while supine. Since it is performed on the yaw plane, it should be more correct to call it "head yaw test" (HYT) while supine.

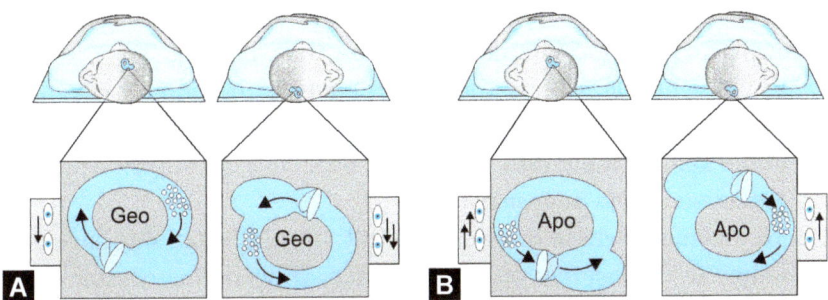

Figs. 6.1A and B: (A) Geotropic horizontal BPPV pathophysiology. (B) Apogeotropic HSC BPPV pathophysiology. (BPPV: Benign paroxysmal positional vertigo; HSC: Horizontal semicircular canal) (this figure shows horizontal BPPV of right side).

Table 6.2: HSC BPPV canalolithiasis nystagmus features.[52]	

Nystagmus' quick phase	• It is a direction changing, bidirectional, bipositional purely horizontal nystagmus:
	  – Geotropic variant: nystagmus beats toward the ground
	  – Apogeotropic variant: nystagmus beats away from the ground

Nystagmus is paroxysmal	• It very rapidly increases, reaches a so called plateau and then slowly decreases • It has a longer duration than the PSC BPPV one: 30/60 second, sometimes longer
Nystagmus' latency	• Its latency is shorter than the PSC BPPV one: 2/3 second, sometimes no latency
Nystagmus' fatigue	• Repetition of the positioning test induces less nystagmus fatigue than the PSC BPPV one. Actually, it is often impossible to proceed with retesting to determine how much the nystagmus is really fatigable because of violent associated neurovegetative symptoms

• Nystagmus' direction	• Sometimes its direction spontaneously reverses while keeping the head in the evocative position:
	  – This last condition is more frequent, if the nystagmus intensity is very strong
	  – It occurs more frequently turning the patient on the affected ear in the geotropic variant
	  – It is sometimes observed turning the patient on the unaffected ear in the apogeotropic variant

(HSC: Horizontal semicircular canal; BPPV: Benign paroxysmal positional vertigo; PSC: Posterior semicircular canal).

As therapeutic maneuvers should be performed toward the healthy side, diagnosing the affected side is critical for successful treatment.

The first described clinical sign in order to identify the impaired side in HSC BPPV is the intensity of the nystagmus evoked by performing HYT while supine: head yaw nystagmus.

The head yaw nystagmus beats with more intensity toward the impaired ear, according to Ewald's second law, which postulates that the response to an excitatory stimulus is always more intense than the one following an inhibitory stimulus (Figs. 6.2A and B), so that:

- In the geotropic variant the affected side is the one on which the nystagmus is more intense in HYT.
- In the apogeotropic variant the affected side is the one on which the nystagmus is less intense in HYT.

New clinical signs to diagnose the HSC BPPV affected side have been described in the last few years. All of them show nonparoxysmal long-lasting nystagmuses, which generally are of low intensity (Table 6.3).

- A nystagmus evoked by bringing the patient down from a sitting position, was first described by Nuti et al. (2005).[7] This is evoked by the

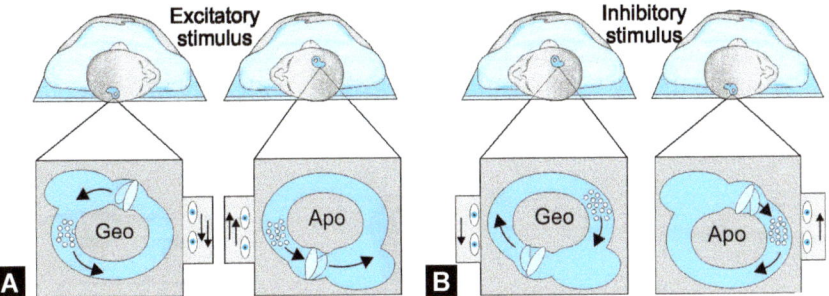

Figs. 6.2A and B: Head yaw test for horizontal BPPV. The head yaw nystagmus beats with more intensity toward the impaired ear (the right one in this figure), according to Ewald's second law, which postulates that the response to an (A) excitatory stimulus is always more intense than the one following an (B) inhibitory stimulus.

Table 6.3: HSC BPPV: rules to diagnose the affected side.	
1.	The direction of the more intense nystagmus in the head yaw test while supine is toward the affected ear
2.	The direction of both the pseudospontaneous nystagmus and the seated supine positioning nystagmus is toward the unaffected ear in the geotropic HSC BPPV
3.	The direction of both the pseudospontaneous nystagmus and the seated supine positioning nystagmus is toward the affected ear in the apogeotropic HSC BPPV

(HSC BPPV: Horizontal semicircular canal benign paroxysmal positional vertigo).

seated supine positioning test (SSPT). When the patient lies supine, having the head flexed 30°, the HSC is on a vertical plane; therefore, due to gravity, the otoliths are pushed downward: when they are in the posterior arm, geotropic variant, they float away from the ampulla. When they are near the cupula, apogeotropic variant, they float toward the ampulla. Therefore, the SSPT evokes a nystagmus beating toward the healthy side in the geotropic variant and toward the affected side in the apogeotropic variant: seated supine positioning nystagmus (Fig. 6.3 and Table 6.3).

- A nystagmus observed in upright position has been described in patients suffering from HSC BPPV. It could be mistaken for a "spontaneous" nystagmus, but it is a direction changing nystagmus because it is strongly modulated by head position, therefore it has been most properly defined as a "pseudospontaneous nystagmus" (PSN).[8] It beats toward the healthy side in geotropic HSC BPPV and toward the affected side in apogeotropic HSC BPPV. It increases if the head is bent 30° backward, disappearing when the head is bent 30° forward (neutral position), and reverses its direction if the head is additionally inclined forward to 60° (Figs. 6.4A to D and Table 6.3). It is sometimes useful to slowly rotate the patient's head horizontally,

because such a maneuver evokes the PSN when it is not evident yet while the head is erect.
- A single theory was postulated to explain both the PSN observed in the upright position, with its modifications induced by slowly flexing

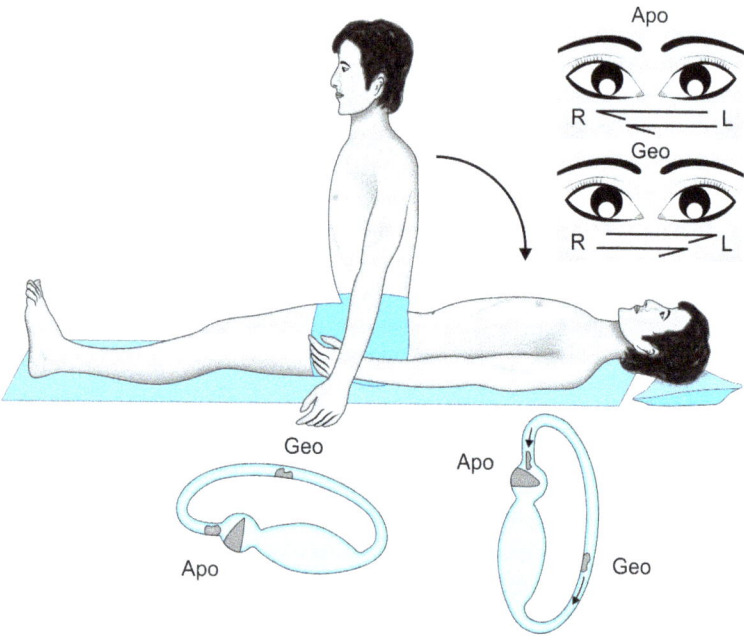

Fig. 6.3: Horizontal BPPV seated supine positioning nystagmus (this figure shows horizontal BPPV of right side).

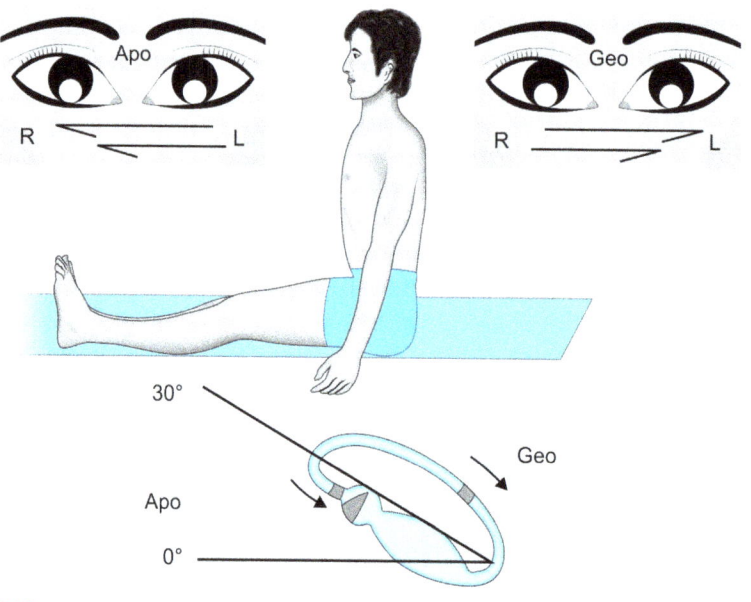

Fig. 6.4A

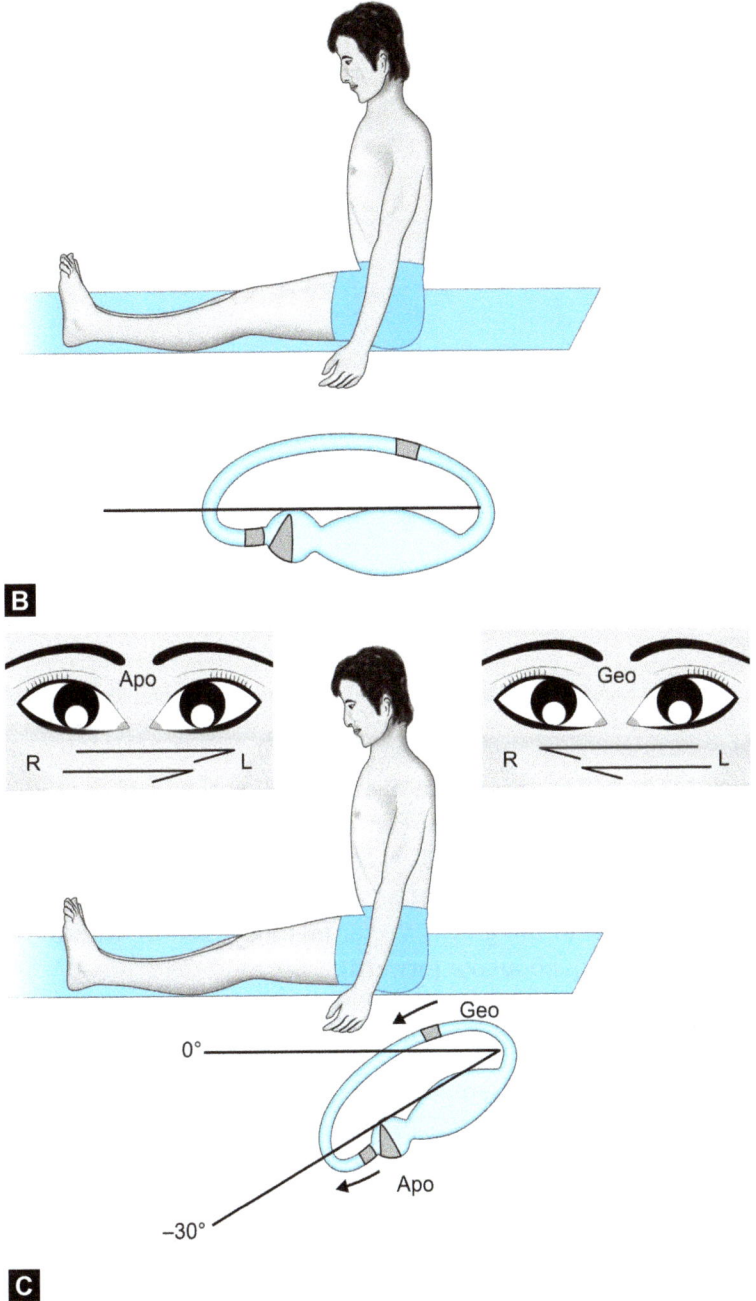

Figs. 6.4B and C

and extending the head (head pitch test—HPT), and the nystagmus induced by the SSPT. Both should be considered as the biological response to a single physical phenomenon: the otoliths gravitate along the inclined plane of the HSC.[8-10] The only variable is the gravity

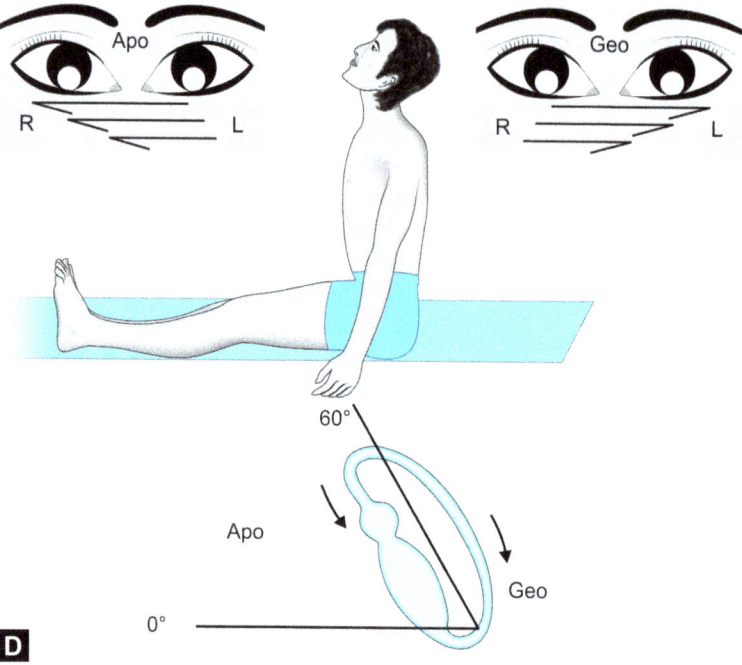

Figs. 6.4A to D: Horizontal BPPV pseudospontaneous nystagmus (this figure shows horizontal BPPV of right side).

vector size, which is active in displacing the otoliths along the HSC. Thus, the acceleration due to gravity on the debris varies from zero (neutral point) when the HSC is orthogonal to the gravity axis (head flexed 30° forward in upright position), to the maximum when the HSC is parallel to the gravity vector (supine position, with the head straight and bent about 30° forward).

DIFFERENTIAL DIAGNOSIS

Persistent horizontal nystagmus in the upright position can be observed in patients suffering from HSC BPPV and it can be misinterpreted as spontaneous nystagmus due to any cause of acute vestibular imbalance such as vestibular neuritis (VN).[10] The PSN, in fact, can be sometimes very intense. This last condition is more frequent in patients observed with a very short delay after the symptom onset, <12 hours. It can cause the misdiagnosis of acute unilateral vestibular loss (VN). The differential diagnosis is based on two points:

1. Pseudospontaneous nystagmus shows poor or no torsional component
2. Pseudospontaneous nystagmus reverses its beating direction by flexing and extending the patient's head while sitting: positive head pitch test.

Table 6.4: HSC BPPV liberatory techniques.	
Type of applied acceleration	Maneuver

• Angular acceleration
• Negative inertia
	• Barbecue rotation:
	  – Lempert (270°)
	  – Baloh (360°)
	  – Vannucchi-Asprella (450° or more)

• Linear acceleration • Positive inertia	• Gufoni maneuver
• Gravitational sedimentation	• Forced prolonged position (Vannucchi)
• Angular and linear accelerations plus gravity action (mixed maneuver)	• Asprella maneuver

We suggest to check the horizontal nystagmus in all patients suffering from acute vertigo by performing the HPT while sitting: if the nystagmus does not change its beating direction it is a direction fixed nystagmus due to VN, if the nystagmus reverses its beating direction it is direction changing nystagmus due to HSC BPPV (PSN).

When a persistent horizontal nystagmus is observed in patients suspected of peripheral vertigo, immediately performing the HPT while sitting would help provide the correct differential diagnosis between the PSN and the spontaneous nystagmus. The HPT would be suggested for screening purposes and, including it as routine evaluation of the patient with acute vertigo, could save time and money by reducing unnecessary and expensive examinations and avoidable requests for hospitalization.

THERAPY

Many therapeutic techniques have been proposed for HSC BPPV, all of them aim to achieve the ampullofugal endocanalar progression of the otoconial debris either by (Table 6.4):
- Angular accelerations (barbecue rotation techniques, Vannucchi-Asprella maneuver)
- Gravitational sedimentation [Vannucchi forced prolonged position (FPP)]
- Linear accelerations (Gufoni liberatory maneuver)
- Angular and linear accelerations plus gravity action (mixed maneuver—Asprella maneuver).

The barbecue rotation techniques work by negative inertia. They are done performing abrupt rotations of the patient's head in steps of 90° toward the healthy side while supine, thus moving the debris in the direction opposite to the head rotation.[44] According to Lempert (1996), the head is rotated three times toward the healthy side, thus applying an overall 270° rotation (Figs. 6.5A to F).[11]

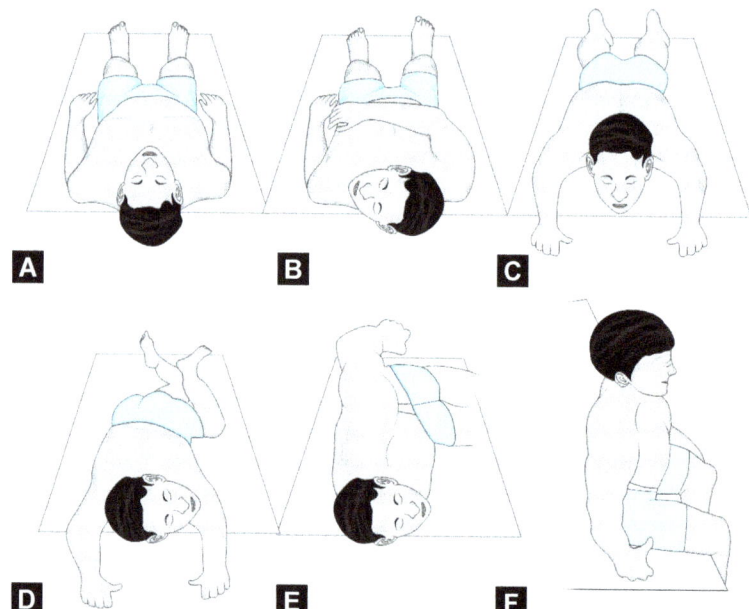

Figs. 6.5A to F: Barbecue rotation technique according to Lempert for right horizontal BPPV. Head is rotated 90° three times toward the healthy side, thus applying an overall 270° rotation.

The Vannucchi-Asprella maneuver (Figs. 6.6A to D): It is a variant of the barbecue maneuvers.[12] It can at once solve both geotropic and apogeotropic forms, as well as often converting apogeotropic into geotropic forms.[36,37,57] In addition, it is easier to be performed than any other barbecue maneuver. In fact, it avoids movements from supine to prone and vice versa. As in the typical barbeque maneuver, the patient's head is quickly rotated 90° toward the healthy side, while supine, then keeping the head turned in this way, he/she sits-up and slowly brings the head back in line with the body. This sequence of movements is repeated five times or more, as long as it does not provoke nystagmus or vertigo. It is important to perform this maneuver under videonystagmoscopic monitoring in order to check if the nystagmus is still beating toward the healthy side immediately after each step. Such a nystagmus denotes that the otolithic mass is moving toward the utricle.[39] A nystagmus beating toward the affected ear means the debris are floating toward the ampulla so the maneuver is being ineffective. The absence of nystagmus finally suggests that the canal has been rid of debris.

Vannucchi FPP: In the geotropic HSC BPPV, the patient is instructed to lie overnight, approximately 12 hours, on the healthy side, one or more times.[13] In this position the affected ear is the uppermost one, with debris in the downward-facing nonampullary arm (Fig. 6.7). Due to gravity, the

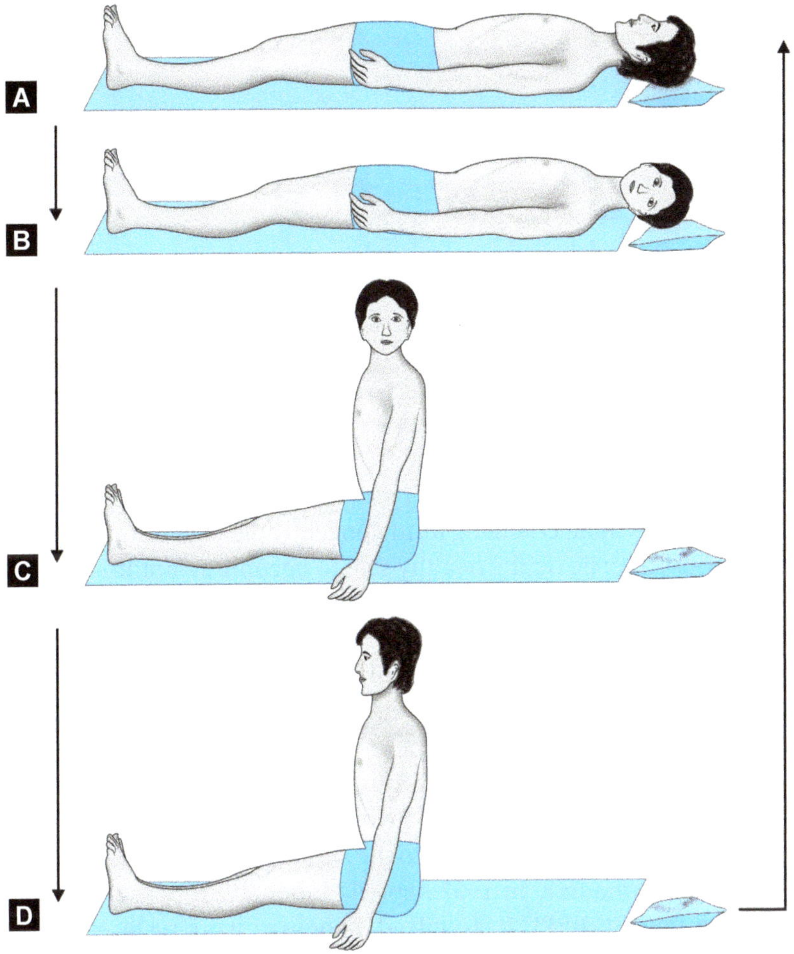

Figs. 6.6A to D: Vannucchi-Asprella maneuver for right horizontal BPPV.

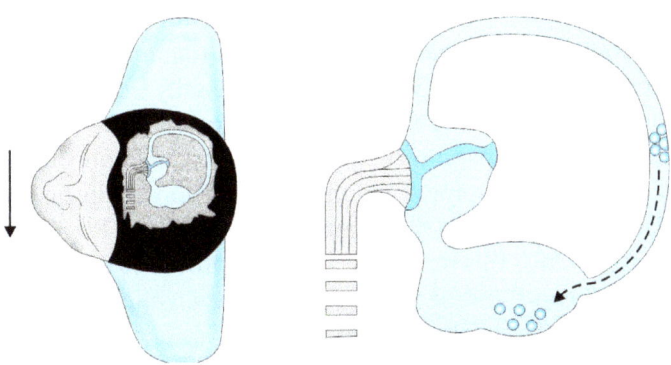

Fig. 6.7: Vannucchi forced prolonged position for right geotropic horizontal BPPV.
Source: Modified from Vannucchi P, Giannoni B, and Pagnini P. Treatment of horizontal semicircular canal benign paroxysmal positional vertigo. J Vestib Res. 1997;7(1):1-6.

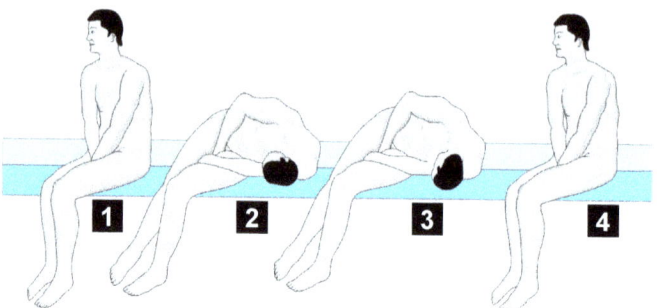

Fig. 6.8: Gufoni maneuver for right geotropic horizontal BPPV.

debris gradually moves into the utricle. Forced prolonged position can be used in the apogeotropic form, but in this case the patient must lie on the affected side; in this way the debris moves from the anterior to the posterior arm of the canal, changing from apogeotropic to geotropic form. The patient must then lie on the healthy side to become symptom-free.

Gufoni maneuver: It works by positive inertia. The maneuver consists of the following steps: (1) the patient sits on the edge of the bed; (2) the patient suddenly lies down on one side that is the healthy one for geotropic HSC BPPV and the affected one in the apogeotropic form; (3) the head is rotated 45° downward and so kept for 2-3 minutes. In this position the outlet of the HSC in the geotropic form, and the ampulla in the apogeotropic one, are vertically oriented favoring the debris to gravitate down; and (4) the patient finally returns to the sitting position (Fig. 6.8).

Asprella maneuver: In 1997 Asprella Libonati proposed a liberatory maneuver for HSC BPPV. It is a mixed maneuver, working by angular and linear brisk accelerations plus gravity action, and combining two rapid body positionings and a brisk head rotation followed by a brief forced position sustained for half an hour (Figs. 6.9A to F). The patient sits with his/her legs dangling on the edge of the bed in front of the examiner (Fig. 6.9A); patient's head is rotated 90° toward the unaffected side (Fig. 6.9B); the patient is quickly brought down on the healthy side reaching the bed face-down (Fig. 6.9C); the patient is tilted on the opposite side with a rapid and unique movement so reaching the face-up position (Fig. 6.9D); the patient assumes the supine position (Fig. 6.9E) and finally his/her head is rapidly rotated 90° toward the unaffected side, this position is held for 30 minutes (Fig. 6.9F). This maneuver has been proved to be effective in 82% of treated patients[12] and has been proposed as an alternative when other techniques have been found ineffective.

Geo-Apogeo conversion: The transformation of the nystagmus from apogeotropic into geotropic is usually observed during the course of canalolithiasis therapy. A geotropic nystagmus can transform into an

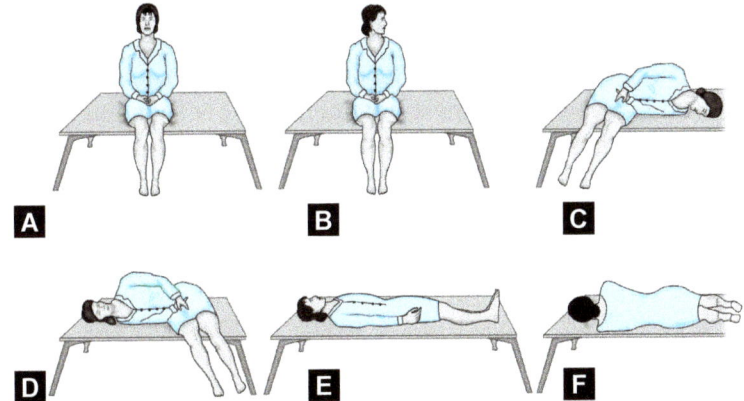

Figs. 6.9A to F: Asprella maneuver for right geotropic horizontal BPPV: (A) the patient sits with his/her legs dangling on the edge of the bed in front of the examiner; (B) patient's head is rotated 90° toward the unaffected side; (C) the patient is quickly brought down on the healthy side reaching the bed face-down; (D) the patient is tilted on the opposite side with a rapid and unique movement so reaching the face-up position; (E) the patient assumes the supine position; and (F) finally his\her head is rapidly rotated 90° toward the unaffected side, this position is held for 30 minutes.

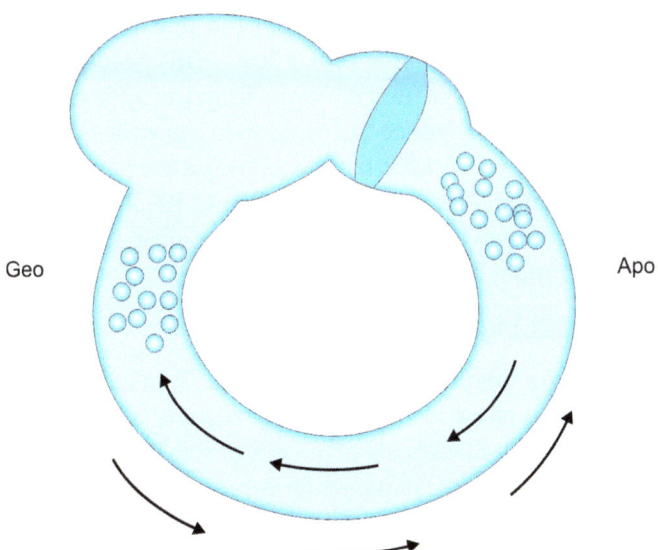

Fig. 6.10: Debris moves from the right lateral semicircular canal (LSC) posterior arm to the anterior one so, transforming a geotropic LSC BPPV into an apogeotropic one and vice versa.

apogeotropic one if the maneuver is performed toward the affected ear by mistake.[40,41] Both these conversions are explained by the migration of the otoconial mass from the anterior HSC arm into the posterior one and in the opposite direction respectively (Fig. 6.10).

POST-TREATMENT COMPLICATIONS

The conversion to another canal involvement (also known as "canal switch") is the most common post-treatment complication encountered after BPPV repositioning therapy.

The debris can move from posterior canal to horizontal canal during treatment of PSC BPPV, this is absolutely the most common conversion observed in BPPV therapy. The conversion from horizontal to posterior canal is less frequent. The canal conversion occurs in about 6–7% of all treated BPPV.[3,14-20] When the conversion from posterior to horizontal canal BPPV occurs, repeating the Dix-Hallpike maneuver results in a dramatically different nystagmus, which is now pure horizontal and usually geotropic. The patient experiences at the same time a violent and stronger vertigo. We must remember that it is the evoked nystagmus and not the kind of the performed maneuver that allows us to properly diagnose which one is the involved semicircular canal. Therefore, if a horizontal paroxysmal nystagmus is evoked performing again the Dix-Hallpike maneuver the correct diagnosis is HSC BPPV. The conversion from PSC to HSC BPPV is more likely to occur if the head is not properly kept 20° extended turning the patient's head from the first to the second position of the canalith repositioning procedure—CRP.[14] Moreover, the head should remain constantly turned 90° away from the affected ear bringing the patient up to seat. To reduce the canal switch, we always use a tiltable headrest table to be certain the head is constantly extended at least 20° down from horizontal plane when carrying out CRP. If particles enter the horizontal canal and an HSC involvement is diagnosed it shall be treated using the proper maneuvers.

Horizontal Canal Light/Heavy Cupula

Acute vertigo is sometimes associated with a steady intensity and persistent direction changing positional nystagmus (PDCPN) beating on the horizontal plane, which is observed either rotating the patient's head from side to side in the yaw plane while supine, or changing its bending angle in the pitch plane in the upright position.[9] It has been suggested that this phenomenon could be caused by a modified density ratio between the HSC cupula and the surrounding endolymph. It was hypothesized that the cupula is lighter than the endolymph (light cupula) in patients showing a geotropic PDCPN, and the cupula is heavier (heavy cupula) when an apogeotropic nystagmus is evoked.[47]

The HSC becomes gravity sensitive because of the difference of specific gravity with the surrounding endolymph, thus generating a direction changing nystagmus showing the following characteristics: gradual in onset and persistent when the position is held, it is not fatigable and it does not show latency. In the upright position: the nystagmus disappears bending the head about 30° forewords—neutral point in pitch plane, the nystagmus reverses its beating direction bending the head 60° forward and it beats again toward the previous direction with the head going back to the erect position, and finally increases by extending the head backward (head pitch test)[2,9] (Fig. 6.11). In the supine position: a PDCPN is evoked on each side, geotropic or apogeotropic respectively. Two neutral

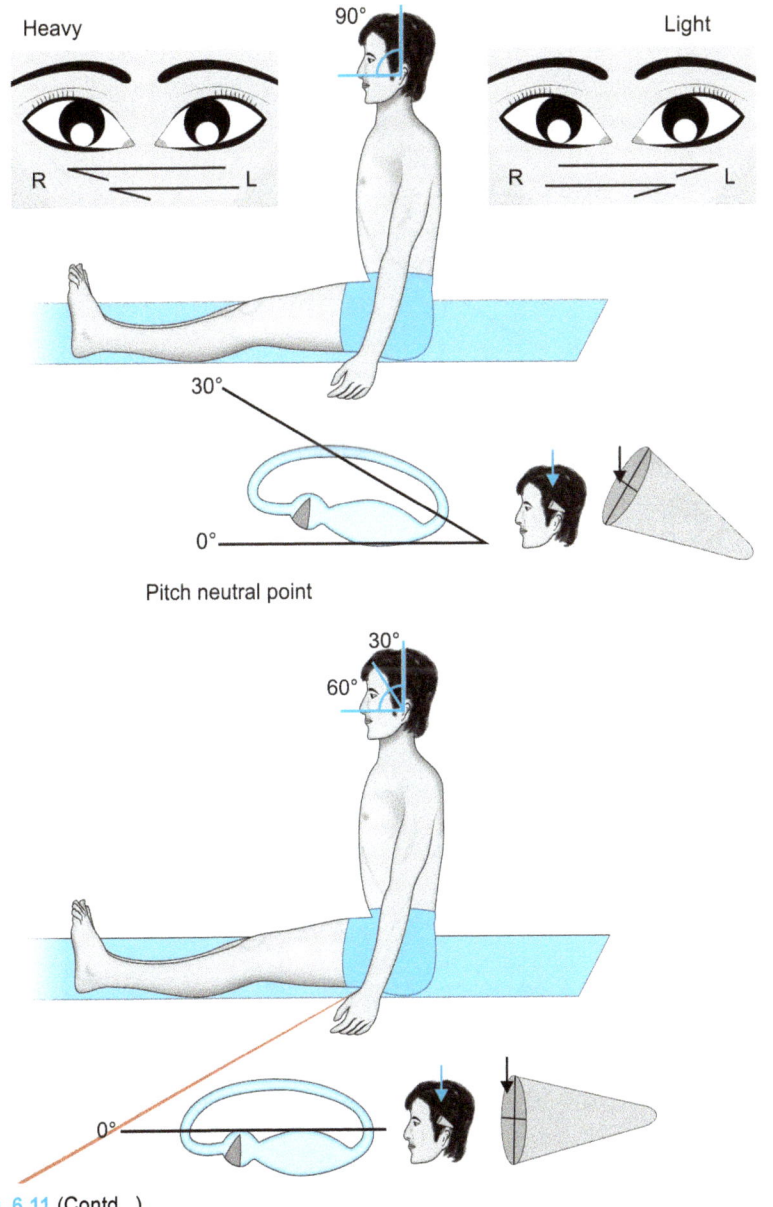

Fig. 6.11 (Contd...)

Contd...

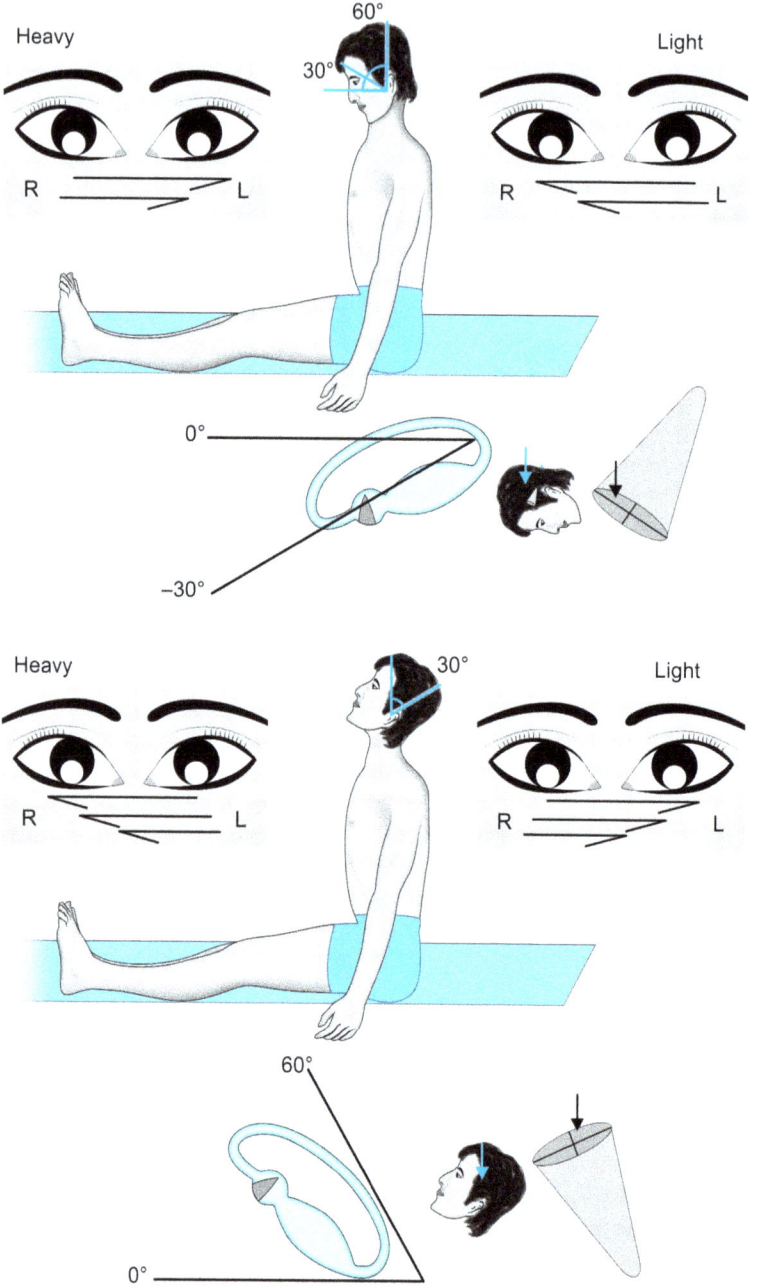

Fig. 6.11: Gravity sensitive cupula of right lateral semicircular canal: Nystagmus modifications obtained by changing the head bending angle in the pitch plane while sitting.

points are identified rotating the head in the yaw plane while supine: the first neutral point with the head rotated about 30° toward the affected ear,

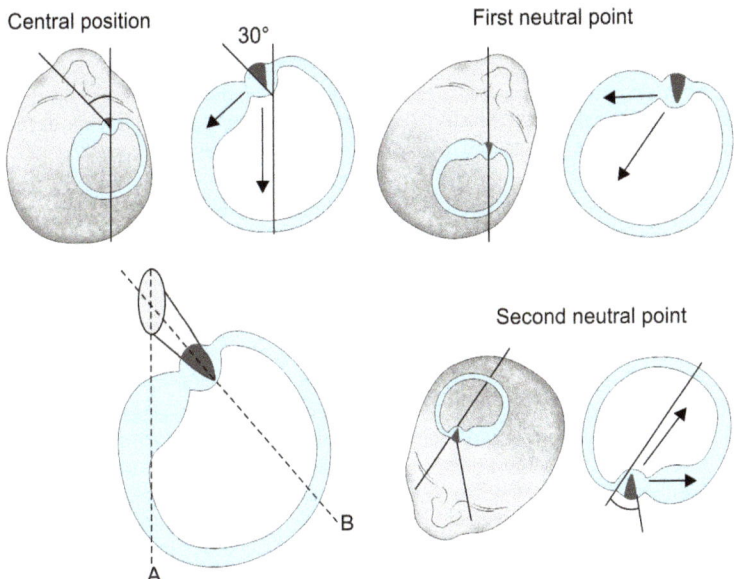

Fig. 6.12: Gravity sensitive cupula of right lateral semicircular canal: Nystagmus modifications obtained by changing the head bending angle in the yaw plane while supine. Cupula faces are roughly comparable to the plane identified by two straight lines: (A) the longer axis of the cupular basis and (B) the straight line running through the center of the cupular basis and its apex.

and the second one in the 180° opposite position. The nystagmus reverses its beating direction once the head is rotated beyond each neutral point in the yaw plane (Fig. 6.12).

Horizontal semicircular canal heavy cupula can be ascribed to otoliths attached to the cupula, cupulolithiasis,[21] or to a transitory modified density ratio between the cupula and the surrounding endolymph.[53,54] This latter condition was frequently observed in patients suffering from migraines whose case history and clinical features are summarized in Tables 6.5 and 6.6.

Central Nervous System Disorders Masquerading as BPPV: Central Positional Vertigo

It is known that central neurological diseases may occur with symptoms and signs suggesting a BPPV diagnosis. In fact, those pathological conditions can evoke positional vertigo associated with nystagmus caused by head movements.[22-24] This group of pathological conditions is known in literature as central positional vertigo (CPV).

Central positional vertigo has been usually ascribed to neurological disorders supported by acquired organic damages within the CNS (Table 6.7).

Table 6.5: PDCPN due to modified relative density ratio of HSC cupula versus endolymph.

Case history	Clinical features

• Acute onset of symptoms, with intense positional vertigo, which is often associated with severe autonomic symptoms
• Patient reports a sudden onset of vertigo often at night, which is intensified by the lateral decubitus position
• Migraine appears in patient's history and/or in his/her family history
• Should be excluded:
  – Any other neurological and/or audiological disorders (e.g. Ménière, vestibular neuritis)
  – Alcohol intake in the previous 10 hours
	• Nystagmus is gradual in onset and persistent when the position is held, it is not fatigable in all the positions in which it is evoked and it does not show latency
	• Horizontal persistent nystagmus observed while sitting with the head erect, reverses its beating direction due to the head pitch test, thus showing that the cupula is gravity sensitive
	• Nystagmus evoked by seated supine positioning maneuver beats toward the same direction of the one observed while sitting with the head erect
	• Persistent direction changing positional nystagmus is evoked on each side while supine, geotropic or apogeotropic. Two neutral points are identified rotating the head in the yaw plane while supine: the first neutral point with the head rotated about 30° toward the affected ear and the second one in the 180° opposite position. The nystagmus reverses its beating direction once the head is rotated beyond each neutral point in the yaw plane
	• The nystagmus evoked by the HYT is usually more intense on one side, beating stronger toward the affected ear
	• Liberatory maneuvers are always ineffective in modifying the nystagmus

(PDCPN: Persistent direction changing positional nystagmus; HSC: Horizontal semicircular canal; HYT: Head yaw test).

Table 6.6: Apogeotropic PDCPN clinical features: heavy cupula due to cupulolithiasis versus nonotolithic cause.

Cupulolithiasis	Nonotolithic
• The time elapsed from symptom onset until otoneurological examination ranges from 2 to 6 weeks • Symptoms are generally fairly well tolerated, without violent vertigo, but with dizziness while upright • HYT is performed inducing poorly or no neurovegetative symptoms • Liberatory maneuvers usually resolve nystagmus and symptoms either previously transforming it into a geotropic one or less frequently with no conversion • The maneuver's effectiveness is increased by using the mastoid vibrator	• Patient's history and/or family history positive for migraine • Sudden and abrupt onset of symptoms for which the patient is usually visited after a short delay, <12 hours • Vertigo is poorly tolerated and usually associated with severe neurovegetative symptoms • Liberatory maneuvers are absolutely inefficient in modifying and resolving both the nystagmus and associated vertigo. Osmotic diuretics has been found effective in solving both vertigo and nystagmus after about 1 hour

(PDCPN: Persistent direction changing positional nystagmus; HYT: Head yaw test).

Table 6.7: CPPV classification.	
CPPV due to organic CNS damage	CPPV due to nonorganic CNS disorder or CNS malformation

Cerebellar or brainstem damage:
• Tumors within the cerebellum:
  – Primary or secondary tumor
• Vascular damage:
  – Ischemic stroke of the nodule
  – Infarction dorsolateral to the fourth ventricle
  – More rarely hemorrhage localized to the vermis
• Degenerative or demyelinating lesion localized to:
  – Dorsal vermis
  – Nodule
  – Dorsolateral area to the fourth ventricle
  – Solitary brachium conjunctivum plaque (monosymptomatic MS onset with positional vertigo)
	Nonorganic CNS disorder:
	• Migraine
	• Positional VM
	CNS malformation:
	• Craniovertebral junction abnormalities including Arnold-Chiari and syringomyelia
	• Enlarged vestibular aqueduct syndrome with dehiscence of the jugular bulb

(CPPV: Central paroxysmal positional vertigo; CNS: Central nervous system; VM: Vestibular migraine).

Impairment of cerebellum or brainstem due to:
- Primary or secondary tumor
- Vascular damage, mainly ischemic stroke and more rarely localized hemorrhage
- Degenerative or demyelinating lesions.

The CNS damage is generally located in cerebellar vermis or nodule, dorsolateral area to the fourth ventricle, brachium conjunctivum. All these CNS damages more frequently evoke vertical positional nystagmus and in so doing they mimic PSC and/or ASC BPPV, they can also provoke horizontal positional nystagmus and in so doing they mimic HSC BPPV. The positional nystagmus due to CPV is always atypical for BPPV,[24] in fact:
- It shows long duration (>2 minutes) or it is persistent (it lasts as long as the position is held)
- It shows poor or no latency and no fatigue due to repeated positioning
- It may change its beating direction while assuming the same position (Nylen III), therefore it is not ascribable to the stimulation of a single channel aligned with the plane along which the positioning movement occurs and is repeated
- It sometimes shows atypical morphological features, e.g. oblique
- The associated neurovegetative symptoms are often intense, even in the presence of a low-intensity nystagmus
- A positional nystagmus not associated with intense vertigo suggests a central origin

- Vertigo and positional nystagmus are not solved or modified by any maneuvers albeit carried out with mastoid vibrator
- Some cerebellar neurological signs can be observed such as ataxia, dysmetria, alterations in saccades or smooth pursuit, impaired visual suppression test, gaze evoked nystagmus, and other neurological symptoms such as cranial nerve deficits.

Even one of the above clinical characters and especially the non-responsiveness to any liberatory maneuvers suggests we need studying CNS by magnetic resonance imaging and/or computed tomography (CT). Imaging usually reveals the CNS lesion: dorsolateral to the fourth ventricle, cerebellar dorsal vermis or flocculus (primary or secondary tumor, hemorrhagic or ischemic vascular lesion, demyelinating plaque).[55,56]

There is a second group of diseases that can also mimic BPPV, with attacks of positional vertigo and nystagmus, which is due to central disorders in absence of acquired organic CNS lesions (see Table 6.7):
- Malformations of the craniocervical junction associated with Arnold-Chiari and syringomyelia.
- Enlarged vestibular aqueduct (EVA), associated with dehiscence of the jugular bulb.[2,9,25,26]
- Vestibular migraine (VM) with "positional" crisis: gravity sensitive cupula.

Central paroxysmal positional vertigo (CPPV) due to craniocervical junction malformations (Arnold-Chiari, syringomyelia) is usually associated with other neurological symptoms such as cerebellar ataxia, dysmetria, hyposthenia, segmental amyotrophy, lower extremity spastic hypertonia, paresthesia and dysesthesia, loss of temperature sensitivity, sphincter incontinence, headache enhanced by maneuvers increasing intracranial pressure, such as coughing, Valsalva maneuver or head hanging position (e.g. Dix-Hallpike maneuver).[49] Nevertheless, CPPV may only show a positional nystagmus not always associated with objective vertigo and autonomic symptoms for a long time.

A higher incidence of BPPV has been reported in patients suffering from EVA syndrome,[27] it has been explained by a higher otolithic displacement due to utricular macula damage. Enlarged vestibular aqueduct syndrome associated with dehiscence of the jugular bulb can mimic BPPV.[2,9] Positional nystagmus can simulate a multicanalar involvement of the affected side, with no other associated symptoms.[2] Both positional vertigo and nystagmus can be explained by the mechanical stimuli due to increased pressure in cephalic venous system transmitted to the labyrinthine fluids through the dehiscence of the jugular bulb. Any increase in cephalic venous system pressure is provoked by reaching the head hanging position as in performing the Dix-Hallpike or the Epley maneuver.[45] Liberatory maneuvers, albeit repeated more and more time, are always ineffective to solve the positional nystagmus due to EVA plus jugular bulb dehiscence. High-resolution temporal bone CT scan clarifies the diagnosis.

Migraine is the central pathology that most frequently mimics BPPV.

It is well known that VM can typically show positional characters so mimicking BPPV.[28] Many authors published about the nystagmus observed in course of acute migraine attacks as a positional and persistent direction changing nystagmus.[28-30]

The diagnosis of positional VM is particularly complex since it must take into account several steps:
1. Making migraine diagnosis with or without aura according to International Headache Society (IHS) criteria[31]
2. Making VM diagnosis according to the well-known VM classifications[32,33]
3. Making differential diagnosis between BPPV and positional VM.

We must consider the higher incidence of BPPV in migrainous compared to normal population.

The Bárány Society Committee for the Standardization of Vestibular Diseases ("diagnostic criteria for VM" online publication: www.barany-society.nl, and the Consensus Document of the Bárány Society and the International Headache Society 2012)[50] stated the following criteria to properly make the differential diagnosis between BPPV and positional VM:
- Vestibular migraine may present with purely positional vertigo, thus mimicking BPPV
- Direct nystagmus observation during the acute phase may be required for differentiation
- In VM, positional nystagmus is usually persistent and not aligned with a single semicircular canal
- Symptomatic episodes tend to be shorter with VM (minutes to days rather than weeks) and more frequent (several times per year with VM rather than once every few years with BPPV).

In recent years, some authors described the nystagmus findings observed during acute attacks of positional VM and suggested the hypothesis of a pathophysiological mechanism due to a modified density ratio between the ampullary cupula versus the surrounding endolymph of the involved semicircular canal. Epley and Asprella Libonati (2008) reported about some patients suffering from recurrent vertigo with persistent bipositional bidirectional apogeotropic horizontal nystagmus, which was observed turning the head toward each side while supine.[34,38] Later, Asprella Libonati (2010) reported other cases with persistent bipositional bidirectional geotropic horizontal nystagmus.[9] The author hypothesized that the

Table 6.8: Clinical features of positional VM crisis.

History	Nystagmus clinical features

• Acute onset of symptoms, with intense positional vertigo often associated with severe autonomic symptoms
• Acute onset of vertigo, often at night, more intense lying on one side
• History of migraine and/or family history of migraine
• Should be excluded:
   – Any other neurological and/or vestibular diagnosis, e.g. Ménière, vestibular neuritis, BPPV, etc.
   – Alcohol intake in the previous 8/10 hours
	• Nystagmus increases gradually after the position has been reached, and then lasts steady and persistent (long-lasting, even >10 minutes, and does not change its intensity)
	• Nystagmus shows no fatigue and poor or no latency in every positions it is evoked
	• The liberatory maneuvers are always ineffective in modifying and resolving the observed nystagmus with and without mastoid vibrator

(VM: Vestibular migraine; BPPV: Benign paroxysmal positional vertigo).

ampullary cupula of the horizontal canal was involved in both geotropic and apogeotropic variant and that it was lighter than the surrounding endolymph in case of geotropic nystagmus, heavier in case of apogeotropic nystagmus.[48,51] The symptoms' onset is usually rapid, often at night, with intense positional vertigo, associated with severe autonomic symptoms, and no other associated neurological and audiological signs. The positional nystagmus is persistent (not paroxysmal) or at least it persists for a very long time.[38] It shows poor or no fatigue even though the provocative movement is repeated many times, and it has little or no latency. It starts without poor or no delay after the position on each side is reached, and gradually increases reaching its maximal intensity, subsequently it remains unchanged for long periods of observation, in some patients it has been recorded for >10 minutes (Table 6.8).[2] Fixed angles of head inclination with respect to gravity vector where the nystagmus stops and reverses were detected in both upright and supine position; they were defined neutral points.[1,2] Asprella Libonati in 2010 proposed a geometric model of the HSC floating cupola to explain the buoyancy mechanism of the light/heavy cupula due to its modified specific gravity. Later the author[1] reported about 12 patients suffering from migraine according to the IHS criteria 2004 with recurrent attacks of positional vertigo associated with persistent positional nystagmus, which was compatible with a PSC heavy/cupula mechanism. In fact, the Dix-Hallpike test evoked a nystagmus with both vertical and torsional components suggestive of a PSC canalolithiasis. However, the temporal characteristics of the nystagmus differed from those of BPPV, as the nystagmus was persistent with short latency and poor or no fatigue. Neutral points have also been described in these patients, the nystagmus stopped and then changed direction by modifying the patient's head bending angle in the PSC plane, both while sitting and in head hanging position while supine. It has been hypothesized that, according to a gravity sensitive cupula mechanism, the cupular axis is aligned with the gravity vector in the neutral points so reaching a condition of neutral buoyancy where gravity is ineffective in moving the cupula, the cupula deflects to the opposite side turning the head over the neutral point, so the nystagmus reverses its beating direction every time the patient's head is rotated over the neutral point.[1]

It is well known that BPPV can be less frequently caused by a cupulolithiasis mechanism,[35] and that BPPV has higher incidence in migrainous population. Therefore, when we observe an apogeotropic and persistent nystagmus in migrainous patients it is important to discriminate whether the heavy cupula nystagmus is due to otoliths attached to the cupula, cupulolithiasis, or to a transitory modification of the relative density ratio between the cupula and the surrounding endolymph, VM attack.[42] The differential diagnosis between the two above mentioned mechanisms should be primarily based on the effectiveness of liberatory maneuvers in solving both vertigo and positional nystagmus.[43] In addition, a history with BPPV recurrence and the elapsed time from the symptoms onset until the vestibular evaluation may contribute to the cupulolithiasis diagnosis; the latter is usually longer when an otolithic mechanism is supposed, ranging generally from 2 to 6 weeks in our experience.[2]

Recurrent vertigo associated with PDCPN and compatible with VM diagnosis has been observed in large series of patients.[1,2,9] The following characters of the nystagmus suggest a peripheral pathophysiological mechanism due to a modified relative density ratio between the cupula and the surrounding endolymph of the involved semicircular canal:

- The observed oculomotor response has the typical patterns due to excitatory or inhibitory stimulus of the ampullary nerve of the supposed involved canal.
- The same oculomotor response can be reproduced every time the patient's head is moved in the involved canal plane; furthermore, the persistent positional nystagmus stops and reverses reaching the same bending angle of the head with respect to the gravity axis, the so-called neutral points. This positional nystagmus shows poor or no fatigue, therefore it is possible to evoke it many times, searching for the neutral points again and again in the same patient (*see* Table 6.8).[46]

It has been hypothesized that the migraine involved mechanisms acting on the labyrinthine microcirculation can provide a modified localized fluid distribution that alters the buoyancy dynamics of the ampullary cupula, making it temporarily gravity sensitive, either in HSC or in PSC.[9,34]

It is important to differentiate the heavy cupula nystagmus (persistent positional apogeotropic nystagmus) due to an otolithic mechanism (BPPV cupulolithiasis) from positional VM. The BPPV maneuvers, sometimes enhanced by using the mastoid vibrator, can remove otoliths from the cupula solving vertigo and positional nystagmus in case of cupulolithiasis, but they are always ineffective in positional VM.[2]

An acute perturbation of the labyrinthine function due to VM should be considered in the differential diagnosis of acute vertigo, taking into account an acute peripheral disorder related to a heavy/light cupula mechanism.

The positional features of the evoked nystagmuses are essential to make a correct diagnosis and realize which cupula is involved in each patient.

Further studies are needed to test the effectiveness of therapies and focalize better on the interaction mechanism between the labyrinthine function and migraine.

REFERENCES

1. Asprella Libonati G. Benign paroxysmal positional vertigo. In: Carmona S, Asprella-Libonati G (eds.). Neuro-otology, 3rd edition. Buenos Aires; 2011, Akadia Editorial; 2011, pp. 39-64.
2. Asprella Libonati G. Benign paroxysmal positional vertigo and positional vertigo variants. Int J Otorhinolaryngol Clin. 2012;4(1):25-40.
3. Epley JM. Positional vertigo related to semicircular canalolithiasis. Otolaryngol Head Neck Surg. 1995;112:154-61.
4. Asprella-Libonati G. Diagnostic and treatment strategy of the lateral semicircular canal canalolithiasis. Acta Otorhinolaryngol Ital. 2005;25:277-83.
5. Cipparrone L, Corridi G, Pagnini P. Cupulolitiasi. In: V Giornata Italiana di Nistagmografia Clinica. Nistagmografia e patologia vestibolare periferica. Milano: CSS Boots-Formenti; 1985. pp. 36-53.
6. McClure A. Lateral canal BPV. Am J Otolaryngol. 1985;14:30-5.
7. Nuti D, Vannucchi P, Pagnini P. Lateral canal BPPV: which is the affected side? Audiol Med. 2005;3:16-20.
8. Asprella-Libonati G. Pseudo-spontaneous nystagmus: a new clinical sign to diagnose the affected side in lateral semicircular canal benign paroxysmal positional vertigo. Acta Otorhinolaryngol Ital. 2008;28:73-8.
9. Asprella-Libonati G. Gravity sensitive cupula: light/heavy cupula of lateral semicircular canal (LSC). J Vestib Res. 2010;20:208-9.
10. Asprella-Libonati G. Lateral canal BPPV with pseudo-spontaneous nystagmus masquerading as vestibular neuritis in acute vertigo: a series of 273 cases. J Vestib Res. 2014;24:343-9.
11. Lempert T, Tiel-Wilck K. A positional maneuver for treatment of horizontal-canal benign positional vertigo. Laryngoscope. 1996;106:476-78.

12. Asprella-Libonati G, Gufoni M. Vertigine parossistica da CSL: manovre di barbecue ed altre varianti. In: Nuti D, Pagnini P, Vicini C (Eds.). Atti della XIX Giornata di Nistagmografia Clinica. Milano: Formenti; 1999. pp. 321-36.
13. Vannucchi P, Giannoni B, and Pagnini P. Treatment of horizontal semicircular canal benign paroxysmal positional vertigo. J Vestib Res. 1997;7(1):1-6.
14. Epley JM. Caveats in particle repositioning for treatment of canalolithiasis (BPPV). Operat Tech Otolaryngol Head Neck Surg. 1997;8(2):68-76.
15. Herdman SJ, Tusa RJ. Complications of the canalith repositioning procedure. Arch Otolaryngol Head Neck Surg. 1996;122:281-6.
16. Tusa RJ, Herdman SJ. BPPV: controlled trials, contraindications, post-manoeuvre instructions, complications, imbalance. Audiol Med. 2005;3(1):57-62.
17. Bhattacharyya N, Baugh RF, Orvidas L, et al. Clinical practice guideline: benign paroxysmal positional vertigo. Otolaryngol Head Neck Surg. 2008;139 (5 Suppl 4):S47-81.
18. Fife TD, Iverson DJ, Lempert T, et al. Quality Standards Subcommittee, American Academy of Neurology. Practice parameter: therapies for benign paroxysmal positional vertigo (an evidence-based review): report of the Quality Standards Subcommittee of the American Academy of Neurology. Neurology. 2008;70(22):2067-74.
19. Lin GC, Basura GJ, Wong HT, et al. Canal switch after canalith repositioning procedure for benign paroxysmal positional vertigo. Laryngoscope. 2012;122(9):2076-8.
20. Foster CA, Zaccaro K, Strong D. Canal conversion and reentry: a risk of Dix-Hallpike during canalith repositioning procedures. Otol Neurotol. 2012;33(2):199-203.
21. Baloh RW, Yue Q, Jacobson KM, et al. Persistent direction-changing positional nystagmus: another variant of benign positional nystagmus? Neurology. 1995;45(7):1297-301.
22. Büttner U, Helmchen C, Brandt T. Diagnostic criteria for central versus peripheral positioning nystagmus and vertigo: a review. Acta Otolaryngol. 1999;119(1):1-5.
23. Brandt T. Positional and positioning vertigo and nystagmus. J Neurol Sci. 1990;95(1):3-28.
24. Brandt T. Central positional vertigo. In: Vertigo: its multisensory syndromes vertigo: its multisensory syndromes, 2nd edition. London: Springer Verlag; 1999. pp. 291-9.
25. White J, Krakovitz P. Nystagmus in enlarged vestibular aqueduct, a case series. Audiol Res. 2015;5(120): 30-33.
26. Oh AK, Ishiyama A, Baloh R. Vertigo and enlarged vestibular aque-duct syndrome. J Neurol. 2001;248:971-4.
27. Manzari L. Enlarged vestibular aqueduct (EVA) related with recurrent benign paroxysmal positional vertigo (BPPV). Med Hypotheses. 2008;70(1):61-5. Epub 2007 Jun 27.
28. von Brevern M, Radtke A, Clarke AH, et al. Migrainous vertigo presenting as episodic positional vertigo. Neurology. 2004;62:469-72.

29. Neuhauser H, Lempert T. Vestibular migraine. Neurol Clin. 2009;27(2):379-91.
30. Radtke A, von Brevern M, Neuhauser H, et al. Vestibular migraine: long-term follow-up of clinical symptoms and vestibulo-cochlear findings. Neurology. 2012;79(15):1607-14.
31. Headache Classification Subcommittee of the International Headache Society. The International Classification of Headache Disorders, 2nd edition. Cephalalgia. 2004;24 Suppl 1:9-160.
32. Neuhauser H, Leopold M, von Brevern M, et al. The interrelations of migraine, vertigo, and migrainous vertigo. Neurology. 2001;56:436-41.
33. Pagnini P, Verrecchia L, Giannoni B, et al. La vertigine emicranica. Acta Otorhinolaryngol Ital Suppl. 2003;75:19-27.
34. Epley JM, Asprella Libonati G. Endolymphatic density changing positional nystagmus. Abstract Book 25° Barany society Meeting. O2-6, p. 140, Kyoto Japan, March 31-April 3 2008.
35. Nuti D, Yagi T. Benign paroxysmal positional vertigo. In: Eggers SDZ and Zee DS (eds.). Vertigo and imbalance: clinical neurophysiology of the vestibular system handbook of clinical neurophysiology. Elsevier; Amsterdam 2010. pp. 357-70.
36. Asprella-Libonati G. La Terapia della Labirintolitiasi: strategie di intervento individualizzato. In: atti congressuali Aggiornamenti di Vestibologia (eds.). Grunenthal-Formenti: Fiuggi; 2004.
37. Asprella-Libonati G. Lateral semicircular canal benign paroxysmal positional vertigo diagnostic signs. Letter to the Editor. Acta Otorhinolaryngol Ital. 2010;30:222-4.
38. Asprella-Libonati G, Epley JM. Management of positional vertigo: a nystagmus-based approach. Abstract Book 25° Barany society Meeting. S7-1, p. 89, Kyoto Japan, March 31-April 3 2008.
39. Asprella-Libonati G, Gagliardi G, Cifarelli D, et al. "Step-by-step" treatment of lateral semicircular canal canalolithiasis under videonystagmoscopic examination. Acta Otorhinolaryngol Ital. 2003;23:10-5.
40. Bergenius J, Tomanovic T. Persistent geotropic nystagmus—a different kind of cupular pathology and its localizing signs. Acta Otolaryngol. 2006;126(7):698-704.
41. Bertholon P, Tringali S, Faye MB, et al. Prospective study of positional nystagmus in 100 consecutive patients. Ann Otol Rhinol Laryngol. 2006;115(8):587-94.
42. Bisdorff AR, Debatisse D. Localizing signs in positional vertigo due to lateral canal cupulolithiasis. Neurology. 2001;57(6):1085-8.
43. Bisdorff AR, Debatisse D. A new differential diagnosis for spontaneous nystagmus: lateral canal cupulolithiasis. Ann N Y Acad Sci. 2002;956:579-80.
44. Epley JM. New dimensions of benign paroxysmal positional vertigo. Otolaryngol Head Neck Surg. 1980;88(5):599-605.
45. Epley JM. The canalith repositioning procedure: for treatment of benign paroxysmal positional vertigo. Otolaryngol Head Neck Surg. 1992;107(3):399-404.
46. Hiruma K, Numata T. Positional nystagmus showing neutral points. ORL J Otorhinolaryngol Relat Spec. 2004;66(1):46-50.
47. Hiruma K, Numata T, Mitsuhashi T, et al. Two types of direction-changing positional nystagmus with neutral points. Auris Nasus Larynx. 2011;38(1):46-51.
48. Kim HA, Yi HA, Lee H. Apogeotropic central positional nystagmus as a sole sign of nodular infarction. Neurol Sci. 2012;33(5):1189-91.

49. Johkura K. Central paroxysmal positional vertigo: isolated dizziness caused by small cerebellar hemorrhage Stroke. 2007;38(6):e26-7; author reply e28. Epub 2007 Apr 19.
50. Lempert T, Olesen J, Furman J, et al. Vestibular migraine: Diagnostic criteria. J Vestib Res. 2012;22(4):167-72.
51. Nam J, Kim S, Huh Y, et al. Ageotropic central positional nystagmus in nodular infarction. Neurology. 2009;73:1163.
52. Nuti D, Vannucchi P, Pagnini P. Benign paroxysmal positional vertigo of the horizontal canal: a form of canalolithiasis with variable clinical features. J Vestib Res. 1996;6:173-84.
53. Pagnini P, Nuti D, Vannucchi P. Benign paroxysmal vertigo of the horizontal canal. ORL J Otorhinolaryngol Relat Spec. 1989;51:161-70.
54. Pagnini P, Vannucchi P, Nuti D. Le nystagmus apogéotrope dans la vertige paroxystique positionnel bénin du canal sémicirculaire horizontal: une canalolithiase. Revue d'ONO. 1994;31:17-9.
55. Sakata E, Ohtsu K, Itoh Y. Positional nystagmus of benign paroxysmal type (BPPN) due to cerebellar vermis lesions. Pseudo-BPPN. Acta Otolaryngol Suppl. 1991;481:254-7.
56. Shoman N, Longridge N. Cerebellar vermis lesions and tumours of the fourth ventricle in patients with positional and positioning vertigo and nystagmus. J Laryngol Otol. 2007;121(2):166-9. Epub 2006 Oct 24.
57. Vannucchi P, Asprella-Libonati G, Gufoni M. The physical treatment of lateral semicircular canal canalolithiasis. Audiol Med. 2005;3:52-6.

Chapter 7

Anterior Benign Paroxysmal Positional Vertigo

Dario A Yacovino

INTRODUCTION

Although the existence of the anterior canal benign paroxysmal positional vertigo (AC-BPPV) has never been denied, it has been considered a less frequent variant of BPPV by several authors, limiting this condition to the category of clinical "rarity." Nevertheless, epidemiological data recently incorporated have shown that this entity is more common than previously thought and that it could be considerably underdiagnosed.[1]

The lack of uniform clinical diagnostic criteria and the absence of specific positional maneuvers to diagnose this variant of BPPV could be some of the most important reasons for failure in its recognition; hence for its underdiagnosis.

Despite the actual prevalence of AC-BPPV, which is still under study and probably only relevant among specialists, a better understanding of this entity (e.g. the clinical similarity between the positional oculomotor findings observed in AC-BPPV and some potentially more severe central disorders) facilitates the decision-making process in the clinical setting.

In this context, it is essential to resort to a more precise clinical criterion and a diagnostic algorithm.

EPIDEMIOLOGY

Regardless of its actual prevalence, the *sine qua non* condition to "diagnose patients with AC-BPPV is to see patients with BPPV." There is a broad spread of data concerning its actual frequency in the clinical setting that ranges between 1.6% and 21%.[1-3]

It has been postulated that AC-BPPV is a rare entity due to the anatomical position (upper) of the anterior canal (AC) that prevents the mobilization of otoliths into the anterior branch (ampullar) of the canal. Additionally, the posterior branch of the AC descends directly to the common cross and then to the vestibule and it spontaneously clears the particles that have entered, preventing in this way the involvement of the canal. However, this debris moves freely inside the endolymphatic system and can thus migrate to any semicircular canal. Epley used the term "vestibular lithiasis" to include the six semicircular canals: all potentially vulnerable to BPPV.[4]

In 1,075 cases of BPPV,[5] we identified 66 (6.1%) cases of the AC variant using the diagnostic criteria proposed later in this chapter.

With regard to the actual origin, of all AC-BPPV cases we examined (n = 66), de novo cases (i.e. without history of vertigo) occurred in 25 (37.8%) patients and there were 18 (27.2%) cases of AC-BPPV and a history of BPPV without temporal relationship. Finally, canal conversion (or canal switch) from other canals to the anterior semicircular canal after any canalith repositioning maneuvers (CRM) was observed in 23 (34.8%) cases. All but one occurred after the Epley maneuver.

In our experience, canal conversion from other canals to the anterior semicircular canals accounts for roughly a third of all cases of AC-BPPV. Similarly, a canal switch after AC-BPPV treatment is also encountered and, in this context, the PC is almost always affected. According to our observation, de novo AC-BPPV is less common than AC-BPPV with a previous BPPV (canal switch or nonrelated). These features would be used as complementary clinical criteria to differentiate between central and peripheral downbeat nystagmus and vertigo (*see* diagnostic criteria).

HISTORY AND CLINICAL FINDINGS

The different variants of BPPV share common clinical patterns such as attacks of vertigo triggered by positional changes. Typically, symptoms are triggered when lying down, getting up, or rolling over in bed and when raising the head to look at a top shelf (top-shelf vertigo) or lower the head to tie the shoelaces or search for something under the bed. Essentially, this type of vertigo is brief (<30 seconds), although patients usually report that the first episode lasts longer or is more intense than the subsequent ones. This initial severity probably results from the first entry of the particles (otoliths) into the canal that have to travel a longer distance in order to reach the lowermost part of the canal compared to the smaller free movement they have once they are inside. Furthermore, anxiety, fear, and hyperventilation that increase the vestibular response and vertigo are caused by the fact that the attack is sudden (paroxysmal) and occurs at a certain unexpected situation (when waking up in the morning). After several attempts, patients are able to predict the postural pattern of vertigo and develop maneuvers to avoid it that improve tolerance and reduce severity. Finally, the intensity of the symptoms might be a multifactorial component arising from the interaction between peripheral variables (particle size, initial location, affected canal—horizontal vs vertical, etc.)

and the variables inherent in each patient (individual vestibular sensitivity, related psychogenic reaction, etc.).

Based on the author's experience, there are some distinctive features of the involvement of the AC. Patients with AC-BPPV usually refer moderate vertigo, mild vertical oscillopsia, and nausea when tilting their head forward. This typical mild symptomatic pattern is clearly evident in patients who have suffered a switch from another canal to the AC, especially after the Epley maneuver for the treatment of the posterior canal. At the follow-up visit after performing the maneuver, they report that the symptoms have improved but they notice a change in pattern and now they feel dizzy when bending their head forward.

In other AC-BPPV cases examined in our clinic, a tendency to sleep on the stomach or in the fetal position with the nose down and practicing yoga have all been implicated in loading the anterior semicircular canals.[6] Furthermore, Jackson, et al.[1] described a significant association between AC-BPPV and head trauma. We noticed that some patients with AC-BPPV had been recently subjected to many CRM performed on the same day or by inexperienced hands. A reasonable cause could be "iatrogenic" AC-BPPV owing to canal switch.

As experience with AC-BPPV is still evolving, we cannot ascertain the importance of this historical background in the diagnosis of AC-BPPV.

The absence of neurological abnormalities in the physical examination supports the diagnosis of peripheral involvement.

The diagnosis of AC-BPPV is typically based on the observation of predominant positional downbeating nystagmus (pDBN) with a slight torsional component in the Dix-Hallpike maneuvers (DHM). The direction of the torsional component of the nystagmus and the most sensitive positional maneuver to generate the best clinical responses (vertigo) and nystagmus are critical to identify the affected ear.

Purely downbeating nystagmus with lack of a torsional component has been reported in cases of AC-BPPV by Bertholon,[7] who suggests that the torsional component is not always present because of the anatomical orientation of the AC: closer to the sagittal plane (about 41°) than the posterior canal (56°). Therefore, it could be said that the vertical component of the nystagmus would be more reliable than the torsional feature in order to reach the diagnosis of AC-BPPV (Fig. 7.1).

According to the anterior and sagittal location of the AC, the final position of Dix-Hallpike on the right (lowermost) locates the anterior arm of the left AC in a more vertical orientation than the right one, that is better aligned with the force of gravity and therefore better positioned for the mobilization of the otolithic particles generating stronger nystagmus. If it were visible, the torsional component would rotate the upper pole

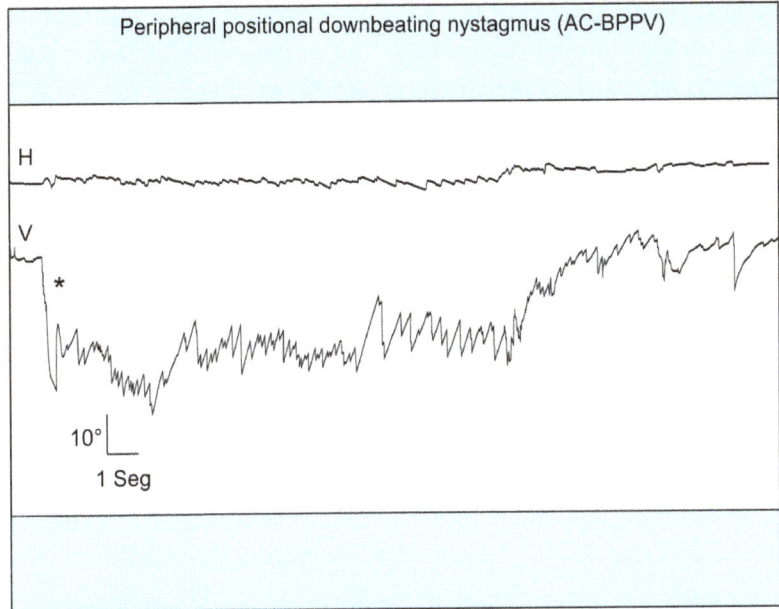

Fig. 7.1: Videonystagmography during the positioning test in a patient with anterior canal benign positional paroxysmal vertigo (AC-BPPV). Positional downbeating nystagmus (pDBN) was induced by the head-hanging position. The evoked pDBN and vertigo disappeared after canalith repositioning maneuvers. (H: Horizontal canal; V: Vertical canal).
*Pointing the head-hanging position maneuver.

of the eye toward the affected ear (to the uppermost), i.e. to the left in this example. The same pattern, but inversely, should be noted in a right AC-BPPV.

Moreover, available reports disagree as to whether nystagmus/vertigo in AC-BPPV with DHM is caused when the affected ear is lower- or uppermost.[7-9] It has recently been reported that the supine head-hanging maneuver (HHM) would be a better approach to trigger nystagmus and vertigo in AC-BPPV cases.[5,10,11] Bertholon and collaborators had previously mentioned that the most sensitive position to detect pDBN in AC-BPPV was the HHM.[7] Cambi also put forth that, in five patients (10%), it was only detectable with this maneuver and not with the Dix-Hallpike test.[10]

In the lithiasis of the AC, the nystagmus is expected to have latency, be transient and reversible (upbeating) when rising from decubitus position. In line with some published works[7,11,12] and the author's experience, the reversal of nystagmus is unsteady and irrelevant for the definitive diagnosis. Cambi, et al. describe it only in 6% of patients.[10] Conversely, we have reported that a second burst of downbeat nystagmus when rising from decubitus position may suggest that the particles migrated through the descending branch of the canal into the common cross and ended in the utricle with the resolution of the symptoms.[13] The latency is also unsteady and can be absent in up to 30% of patients.[10]

Fatigability (habituation) is the fourth typical element expected from the mechanism of canalolithiasis. Nonetheless, fatigability has also been reported in central lesions (cerebellar) not only in animals[14] but also in human beings.[15] Therefore, this clinical feature should not be used as isolated element to determine a topographic lesion (central vs peripheral). The resolution of AC-BPPV after performing the diagnostic HHM can be interpreted as fatigability when it is actually the recovery[5] (see diagnostic criteria).

As with the other variants of BPPV, the AC type can be also self-limited. The time course of positional vertigo episodes in AC-BPPV, without specific treatment, is similar to that of other forms of BPPV. The mean duration was about 10 days, while it ranges from 4 to 16 days in horizontal canal BPPV[16-18] and is about 40 days in PC-BPPV.[16]

DIFFERENTIAL DIAGNOSIS

Central Vestibular Disorders

There are usually no diagnostic doubts when neurologic abnormalities—including the oculomotor system—suggesting central dysfunctions as a consequence of vertigo or nystagmus in a given patient are present. The extensive experience, however, shows that vertigo and pDBN similar to the one caused by AC-BPPV can occasionally be the only detectable abnormalities[19] (Figs. 7.2 and 7.3).

Yee found 2 out of 36 patients with different structural disorders of the posterior fossa whose only abnormality in the positional tests was downbeat nystagmus.[20]

Positional downbeating nystagmus (similar to the one described in AC-BPPV) may be a clinical sign of a central nervous system (CNS) abnormality. It occurs with structural lesions in the vestibulocerebellum (floccular and nodular lesions), vermis dorsolateral, fourth ventricle, and superior cerebellar peduncle and in conditions such as multiple system atrophy, multiple sclerosis, cerebellar degeneration, Chiari malformation, hydrocephalus, and tumors.[7,19,21,22]

The underlying mechanism of nystagmus would be the disruption of the otolith path due to a defect in the cerebellum or in the fibers connecting the cerebellar nucleus with the vestibular nuclei. Other central syndromes might cause vertigo/pDBN in the absence of an evident structural lesion, such as pharmacological[23,24] and alcohol intoxication, paraneoplastic syndrome,[25] or hereditary ataxias.[26]

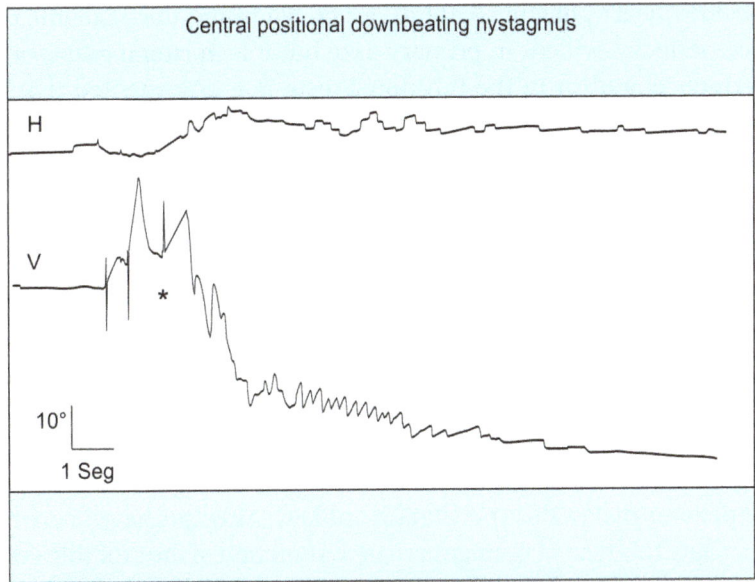

Fig. 7.2: Videonystagmography during the positioning test in a patient with cerebellar disorders (the brain magnetic resonance imaging is shown in Figure 7.3). Positional downbeating nystagmus was induced by the head-hanging position. The evoked pDBN reduced gradually. (H: Horizontal canal; V: Vertical canal).
*Pointing the head-hanging position maneuver.

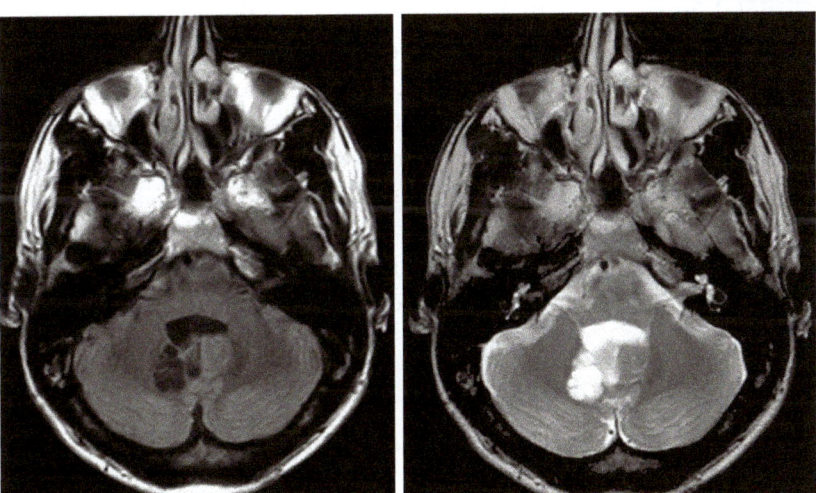

Fig. 7.3: Magnetic resonance imaging of a patient with positional downbeating nystagmus mimicking an anterior canal benign positional paroxysmal vertigo (videonystagmography in Figure 7.1) that did not respond to any reposition maneuver. A cystic tumor lateral to the fourth ventricle was diagnosed.

As clinical pitfall, the first element to determine is the occurrence of some mild downbeat nystagmus in a seated position not only in primary gaze but also in convergence and in lateral gazes with or without fixation.

In the downbeat nystagmus-central vertigo syndrome, the nystagmus may not be perfectly evident in primary gaze but it is in lateral gazes, ocular convergence, and/or in the positional tests. Yee documented that 67% (24 out of 36) of subjects with underlying downbeat nystagmus increased their magnitude of nystagmus during the positional maneuvers.[20]

Peripheral Vestibular Disorders

Bela Buki recently theorized that a slight and prolonged pDNB indistinguishable from AC-BPPV might be expected in the cupulolithiasis of the posterior canal, if the head were placed down; e.g. in the head-hanging maneuver (HHM).[27] In the same way, Cambi et al.[10] postulated that some patients in his series could suffer an atypical form of cupulolithiasis of the posterior canal; however, the absence of reversion and torsional component (characteristic of the involvement of the posterior canal) in most patients makes this speculation unlikely. Attempts have been made to associate this type of nystagmus to a dysfunction of the otolithic system at the peripheral level but there is little evidence of this speculation and a spontaneous recovery as outlined would not be expected.

Using high-resolution three-dimensional magnetic resonance imaging Schratzenstaller et al.[28] found a morphological abnormality at the top of the superior semicircular canal (generating a stop to free floating otoconia) in patients with AC-BPPV resistant to therapy, particularly in patients with previous ear surgery or ear disease.

Pseudovertical multicanal BPPV: In some cases, after a strong burst of BPPV-induced nystagmus, a brief reversal nystagmus may be seen. This is thought to be neurogenic in origin (adaptation). That is, a reversal nystagmus from a left posterior canal BPPV (PC-BPPV) may appear similar to right AC stimulation. This would lead to an erroneous diagnosis of PC and AC-BPPV. However, the underlying mechanism is clearly different and the pDBN component disappears as soon as the PC-BPPV resolves.

pDBN of Unknown Origin

In an undetermined number of patients—about a third in the author's experience—preliminary diagnosed with AC-BPPV on account of the presence of pDBN with mild positional symptoms, the cause cannot be clearly established in the end. They often have a self-limited or fluctuating evolution and minimal or absent impact on everyday life. They do not exhibit abnormalities in the imaging of the CNS or a thorough physical examination and cannot be attributed to any medication. The nystagmus is only visible without fixation by means of video Frenzel or video-oculography and it usually disappears when it is fixated. In general, these patients have a previous history typical of BPPV and, in some cases, migraine. Nevertheless, they do not respond to any type of repositioning maneuver for AC-BPPV.

It remains to be determined whether they are patients with a slight vestibulocerebellar defect associated with migraine,[29] mild cupulolithiasis of the AC, canalolithiasis that has not reached the "critical mass" of particles (due to history of BPPV), or if the nystagmus simply has low pathologic value ("benign").[30]

DIAGNOSTIC CRITERIA FOR AC-BPPV

As mentioned above, one of the major flaws in the management of AC-BPPV is the lack of uniform diagnostic criteria. It has also been stated that, unlike the involvement of other canals due to canalolithiasis, elements such as fatigability, reversion, and latency lack specificity in the case of the most important clinical-topographic marker—the nystagmus. We have postulated somewhat restrictive but, in our opinion, highly specific diagnostic criteria.

Elements that support the diagnosis of AC canalolithiasis:
1. Recurrent attacks of positional vertigo or dizziness
2. Positional downbeat nystagmus with or without a torsional component in DHM and HHM
3. Brief positional nystagmus lasting less than a minute (transient, with obvious ending)
4. Resolution of nystagmus and vertigo after appropriate repositioning maneuver
5. Exclusion of other causes after a thorough physical examination.

Note: Well-documented recent history of BPPV of other canals on the same side with CRM additionally supports the diagnosis of AC-BPPV.

Please note that we have not included any radiological imaging of the CNS but we incorporated the concept of immediate resolution of symptoms and vertigo after an appropriate repositioning maneuver instead. Similarly, a switch to other canal with disappearance of the pDBN caused by the repositioning maneuver for AC-BPPV should be interpreted as a confirmation of the peripheral origin and then of the mechanism of canalolithiasis.

Usually, further vestibular and auditory testing is indicated only when a pre-existing disorder of the inner ear (e.g. vestibular neuritis and Ménière's disease) is suspected.

The diagnostic algorithm shown in Flowchart. 7.1 summarizes the theoretical elements described in the text.

Flowchart 7.1: The graph shows the suggested algorithm for the diagnosis of a case of benign positional paroxysmal vertigo (BPPV). Dix-Hallpike and Roll Test maneuvers are specifically performed for the diagnosis of posterior canal BPPV (PC-BPPV) and horizontal canal (HC), respectively. If both maneuvers are negative, we suggest the head-hanging maneuver (HHM). Finding downbeating nystagmus in that maneuver is a preliminary diagnosis of anterior canal (AC-BPPV). Then a canalith repositioning maneuver (CRM) should be performed (*). Head-hanging maneuver is repeated in order to evaluate the CRM efficacy. In case of negative result, the definitive diagnosis of AC-BPPV is reached. The brain MRI should be performed in case of persistent vertigo and downbeat nystagmus after several CRMs.

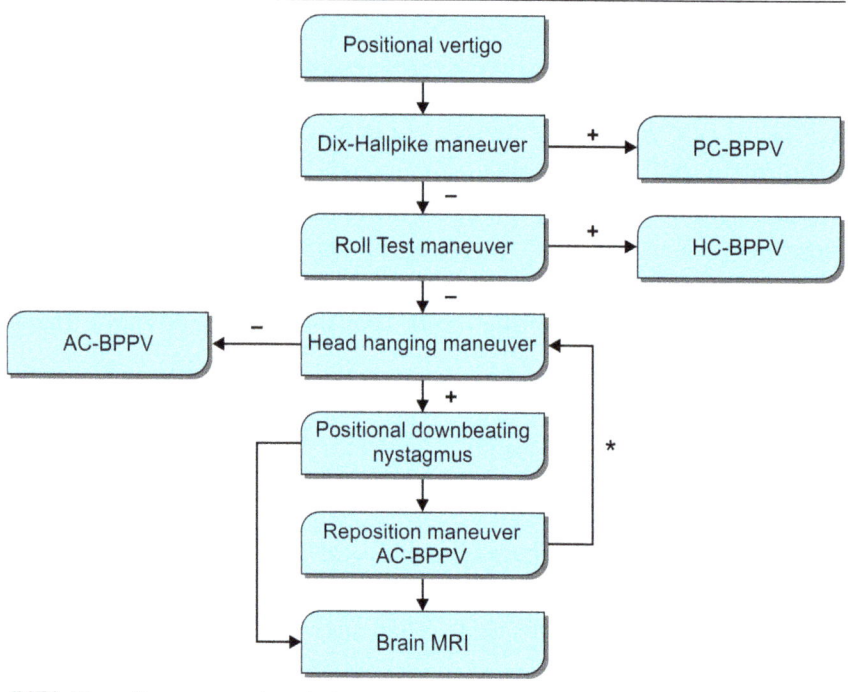

(MRI: Magnetic resonance imaging).

TREATMENT

There have been several noncontrolled studies concerning the treatment of AC-BPPV. Honrubia et al. mentioned a "reverse Epley" postural repositioning procedure.[31] The "reverse Semont" maneuver has also been recommended. As head positions with respect to gravity are identical to those of the Epley maneuver, this procedure is likely to be equally effective. However, there are no published data concerning efficacy.

Kim and associates studied 30 patients using a procedure based on biomechanical principles. The authors found 96.7% efficacy in over 30 patients (12 AC-BPPV and 18 multicanal BPPV).[32]

As precondition to use these reposition maneuvers, it is necessary to identify which (side) AC is affected. Nevertheless, Lopez-Escamez et al.[11]

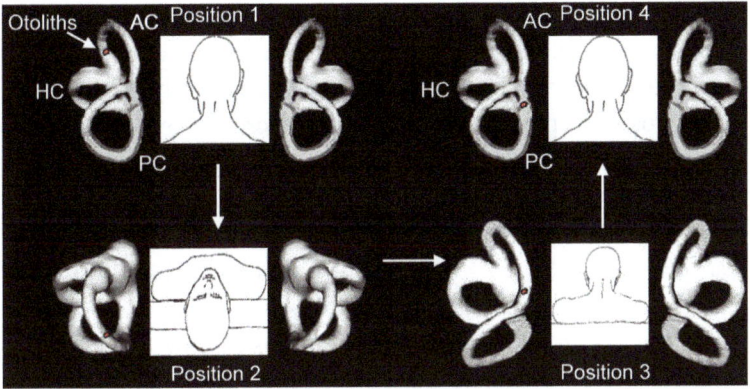

Fig. 7.4: Repositioning maneuver for the anterior canal (AC) benign positional paroxysmal vertigo. Image (point of view) of the subject seen from behind. The left and right labyrinths are located one on each side of the head. The image of the labyrinth was obtained from a reconstruction of a high resolution three-dimensional inner ear magnetic resonance imaging. Otoliths were represented on the left although the same motion path would be expected in the case of an otolith located in the right AC. (PC: Posterior canal; HC: Horizontal canal).

found that bilateral pDBN was triggered by the DHM in 5 out of 14 AC-BPPV patients, with difficulty localizing the affected ear.

Another maneuver for AC-BPPV was described by Rahko (2002).[33] In this maneuver, the patient lies on the healthy side. The head is first tilted downward 45° (position 1), then horizontally (position 2), next upward 45° (position 3) for 30 seconds on each occasion; finally the patient sits up (position 4) remaining well-supported in this position for at least 3 minutes. Fifty-three out of 57 patients were symptom-free after the maneuver. Neither diagnosis nor results were based on nystagmus pattern, nor did the study include a control group or a double blind design.

Crevits described a "prolonged forced position procedure" in two patients with refractory AC-BPPV. Biomechanically, this maneuver differs significantly from the others described because there is an explicit effort to position the AC so that it is nearly upside down, rather than an attempt to position it 45° to one side as in the variants of the Epley maneuver described above. Helminski and Hain (2007) proposed using a "deep DHM" for AC-BPPV treatment without clinical data about its efficacy.[34]

We have reported a specific CRM for AC-BPPV (Fig. 7.4).[3] It consists of four steps with position changes occurring at 30-second intervals (Fig. 7.4). From the head-straight sitting position (position 1), an HHM is performed so that the head is brought to at least 30° below the horizontal, as shown in Figure 7.4 (position 2). During the maneuver, loose otoconia within the AC should move away from the AC cupula, triggering a downbeating nystagmus. After 30 seconds, once vertigo and nystagmus induced by the maneuver cease, the patient's head is moved quickly forward "chin-to-chest" while still supine (position 3), with the vertex near the vertical axis. After another 30 seconds have elapsed, head and body are brought into the sitting position (position 4), remaining there for another 30 seconds. In cases of failure or incomplete remission of symptoms, we would advise repeating it several times and waiting a longer period in the initial head-hanging position, as well as between positions. If it still does not work, we suggest completing the work up to ruling out other reasonable causes like central positional vertigo (e.g. nodulus lesion).[35]

According to our observations, this repositioning maneuver works symmetrically for unilateral AC-BPPV (regardless of which side is affected); therefore, identifying the affected ear should not be critical under these conditions.

Efficacy of the maneuver: In the case of our 60 patients[5] who were initially diagnosed with AC-BPPV, treated with CRP, and followed up, 41 (68.3%) resolved after one to three maneuvers and 19 (31.6%) switched to other canals (to PC-BPPV in 18 cases and to horizontal canal in one) at a follow-up visit. In 2 (3.3%) out of 60 patients, a "double canal switch" (posterior to anterior to posterior) occurred. The bidirectional vertical canal involvement could be explained by the spatial orientation of the common cross during each maneuver acting as unidirectional selector.[5]

A recurrent, refractory, and recalcitrant pattern of vertigo associated with pDBN should alert on a possible central origin of symptoms that should be completed with an appropriate workup.

In well-documented cases of AC-BPPV that are symptomatic and resistant to treatment, there are isolated reports about the potential usefulness of the surgical plugging of the AC,[36] though the treatment is limited to very few cases.

CONCLUSION

According to our review and experience, AC-BPPV is not a rare condition presented with pDBN. The foremost differential diagnosis of AC-BPPV is central positional vertigo. The most restrictive diagnostic criterion of AC-BPPV, including resolution of vertigo and nystagmus after a canalith repositioning procedure as the main point, is the best pragmatic diagnostic criterion. The absence of the torsional component does not rule out AC involvement. Patients with positional vertigo and a negative DHM or downbeating nystagmus complete the examination with the HHM and follow the procedure to treat AC-BPPV.

REFERENCES

1. Jackson LE, Morgan B, Fletcher JC, Jr, et al. Anterior canal benign paroxysmal positional vertigo: an underappreciated entity. Otol Neurotol. 2007;28(2):218-22.
2. Korres SG, Balatsouras DG. Diagnostic, pathophysiologic, and therapeutic aspects of benign paroxysmal positional vertigo. Otolaryngol Head Neck Surg. 2004;131(4):438-44.
3. Yacovino DA, Hain TC, Gualtieri F. New therapeutic maneuver for anterior canal benign paroxysmal positional vertigo. J Neurol. 2009;256(11):1851-5.
4. Epley JM. Human experience with canalith repositioning maneuvers. Ann N Y Acad Sci. 2001;942:179-91.
5. Yacovino DA, Hain TC, Olivier MA, et al. Anterior canal benign paroxysmal vertigo in practice: where does it come from and where does it go? J Vestib Res. 2014;24(2-3):213.
6. Zapala DA. Down-beating nystagmus in anterior canal benign paroxysmal positional vertigo. J Am Acad Audiol. 2008;19(3):257-66.
7. Bertholon P, Bronstein AM, Davies RA, et al. Positional down beating nystagmus in 50 patients: cerebellar disorders and possible anterior semicircular canalithiasis. J Neurol Neurosurg Psychiatry. 2002;72(3):366-72.
8. Brandt T, Steddin S, Daroff RB. Therapy for benign paroxysmal positioning vertigo, revisited. Neurology. 1994;44(5):796-800.
9. Herdman SJ, Tusa RJ. Complications of the canalith repositioning procedure. Arch Otolaryngol Head Neck Surg. 1996;122(3):281-6.
10. Cambi J, Astore S, Mandala M, et al. Natural course of positional down-beating nystagmus of peripheral origin. J Neurol. 2013;260(6):1489-96.
11. Lopez-Escamez JA, Molina MI, Gamiz MJ. Anterior semicircular canal benign paroxysmal positional vertigo and positional downbeating nystagmus. Am J Otolaryngol. 2006;27(3):173-8.
12. Ogawa Y, Suzuki M, Otsuka K, et al. Positional and positioning down-beating nystagmus without central nervous system findings. Auris Nasus Larynx. 2009;36(6):698-701.
13. Luis L, Costa J, Yacovino D. A Pragmatic Strategy for the Evaluation and Management of Anterior Canal Benign Positional Vertigo. Otol Neurotol. 2015. 10.1097/MAO.0000000000000783
14. Allen G, Fernandez C. Experimental observations in postural nystagmus. I. Extensive lesions in posterior vermis of the cerebellum. Acta Otolaryngol. 1960;51:2-14.
15. Kattah JC, Kolsky MP, Luessenhop AJ. Positional vertigo and the cerebellar vermis. Neurology. 1984;34(4):527-9.
16. Imai T, Ito M, Takeda N, et al. Natural course of the remission of vertigo in patients with benign paroxysmal positional vertigo. Neurology. 2005;64(5):920-1.
17. Imai T, Takeda N, Ito M, et al. Natural course of positional vertigo in patients with apogeotropic variant of horizontal canal benign paroxysmal positional vertigo. Auris Nasus Larynx. 2011;38(1):2-5.
18. Nuti D, Vannucchi P, Pagnini P. Benign paroxysmal positional vertigo of the horizontal canal: a form of canalolithiasis with variable clinical features. J Vestib Res. 1996;6(3):173-84.

19. Lea J, Lechner C, Halmagyi GM, et al. Not so benign positional vertigo: paroxysmal downbeat nystagmus from a superior cerebellar peduncle neoplasm. Otol Neurotol. 2014;35(6):e204-5.
20. Yee RD. Downbeat nystagmus: characteristics and localization of lesions. Trans Am Ophthalmol Soc. 1989;87:984-1032.
21. Brandt T. Positional and positioning vertigo and nystagmus. J Neurol Sci. 1990;95(1):3-28.
22. Yabe I, Sasaki H, Takeichi N, et al. Positional vertigo and macroscopic downbeat positioning nystagmus in spinocerebellar ataxia type 6 (SCA6). J Neurol. 2003;250(4):440-3.
23. Choi JY, Park YM, Woo YS, et al. Perverted head-shaking and positional downbeat nystagmus in pregabalin intoxication. J Neurol Sci. 2014;337(1-2):243-4.
24. Oh SY, Kim JS, Lee YH, et al. Downbeat, positional, and perverted head-shaking nystagmus associated with lamotrigine toxicity. J Clin Neurol. 2006;2(4):283-5.
25. Choi SY, Park SH, Kim HJ, et al. Paraneoplastic downbeat nystagmus associated with cerebellar hypermetabolism especially in the nodulus. J Neurol Sci. 2014;343(1-2):187-91.
26. Kattah JC, Gujrati M. Familial positional downbeat nystagmus and cerebellar ataxia: clinical and pathologic findings. Ann N Y Acad Sci. 2005;1039:540-3.
27. Buki B. Benign paroxysmal positional vertigo—toward new definitions. Otol Neurotol. 2014;35(2):323-8.
28. Schratzenstaller B, Wagner-Manslau C, Strasser G, et al. Canalolithiasis of the superior semicircular canal: an anomaly in benign paroxysmal vertigo. Acta Otolaryngol. 2005;125(10):1055-62.
29. Polensek SH, Tusa RJ. Nystagmus during attacks of vestibular migraine: an aid in diagnosis. Audiol Neurootol. 2010;15(4):241-6.
30. Bisdorff AR, Sancovic S, Debatisse D, et al. Positional nystagmus in the dark in normal subjects. Neuro-Ophthalmol. 2000;24(1):283-90.
31. Honrubia V, Baloh RW, Harris MR, et al. Paroxysmal positional vertigo syndrome. Am J Otol. 1999;20(4):465-70.
32. Kim YK, Shin JE, Chung JW. The effect of canalith repositioning for anterior semicircular canal canalithiasis. ORL J Otorhinolaryngol Relat Spec. 2005;67(1):56-60.
33. Rahko T. The test and treatment methods of benign paroxysmal positional vertigo and an addition to the management of vertigo due to the superior vestibular canal (BPPV-SC). Clin Otolaryngol Allied Sci. 2002;27(5):392-5.
34. Helminski JO, Hain TC. Evaluation and treatment of benign paroxysmal positional vertigo. Ann Long Term Care. 2007; 15(6):33–39.
35. Fernandez C, Alzate R, Lindsay JR. Experimental observations on postural nystagmus. II. Lesions of the nodulus. Ann Otol Rhinol Laryngol. 1960;69:94-114.
36. Brantberg K, Bergenius J. Treatment of anterior benign paroxysmal positional vertigo by canal plugging: a case report. Acta Otolaryngol. 2002;122(1):28-30.

Chapter 8

Residual Dizziness after Successful Canalith Repositioning Procedures for Benign Paroxysmal Positional Vertigo

Alev Uneri, Ayse Uneri

OVERVIEW

Dizziness and vertigo are among the most common symptoms causing patients to visit a physician; however, the epidemiology of dizziness and vertigo is still a small and developing field, with a large potential impact on patient care. Dizziness, apart from the obvious economic, has dire effects on the working population. Falling can be a direct consequence of dizziness in dizziness/vertigo patients; the risk is serious and much more common in the elderly population with additional, mostly age-related, deficits and medical problems.[1,2] We need to consider residual dizziness (RD) after canalith repositioning procedures (CRP) for benign paroxysmal positional vertigo (BPPV) in this context. Unfortunately, epidemiologic data on the prevalence of specific dizziness such as RD are scarce and are based primarily on selected case series or not explicitly defined diagnostic criteria.

Residual dizziness after CRP is a residual nonspecific dizziness such as the sensation of floating or light-headedness, after resolving the BPPV by CRP. To define dizziness as RD after successful CRP, typical nystagmus and vertigo of BPPV must have been resolved.

As early as 4 years after Epley's original article,[3] Shepard and Telian[4] reported that 28% of patients with pure BPPV and 70% with secondary BPPV had residual symptoms or a positive Dix-Hallpike test after CRP. Regarding literature published to this day, reported prevalence of RD after successful CRP varies from 22 to 74%.[5,6]

Canalith repositioning procedures, with several modifications since Epley's original description,[3] has become a first choice of therapy due to its easy application, noninvasive nature, and obvious effectiveness at relieving vertigo. Even though the efficiency of CRP in clinical practice has been questioned because of the high rate of spontaneous resolution of symptoms in patients who receive no treatment, meta-analysis show that CRP treatments appear consistent and strong.[7] With appropriate CRPs depending on the affected canal, success rates are as high as 90–99%.[8-11] Nevertheless, more than half of the subjects report nonpositional, persistent dizziness and imbalance after resolving the typical nystagmus and vertigo by CRP. While causal factors are still under debate, the elderly groups experience it more often.[8,12,13]

DIAGNOSTIC EVALUATION

Residual dizziness that we may call an unresolved symptom, commonly cause a sense of impaired overall health and a reduced quality of life with both physical and psychological impairments. Prolonged RD, especially in elderly, has additional adverse physical, psychological and social consequences; it increases the possibility of falling as well as the fear of it. Fear of falling normally decreases daily living activities and it may reduce participation in social activities, which may lead to depression.[14,15]

In the analysis of symptom characteristics, the most common residual symptoms are continuous or intermittent light-headedness, floating sense, vertigo without positional and/or rotational components and unsteadiness.[12,16]

These residual symptoms are hard to detect with conventional vestibular function tests. Questionnaires as dizziness handicap inventory, visual analog scale or activities-specific balance confidence scale for RD are widely used to quantify subjective symptoms and to evaluate treatment results.[7,14]

Although these questionnaires may be helpful to understand the patient's existing symptoms, the diagnostic procedure must consist of a detailed clinical history, a neuro-otologic examination, and more importantly videonystagmography (VNG).[17] Detection of nystagmus is crucial for the diagnosis in dizziness/vertigo patients. Videonystagmography goggles uses the infrared camera in total darkness, it allows eliminating gaze fixation, thus uncovers even the weakest nystagmus, therefore nystagmus's existence can be confirmed and recorded at the same time by VNG. If VNG is not achievable, a Frenzel goggle may help to reveal residual nystagmus but not at the same accuracy as with VNG, still it is much better than examination by naked eye only.

To expose a nystagmus is essential in vestibular disorders. One of the main practical results of the discovery of a nystagmus in RD patients is to detect concurrent vestibular disorder.

Vestibular disorders, such as vestibular migraine (VM), may have extended, complicated and entangled medical histories with episodic vertigo attacks including BPPVs, acute vestibular spells, prolonged or intermittent dizziness periods. These symptom clusters may easily be misdiagnosed as one of their symptomatic scene or as a psychological vertigo/dizziness disorder if only deciding with history of symptoms, without detecting the nystagmus. Therefore, revealing nystamus always helps to distinguish diagnoses, especially in prolonged dizziness such as RD after successful CRPs.

There is also a lack of consensus about the timing of the control examination for RD also. Some researchers begin to evaluate RD in their patients as soon as the next day with Dix-Hallpike maneuver or questionnaires while others evaluate them after 2 weeks or 1 month later.[5] In our institutes, we chose to wait at least 1 week to see whether CRP was successful or not, and suggested mild head movement restrictions until the control examination.

THEORIES OF PATHOGENESIS

Several hypotheses exist for RD after successful CRP throughout the literature.

Inner ear problems, mainly semicircular canal-otolith problems are the most common explanation model accepted by many authors. Persistence of debris in the semicircular canal which is insufficient to provoke noticeable positional nystagmus or an utricular dysfunction, considered responsible as the underlying cause of RD.[18-20] This hypothesis proposes that remaining otoconial debris due to incomplete repositioning could produce mild positional dizziness, but it is not able to deflect the cupula to the degree needed to provoke overt positional nystagmus. If this hypothesis is true, RD after CRPs must be seen only by certain head positions like Dix-Hallpike maneuver, but that's not the case. They are generally in continuous nature, which worsens with head movements like all other vestibular dizziness disorders.

Many researchers believed that BPPV is not only a disorder of the semicircular canals, but also a disorder of the otoliths; otolith dysfunction or unequal weight distribution of the two utricles on the macule could explain RD in some patients.[21] More recently, supporting previously reported utricular dysfunction in BPPV patients, Seo et al. reported 84.5% reduced ocular vestibular-evoked myogenic potential measurements that indicate abnormal function of the utricle in patients with BPPV.[22] If RD is looked at through this point of view, it is easy to assume that utricular problem might create RD after successful CRP. However as all other hypothesis, this hypothesis needs more supportive data.

While some studies validate that a long duration of vertigo before CRPs was associated with an increased risk of RD, others did not find any association between the duration of vertigo and the presence of RD. Small sample sizes and different inclusion criteria may explain the discrepancy between the studies.[18,21]

Several researchers claim that residual symptoms after BPPV episodes are a cause of psychological anxiety or fear of dizziness recurrence.

Furthermore, loss of confidence or deterioration of overall physical condition may be caused by the residual symptoms.[23] Although relationship between anxiety disorders and vertigo is still under debate, anxiety and dizziness are comorbid symptoms in a larger percentage of patients than would be expected from chance alone, and among patients presenting dizziness, psychiatric disorders are elevated to 5-15 times the rate of the general population. Dizziness is suggested as a part of the symptom cluster of other anxiety disorders, such as "generalized anxiety disorder" by many researchers.[24-26]

Clinical evidence for the link between vestibular and anxiety disorders can also be supported by the "Selective serotonin reuptake inhibitor (SSRI) discontinuation syndrome," characterized by dizziness >50% of cases following the abrupt interruption of SSRI therapy.[27]

A rather enticing hypothesis for RD after successful CRP is unusual neural connections. Objective signs of balance dysfunction, visual motion sensitivity and presence of anxious temperament are well documented in the literature on comorbid anxiety and balance disorders.[28] In this context, Coelho and Balaban indicated "uncommon arrangement of visual and vestibular stimuli might exceed the capacity to integrate multimodal information, creating a sensory conflict that either generates the typical motion sickness physiological responses, or, in different circumstances (and in different people) might give rise to a fearful or phobic response."[29]

In longer follow-ups, treated BPPVs tend to recur. The recurrence rate at 1 year is estimated 15% and 37% at 5 years on the Kaplan-Meier curve.[30,31] It has been shown that in frogs, otoconia dissolves more slowly if the calcium level rise in endolymph. Furthermore if female rats become osteoporotic artificially, this change leads to ultrastructural changes in otoliths.[30,32]

New studies associate between reduced bone mineral density (BMD) and development/recurrence of BPPV. Additionally, low levels of vitamin D were related to development of BPPV, while very low levels were associated with recurrence of BPPV. The co-occurrence of two morbidities is not by itself supportive of a relationship, but the cumulating studies correlating between BPPV and both vitamin D deficiency and low BMD indicate the investigation and treatment of those disorders in cases with recurrent BPPV.[33] Yu et al. analyzed seven studies in 2014 and showed that most of the studies demonstrate a correlation between osteoporosis (osteopenia) and the occurrence and recurrence of BPPV, especially in older women.[34]

It is known that the major process involved in the spontaneous recovery of BPPV episodes is the capability of the endolymph to dissolve dislodged otoconia. Increased free calcium concentration due to estrogen deficiency may decrease the capability of the endolymph for resolving otolithic debris even after successful CRP; this might result in prolonged dizziness such as RD; however, I have not come across any publication supporting or investigating this possibility.

A concurrent vestibular disorder with BPPV might be the very likely explanation for persistent RD after successful CRP. Pollak et al. found that the prevalence of persistent dizziness was significantly higher in patients with BPPV and additional peripheral or central vestibular dysfunction.[5] Another vestibular lesion, similarly causing vertigo and/or dizziness with positional triggers, very likely coexists with BPPV. In this group, it is usually possible to distinguish, on the history alone, that underlying or concurrent vestibular disorder exists. These patients have a significantly higher prevalence of ongoing symptoms, including positional vertigo without specific nystagmus or persistent dizziness.[5] Therefore, patients with any kind of a peripheral and/or a central vestibular disorder (CVD) will probably have RD after successful CRP.

Vestibular neuronitis (VN) can be considered under "concurrent vestibular disorder" label in RD after successful CRP. Gacek[35] demonstrated the degeneration of the saccular ganglion in two temporal bones of patients with posterior canal BPPV and suggested that BPPV can coexist with VN. Balatsouras et al.[36] reported that they found a prevalence of 5.2% of BPPV secondary to VN in their patients. Although there is not any publication in the literature showing correlation between RD after successful CRP and VN, it could be at least implied that some of the RDs may have VN background. Still, there are a few weaknesses within this hypothesis. Initially, as Gacek[37] himself reported symptoms of some of the VN patients may be indistinguishable from those called VM. Even though there has been no pathological correlation described to support VM syndrome, considering the coincidences of migraine and vertigo, yet the probability of VM as underlying cause of RD is undeniable.

Regarding this concept, VM must be the most common coexisting vestibular disorders with BPPV.[38] In 2004, we found 54.8% of the 476 BPPV patients had history of migraine headaches.[39] This is three times the incidence of migraine in the general population and correlates with the series reported by Ishiyama et al.[40] Although the relationship between migraine and vertigo/dizziness, thereby BPPV, is poorly understood, the connection has been known since Liveing's publication.[41]

Many researches indicate the large overlap between migraine pathways and vestibular pathways, which is coherent with the interpretation of VM is a migraine variant with vestibular manifestations.[42,43] More precisely, all mechanisms that have been implicated for migraine are all comprised central vestibular pathways and the inner ear.[44,45] Moreover, some VM patients complain from nearly persistent dizziness with recurrent exacerbations as BPPV attacks. We followed up 600 patients with the diagnosis of VM up to 9 years and noted changes and overlapping features of the vestibular manifestations over time ranging from episodic, recurrent or short lasting vertigo spells, BPPV episodes to constant feeling of dizziness or unsteadiness even after years of symptom-free intervals. The predominant symptoms reported by 63% patients were chronic dizziness, imbalance and unsteadiness. Symptoms occurred prior to the onset of headache, during a headache, or, as was common, during a headache-free interval. All this information and proposed mechanisms infer that a huge proportion of RD cases after successful CRPs might be the outcome of underlying VM.

Another hypothesis for the RD after successful CRPs is delayed central adaptation after particle repositioning procedure. Although some researchers mentioned this probability, there is no presented study questioning this.[16,46]

Finally, the possibility of a concomitant CVD should not be overlooked. An unnoticed CVD, which causes dizziness in a BPPV patient, can easily be misdiagnosed as RD after a CRP. Central vestibular disorders are the result of lesions of central vestibular pathways. These lesions might be caused by vascular events, tumors, and degenerative processes as well as by multiple sclerosis, or, more rarely vestibular epilepsy. Central vestibular disorders are reported as the third and fourth most frequent forms of vertigo in some neurological dizziness units, but this high incidence is possibly the result of different forms of migraine such as basilar or VM are included in CVDs.[47,48]

MANAGEMENT

A significant percentage of patients with BPPV are more likely to have associated vestibular pathology; therefore, patients with RD after successful CRPs might be candidates for detailed examination and vestibular function testing. After completing these requirements if a concurrent disorder is discovered, the treatment must be defined according to this condition, such as VM, vestibular neuritis, or anxiety disorder.

There is very little publication concerning RD after successful CRPs in the literature, and very little is written about the treatment as anticipated. What is found as different approaches to treat RD are the following: Kim et al.[49] tried vestibular suppressants in their research and found it significantly effective, while Jung's study[14] suggested that adjuvant antianxiety medication might be helpful for RD after a successful CRP, and Deng et al.[46] proposed a traditional Chinese medicine, Danhong injection. They assumed that Danhong injection's benefit might be due to its antioxidant activity and improving microcirculation.

If there is not any explanatory origin for the RD, logical approach might be to give home exercises such as Brandt-Daroff exercises (or any other vestibular home exercise program) with the intention of vestibular compensation, therefore giving vestibular suppressants that simultaneously suppress vestibular compensation does not appear to be a rational choice for RD patients. Vestibular compensation with exercise, aims to use of the visual, proprioceptive and vestibular inputs involved in the postural control and might help to strengthen strategy of equilibrium or accelerate the compensation process.

CONCLUSION

In summary, RD after successful CRP is a burdensome, yet very common problem nevertheless its consideration is very sporadic. Residual dizziness can persist for weeks, months, or even years, and in some patients, dizziness may be more frustrating than the BPPV.

Condemned to live with an unsolved "dizziness problem" might be sufficient to create anxiety in many patients. Incomplete diagnosis, possibly due to missing technologic aids, and most importantly not spending adequate time with a patient to get the thorough history of the disorder, makes it impossible to understand the problem and the patient.

Even today, many controversies and arguments are still going on about etiology, classification and understanding about BPPV, the same as for other vestibular disorders; consequently, complete understanding and treatment of the RD after successful CRP is still on hold.

I believe that a better understanding in peripheral vestibular disorders will come with a larger and a holistic perspective. To separate vestibular system from nervous system and to try to find out an etiology solely in the inner ear or peripheral part of vestibular system is possibly our biggest burden about this subject.

Most of the different classifications and disarrays are coming from short follow-up periods and many vestibular disorders are probably developing from genetic and epigenetic factors working together. If we can able to follow-up patients long enough, we will probably see many different forms of vestibular problems on the same patient.

REFERENCES

1. Maarsingh OR, Dros J, Schellevis FG, et al. Dizziness reported by elderly patients in family practice: prevalence, incidence, and clinical characteristics. BMC Family Pract. 2010;11:2.

2. Neuhauser HK, Radtke A, von Brevern M, et al. Burden of dizziness and vertigo in the community. Arch Inter Med. 2008;168(19):2118-24.
3. Epley JM. The canalith repositioning procedure: for treatment of benign paroxysmal positional vertigo. Otolaryngol Head Neck Surg. 1992;107:399-404.
4. Shepard NT, Telian SA. Practical management of the balance disorder patient. San Diego: Singular Publishing Group; 1996.
5. Pollak L, Davies RA, Luxon LL. Effectiveness of the particle repositioning maneuver in benign paroxysmal positional vertigo with and without additional vestibular pathology. Otol Neurotol. 2002;23(1):79-83.
6. Prokopakis EP, Lachanas VA, Christodoulou PN, et al. Dizziness after canalith repositioning procedure for benign paroxysmal positional vertigo. Auris Nasus Larynx. 2007; 34(3): 435.
7. Lee NH, Kwon HJ, Ban, JH. Analysis of residual symptoms after treatment in benign paroxysmal positional vertigo using questionnaire. Otolaryngol Head Neck Surg. 2009;141(2):232-6.
8. Gordon CR, Gadoth N. Repeated vs single physical maneuver in benign paroxysmal positional vertigo. Acta Neurol Scand. 2004;110:166-9.
9. Woodworth BA, Gillespie MB, Lambert PR. The canalith repositioning procedure for benign positional vertigo: a meta-analysis. Laryngoscope. 2004; 114(7):1143-6.
10. White J, Savvides P, Cherian N, et al. Canalith repositioning for benign paroxysmal positional vertigo. Otology & Neurotology. 2005;26(4):704-10.
11. Dornhoffer J, Colvin G. Benign paroxysmal positional vertigo and canalith repositioning: clinical correlations. Am J Otolaryngol. 2000;21(2):230-3.
12. Teggi R, Giordano L, Bondi S, et al. Residual dizziness after successful repositioning maneuvers for idiopathic benign paroxysmal positional vertigo in the elderly. Eur Arch Otorhinolaryngol. 2011;268(4):507-11.
13. Oghalai JS, Manolidis S, Barth JL, et al. Unrecognized benign paroxysmal positional vertigo in elderly patients. Otolaryngol Head Neck Surg. 2000;122(5):630-4.
14. Jung HJ, Koo J-W, Kim CS, et al. Anxiolytics reduce residual dizziness after successful canalith repositioning maneuvers in benign paroxysmal positional vertigo. Acta Otolaryngol. 2012;132(3):277-84
15. Pritcher MR, Whitney SL, Marchetti GF, et al. The influence of age and vestibular disorders on gaze stabilization: a pilot study. Otol Neurotol. 2008;29:982-8.
16. Teggi R, Quaglieri S, Gatti O, et al. Residual dizziness after successful repositioning maneuvers for idiopathic benign paroxysmal positional vertigo. ORL J Otorhinolaryngol Relat Spec. 2011;75(2):74-81.
17. Maslovara S, Vešligaj T, Butković Soldo S, et al. Importance of accurate diagnosis in benign paroxysmal positional vertigo (BPPV) therapy. Med Glas. 2014;11(2):300-6.
18. Seok JI, Lee HM, Yoo JH, et al. Residual dizziness after successful repositioning treatment in patients with benign paroxysmal positional vertigo. J Clin Neurol (Seoul, Korea).2008; 4(3):107-10.
19. Von Brevern M, Schmidt T, Schonfeld U, et al. Utricular dysfunction in patients with benign paroxysmal positional vertigo. Otol Neurotol. 2006;27:92-6.
20. Hong SM, Park MS, Cha CL, et al. Subjective visual vertical during eccentric rotation in patients with benign paroxysmal positional vertigo. Otol Neurotol. 2008;29(8):1167-70.

21. Kim HA, Lee H. Autonomic dysfunction as a possible cause of residual dizziness after successful treatment in benign paroxysmal positional vertigo. Clin Neurophysiol. 2014;125(3):608-14.
22. Seo T, Saka N, Ohta S, et al. Detection of utricular dysfunction using ocular vestibular evoked myogenic potential in patients with benign paroxysmal positional vertigo. Neurosci Lett. 2013;550:12-6.
23. Mendel B, Bergenius J, Langius A. Dizziness symptom severity and impact on daily living as perceived by patients suffering from peripheral vestibular disorder. Clin Otolaryngol Allied Sci. 1999;24:286-93.
24. Jacob RG, Furman JM. Psychiatric consequences of vestibular dysfunction. Curr Opin Neurol. 2001;14:41-6.
25. Staab JP. Chronic dizziness: the interface between psychiatry and neuro-otology. Curr Opin Neurol. 2006;19:41-8.
26. Pollak L, Klein C, Rafael S, et al. Anxiety in the first attack of vertigo. Otolaryngol Head Neck Surg. 2002;128:829-34.
27. Black K, Shea C, Dursun S, et al. Selective serotonin reuptake inhibitor discontinuation syndrome: proposed diagnostic criteria. J Psych Neurosci. 2000;25(3):255-61.
28. Balaban CD. Migraine, vertigo and migrainous vertigo: links between vestibular and pain mechanisms. Journal of Anxiety Disorders. 2011;15(1-2):53-79.
29. Coelho CM, Balaban CD. Model visuo-vestibular contributions to anxiety and fear. Neurosci Biobehav Rev. 2015;48:148-59.
30. Jeremy H. Benign paroxysmal positional vertigo (BPPV): history, pathophysiology, office treatment and future directions, International Journal of Otolaryngology. 2011;2011: Article ID 835671.
31. Nunez RA, Cass SP, Furman JM. Short- and long-term outcomes of canalith repositioning for benign paroxysmal positional vertigo. Otolaryngol Head Neck Surg. 2000;122:647-52.
32. Vibert D, Sans A, Kompis M, et al. Ultrastructural changes in otoconia of osteoporotic rats. Audiol Neurotol. 2008;13(5):293-301.
33. Talaat HS, Abuhadied G, Talaat, et al. Low bone mineral density and vitamin D deficiency in patients with benign positional paroxysmal vertigo. Eur Arch Otorhinolaryngol. 2015;272(9):2249-53.
34. Yu S, Liu F, Cheng Z, et al. Association between osteoporosis and benign paroxysmal positional vertigo: a systematic review. BMC Neurol. 2014;14:110.
35. Gacek RR. A perspective on recurrent vertigo. ORL J Otorhinolaryngol Relat Spec. 2013;75(2):91-107.
36. Balatsouras DG, Koukoutsis G, Ganelis P, et al. Benign paroxysmal positional vertigo secondary to vestibular neuritis. Eur Arch Otorhinolaryngol. 2014; 271(5):919-24.
37. Gacek RR. Pathology of benign paroxysmal positional vertigo revisited. Ann Otol Rhinol Laryngol. 2003;112:574-82.
38. Furman JM, Balaban CD. Vestibular migraine. Ann New York Acad Sci. 2015; 1343:90-6.
39. Uneri A. Migraine and benign paroxysmal positional vertigo: an outcome study of 476 patients. Ear Nose Throat J. 2014;83(12):814-5.

40. Ishiyama A, Jacobson KM, Baloh RW. Migraine and benign positional vertigo. Ann Otol Rhinol Laryngol. 2000;109(4):377-80.
41. Liveing E. Observations on megrim or sick-headache. Br Med J. 1872;1(588):364-6.
42. Balaban CD, Jacob RG, Furman JM. Neurologic bases for comorbidity of balance disorders, anxiety disorders and migraine: neurotherapeutic implications. Exp Rev Neurother. 2011;11(3):379-94.
43. Balaban CD, Thayer JF. Neurological bases for balance-anxiety links. J Anxiety Dis. 2001;15(1-2):53-79.
44. Ho TW, Edvinsson L, Goadsby PJ. CGRP and its receptors provide new insights into migraine pathophysiology. Nat Rev Neurol. 2010;6(10):573-82.
45. Furman JM, Marcus DA, Balaban CD. Vestibular migraine: clinical aspects and pathophysiology. Lancet Neurol. 2013;12(7):706-15.
46. Deng W, Yang C, Xiong M, et al. Danhong enhances recovery from residual dizziness after successful repositioning treatment in patients with benign paroxysmal positional vertigo. Am J Otolaryngol. 2014;35(6):753-7.
47. Brandt T, Strupp M. Migraine and vertigo: classification, clinical features, and special treatment considerations. Headache Curr. 2006;3(1):12-9.
48. Dieterich M. Central vestibular disorders. J Neurol. 2007;254(5):559-68.
49. Kim MB, Lee HS, Ban JH. Vestibular suppressants after canalith repositioning in benign paroxysmal positional vertigo. Laryngoscope. 2014;124(10):2400-03.

Chapter 9

Complex Forms of Benign Paroxysmal Positional Vertigo

9A: CUPULOLITHIASIS

Essam Saleh, Alfarghal Mohamad

OVERVIEW

Although the majority of cases of benign paroxysmal positional vertigo (BPPV) are believed to be due to canalithiasis, the presence of free-floating otoconia in the endolymph of the semicircular canals, in some cases, is still believed to result from cupulolithiasis. In the latter case, otoconia, which have specific gravity greater than endolymph, adhere to the cupula of the posterior or lateral canal rendering the cupula gravity sensitive.[1] The term cupulolithiasis was first suggested by Schuknecht who identified basophilic staining mass attached to the cupula of posterior canals in temporal bones of patients with BPPV.[2,3]

PATHOGENESIS

Otoconia are composed of calcium carbonate crystals. They are tightly bound to the proteinaceous layer of the otolithic membrane. The otoconia are detached from the utricular macula mostly as a result of degeneration. Causes of otoconia detachment are idiopathic in 50% of cases, post-traumatic, postvestibular neuronitis, and after aminoside treatment. Otoconia detachment is also associated with Ménière's disease and unilateral inner ear disease such as unilateral sensorineural hearing loss (Karlberg et al. 2000).[4] Idiopathic BPPV has also been noticed in osteoporotic/osteopenic patients.[5]

Normally, the cupula has the same specific gravity as endolymph. On the other hand, otoconia have a specific gravity of 2.7 which is greater than endolymph. When they adhere to the cupula of the semicircular canal they render it gravity sensitive. The canal is transferred from a sensor of rotatory acceleration into a transducer of linear or angular acceleration. Certain head movements may then produce inappropriate endolymph-cupula displacement, causing nystagmus and vertigo. The latency before the onset of nystagmus reflects the inertia of the otoconial mass and the cupula, and the fatigability is presumably caused by dispersal of the debris attached to the cupula or even to the central vestibular adaptation.[6]

Squiresa et al.,[7] in a study on a mathematical model on BPPV, concluded that canalithiasis is a stronger mechanism than cupulolithiasis; therefore, multiple and/or larger otoconia are necessary to produce the same response in cupulolithiasis than in canalithiasis. As explained by House and Honrubia[8] in cupulolithiasis, particles act directly on the surface of the cupula which has a large surface area and hence the need for a much greater number of particles to induce nystagmus. This may explain why this condition is less common than canalithiasis.

POSTERIOR CANAL CUPULOLITHIASIS

Incidence

The majority of cases of posterior canal BPPV are believed to result from canalithiasis. The incidence of cupulolithiasis is not exactly known. It is mostly reported as less common, infrequent, or rare. Imai et al.[9] studied nystagmus in 111 cases of posterior canal BPPV using three-dimensional analysis and found 8 cases (7.2% of total) to have nystagmus consistent with cupulolithiasis.

Clinical Picture

In general, symptoms in patients with cupulolithiasis are not grossly different from other cases of posterior canal BPPV. However, examination of the nystagmus shows that latency, nystagmus short duration (<1 minute), and refractoriness might be absent in cupulolithiasis.[10] Imai et al.[9] showed that the time constant of this group lasted >40 seconds in comparison to <20 seconds in canalithiasis group. Moreover, the vertical-torsional positional nystagmus disappeared when the head was overextended or when the axis of the cupula of the posterior semicircular canal (PSCC) was aligned with gravity. Ichijo[11] set criteria for the diagnosis of posterior canal cupulolithiasis. These included a torsional-vertical upbeating nystagmus on Dix-Hallpike that lasts >1 minute. The nystagmus may or may not show a mild reversal in the sitting position. In the nose-down position, a torsional-vertical (downbeating) nystagmus occurs and lasts >1 minute while in the supine position, a torsional/vertical (upbeating) nystagmus occurs and lasts >1 minute.

Treatment

We use Epley's maneuver[12] with head shaking to facilitate detachment of the otolith debris from the cupula. In case of failure on follow-up, Semont's maneuver is performed.[13]

Differential Diagnosis

Positional/positioning nystagmus can occur in central conditions. In some cases of central etiology, nystagmus persists as long as the head is kept in the provoking position with the absence of vertigo. The lack of vertigo points out to a central cause of the condition. However, in other central conditions, both positional nystagmus and vertigo are present. These cases can be difficult to distinguish from BPPV of peripheral origin particularly from cupulolithiasis cases. The most important distinctive feature is that in peripheral disorders the resulting nystagmus always beats in the direction of the expected eye movements if the affected semicircular canal is optimally stimulated. Stimulation of the posterior canal would produce a mixed upbeat and torsional nystagmus. A pure positional, torsional, or upbeat or downbeat nystagmus is almost always of a central origin. Moreover, central disorders can have abnormal neurological signs, cerebellar manifestations, or oculomotor signs as saccadic pursuit and gaze evoked nystagmus, which might facilitate the diagnosis. However, a few central cases might have completely normal neurological examination.[14] The course of the disease and the remission with repositioning maneuver are strongly suggestive of peripheral etiology.[10,15]

LATERAL CANAL CUPULOLITHIASIS

Pathophysiology

Lateral canal BPPV can present either as a geotropic or an apogeotropic form. According to Ewald's law, the response to an excitatory stimulus is more intense than that of the inhibitory one. Therefore, in the geotropic form, nystagmus beats toward the undermost ear on the supine lateral roll test while in the apogeotropic form nystagmus beats toward the uppermost ear. Apogeotropic lateral canal BPPV can be due to otoconia adhering either to the utricular side or the canal side of the macula (cupulolithiasis), or to free debris floating in the anterior arm of the lateral canal (canalithiasis) (Fig. 9A.1). It is not possible, based on the clinical picture, to differentiate cases according to the cause of the apogeotropic nystagmus.

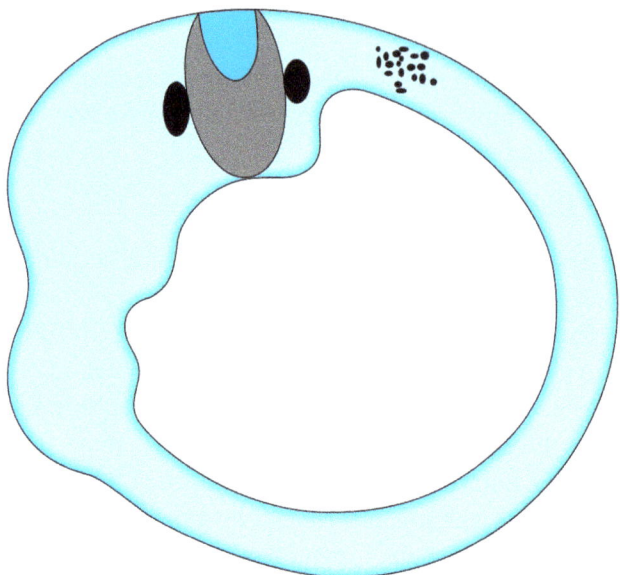

Fig. 9A.1: Pathophysiologic mechanisms for apogeotropic lateral semicircular canal benign paroxysmal positional vertigo; either canalithiasis of the anterior arm of the canal or cupulolithiasis of either side of the cupula.

Incidence

Lateral canal BPPV account for 6–33% of all cases of BPPV.[16,17] Most series report an incidence between 10% and 20%.[18] Cupulolithiasis cases are less frequent and account for 26.1–41% of all cases of lateral canal BPPV.[18,19]

Clinical Picture

Patients usually complain of positional vertigo that occurs when they turn their head or the whole body toward either side during the supine position. Unlike posterior canal BPPV, the vegetative symptoms like nausea and vomiting are more intense. On the supine lateral roll test, turning the head to the affected side leads to ampullofugal deviation of the cupula with a resultant apogeotropic nystagmus (beating toward the uppermost ear). On turning the head toward the normal side, a resultant ampullopetal movement of the cupula occurs and a stronger apogeotropic nystagmus occurs. Therefore, nystagmus is stronger when the head is turned toward the healthy side than when it is turned toward the diseased side. Nystagmus is without latency; its duration is prolonged; and fatigability is absent or much less when compared to posterior canal BPPV.

Riga et al.[20] in a reviewed literature, found that in 9.7% cases of apogeotropic variant of lateral canal BPPV, a symmetrical nystagmus is obtained when the head is turned to either side and the patient is in the supine position. In cases with controversial side determination, secondary procedures to determine the affected side were suggested by different authors (Figs. 9A.2 to 9A.4). These tests included the following.

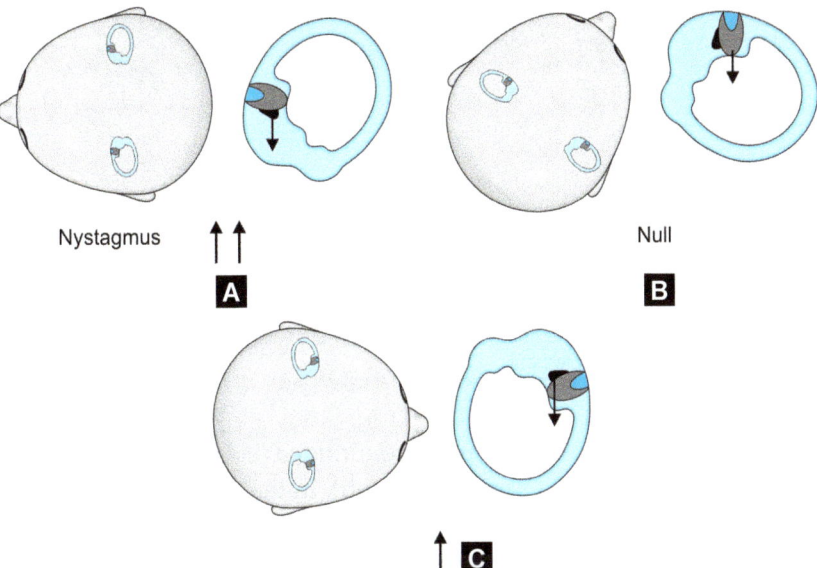

Figs. 9A.2A to C: Apogeotropic benign paroxysmal positional vertigo of the right lateral semicircular canal: (A) Nystagmus is stronger when the head is turned toward the healthy ear and is (C) weaker when it is turned to the affected ear. The null point where nystagmus stops before it reverses direction (B) is while head is still toward the side of the lesion (right side in this case).

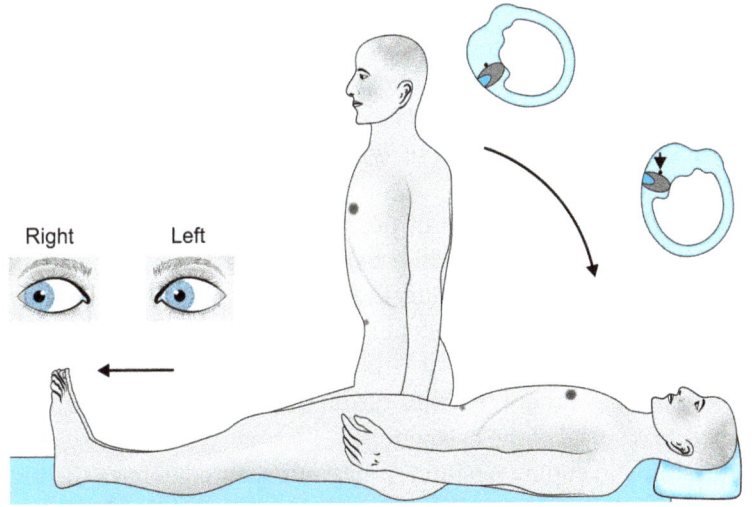

Fig. 9A.3: Right apogeotropic lateral semicircular canal benign paroxysmal positional vertigo. Sit to supine positioning leading to nystagmus beating toward the affected ear.

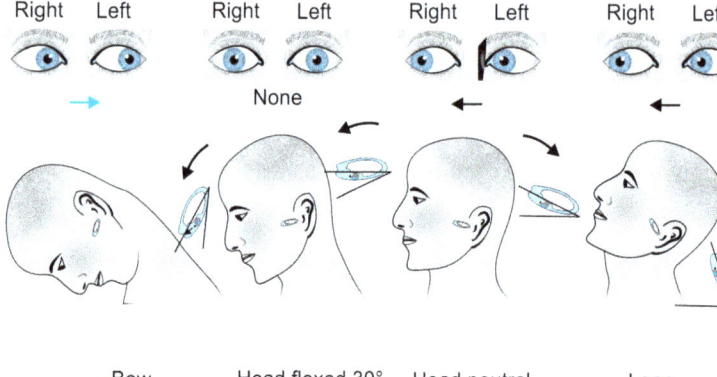

Fig. 9A.4: Right apogeotropic lateral semicircular canal benign paroxysmal positional vertigo. In the neutral position, the patient experiences pseudospontaneous nystagmus beating toward the affected ear. When the head is flexed 30°, the nystagmus stops. Further 60° bending of the head (bow test) the nystagmus reverses direction beating toward the left ear. If from the neutral position, the head is bent 45° backward (Lean test) nystagmus increases still beating toward the affected ear.

1. Nystagmus when moving from the sitting to the supine position and when the head is not turned (nose up). In the apogeotropic variant, nystagmus beats toward the affected side.[21]
2. *Pseudospontaneous nystagmus*:[22] This is a spontaneous nystagmus that occurs while the patient is seated in the neutral position. The reason for this nystagmus is the 30° inclination the lateral canal makes with the horizontal plane and hence the cupula, being gravity sensitive to the adherent otoconia, constantly deviates causing nystagmus moving toward the affected side. Nystagmus stops if the head is flexed 30° forward, as in this position the lateral canal is aligned with the horizontal plane and the gravity effect is nullified.
3. *Nystagmus during bowing and leaning*: When the head is bowed forward >90° the nystagmus is away from the side of the lesion while a backward lean of 45° produces a reverse nystagmus beating toward the side of the lesion.[23]
4. *The null point*: Recording of positions was nystagmus ceased.[23] In the supine position when the head is toward one side and slowly turning toward the other side, there comes a point where nystagmus completely stops. This occurs at an angle of ~20°–30° with the neutral position while the head is still toward the affected side in the apogeotropic variant. Further turning of the head to the other side leads to reversal of the nystagmus.

The sitting to supine position nystagmus seemed to have the highest specificity and the lowest false-negative results while the bow-lean nystagmus was the least reliable in this context.[20] Table 9A.1 shows the

Table 9A.1: Localizing signs for identification of the affected side in apogeotropic variant of lateral semicircular canal benign paroxysmal positional vertigo.

Positional test	Nystagmus direction
Sit to supine	Toward the affected side
Spontaneous (pseudo) nystagmus	Toward the affected side
Null point	Toward the affected side
Bow and lean tests • Lean (up) • Bow (down)	 Toward the affected side Away from the affected side

direction of nystagmus in the apogeotropic variant in different methods used for localization of the side of the lesion.

A simple algorithm of positioning maneuvers for localizing the side of the disease is as follows:[24]

1. While in the sitting position, the patient is observed for any pseudospontaneous nystagmus. The patient is brought from the sitting to the supine position and any nystagmus is noticed (sitting to supine or lying-down nystagmus).
2. Then the head is rotated to either side and apogeotropic nystagmus intensity on each side is determined.
3. If the side could not be still determined, while in the supine position, the head is slowly rotated from one side to the other until nystagmus stops and with further rotation it reverses (null point determination).
4. If still not determined, the patient is brought to the sitting position and the head is further bent forward (bowing nystagmus).

DIAGNOSIS

Diagnosis is typically made in the following cases:[22,24]
1. The patient has a history of brief episodes of positional vertigo.
2. Direction-changing horizontal nystagmus beating toward the upper ear when on the supine position and the head is turned to either side.
3. Absence of identifiable central nervous system is the cause for this nystagmus.

Differential Diagnosis

Certain central lesions might produce positional apogeotropic nystagmus that might mimic apogeotropic variant lateral semicircular canal (LSC) BPPV. In the central lesion, a spontaneous nystagmus is present during the sitting position and its intensity is equal to that when the patient is brought to the supine position. In the LSC BPPV, the intensity of the supine nystagmus is stronger than pseudospontaneous nystagmus (if present) when the patient is in the sitting position.[25] Vestibular migraine can also give rise to apogeotropic horizontal positional nystagmus that is difficult to differentiate from LSC cupulolithiasis. History of migraine attacks and the lack of response to repositioning maneuvers may help establish the diagnosis.[26] Rarely, vestibular schwannoma can also present with apogeotropic nystagmus that is refractory to therapy. Atypical nystagmus and abnormal audiological testing may raise suspicion.[27] In these patients, vertigo may subside with time but nystagmus usually persists.

Treatment

Apogeotropic variant of LSC BPPV is more difficult to treat than geotropic variant. As previously explained, the apogeotropic form can be due to either canalithiasis of the anterior arm of the canal or cupulolithiasis. Cupulolithiasis forms need maneuvers that detach the adherent otoconia from the cupula. Moreover, the otolith can attach to either side of the cupula (canal side or utricular side). Repositioning maneuvers performed toward the diseased side, for example, can detach the debris from the canal side but would have no effect on the debris of the utricular side.

Different maneuvers have been proposed for the treatment of LSC apogeotropic BPPV. The 270° barbecue maneuver toward the healthy side was proposed by Lempert.[28] Other authors suggested a 360° barbecue maneuver departing from the healthy side.[29,30]

The Vannucchi-Asprella maneuver is a modification of the barbecue maneuver. When the patient is in supine position, the head is quickly turned 90° to the healthy side. The patient is brought to the sitting position with the head still rotated and then head is slowly turned back to the neutral position. The maneuver is repeated 5-8 times at the same session.[31]

Vannucchi et al.[32] proposed the technique of "forced prolonged position" (FPP), which consists of forced immobility on the affected side for 12 hours.

Gufoni et al.[33] used a therapeutic maneuver that is a form of a modified Semont's maneuver. This maneuver was performed with the patient beginning in the sitting position and lying quickly to the affected side in the apogeotropic variant and then rotating the head 45° downward, maintaining the position for 2-3 minutes, then the patient is brought to the sitting position again.

Kim et al.[34] used a modified barbecue maneuver that includes a step aiding utricular otoconia to deposit.

Head shaking has also been proposed as a nonspecific maneuver with some degrees of success. The rapid alternating movements lead to detachment of the otoconia from the cupula.[24]

Table 9A.2: Common maneuvers performed for cupulolithiasis of the lateral semicircular canal.

Maneuver	Direction	Conversion to canalithiasis	Direct cure
Barbecue	Healthy side	+	+
Asprella Libonati	Healthy side	++	–
Gufoni	Diseased side	++	+++
Forced prolonged position	• Diseased side • Healthy side	+ –	++ +
Head rotations	Nonspecific	+	±
Head shaking	Nonspecific	+	+

(–: Not effective; ±: Questionable efficacy; +: Reflect degree of effectiveness).

The results of these maneuvers vary according to different authors and range from 20.2 to 81.3%. The FPP and the Gufoni maneuver seem to have better results though results among different authors again vary widely (Table 9A.2).[20]

Our current treatment strategy is as follows:

An attempt is first made to transform the apogeotropic nystagmus to geotropic nystagmus. This is done by head shaking in the horizontal plane followed by a barbecue maneuver to the healthy side. After that, the patient is retested and if conversion occurs, treatment proceeds as for the geotropic lateral canal BPPV. If apogeotropic nystagmus persists, FPP on the diseased side is advised for 8–12 hours. These maneuvers would help shift free debris from the anterior to the posterior arm of the lateral canal or in cupulolithiasis where debris are on the canal side, they would possibly dislodge the particles into the canal. Patients are then assessed next day and if apogeotropic nystagmus persists, barbecue maneuver is again performed to the healthy side followed by FPP. These cases are probably due to particles sticking to the utricular side of the cupula. When the patient sleeps on the healthy side, the contralateral diseased cupula is located uppermost and the gravitational force tends to dislocate the particles into the vestibule (Fig. 9A.5). In obese or pregnant patients who cannot tolerate the barbecue maneuver, and for cases with persistent disease, the Gufoni maneuver is to be performed. In cases with excessive vegetative symptoms, which are more frequently encountered when compared to the posterior canal BPPV, or with marked cervical spondylosis, the FPP can be utilized alone. Because of the severity of symptoms and the need to modify the treatment according to the results (e.g. transformation to geotropic or in case of utricular versus canal side otoconia) we always prefer to reassess all the patients one day following therapeutic maneuvers.

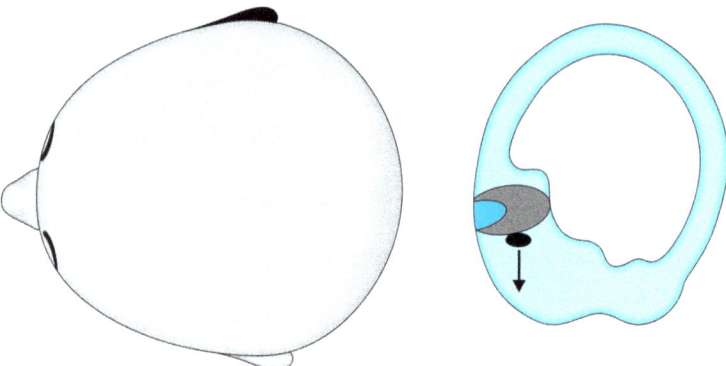

Fig. 9A.5: Right apogeotropic lateral semicircular canal benign paroxysmal positional vertigo on the utricular side. Forced prolonged position to the healthy side leads to dislodgment of the otoconia to the vestibule.

Natural Course

The natural course of the lateral canal BPPV is short. Imai et al.[9] found the average time taken from the onset of the disease to complete remission to be 13 days for the apogeotropic variant.

REFERENCES

1. Korres SG, Balatsouras DG. Diagnostic, pathophysiologic, and therapeutic aspects of benign paroxysmal positional vertigo. Otolaryngol Head Neck Surg. 2004;131:438-44.
2. Schuknecht HF. Cupulolithiasis. Arch Otolaryngol. 1969;90:113-26.
3. Moriarty B, Rutka J, Hawke M. The incidence and distribution of cupulae deposits in the labyrinth. Laryngoscope. 1992;102:56-9.
4. Karlberg M, Hall K, Quickert N, et al. What inner ear diseases cause benign paroxysmal positional vertigo? Acta Otolaryngol. 2000;120:380-5.
5. Vibert D, Sans A, Kompis M, et al. Ultrastructural changes in otoconia of osteoporotic rats. Audiol Neurotol. 2008;13:293-301.
6. Baloh, RW. Clinical features and pathophysiology of posterior canal benign positional vertigo. Audiol Med. 2005;3:12-5.
7. Squiresa TM, Weidmanb MS, Hainc TC, et al. A mathematical model for top-shelf vertigo: the role of sedimenting otoconia in BPPV. J Biomech. 2004;37:1137-46.
8. House MG, Honrubia V. Theoretical models for the mechanisms of benign paroxysmal positional vertigo. Audiol Neurotol. 2003;8:91-9.
9. Imai T, Takeda N, Ito M, et al. 3D analysis of benign positional nystagmus due to cupulolithiasis in posterior semicircular canal. Acta Otolaryngologica. 2009;129:1044-9.
10. Soto-Varela A, Rossi-Izquierdo M, Sanchez-Sellero I, et al. Revised criteria for suspicion of non-benign positional vertigo. QJM. 2013;106:317-21.

11. Ichijo H. Cupulolithiasis of the posterior semicircular canal. Am J Otolaryngol Head Neck Surg. 2013;34:458-63.
12. Epley JM. The canalith repositioning procedure for treatment of benign paroxysmal positional vertigo. Otolaryngol Head Neck Surg. 1992;107:399-404.
13. Semont A, Freyss G, Vitte E. Benign paroxysmal positional vertigo and provocative manoeuvres. Ann Otolaryngol Chir Cervicofac. 1989;106:473-6.
14. Buttner U, Helmchen Ch, Brandt TH. Diagnostic criteria for central versus peripheral positioning nystagmus and vertigo: a review. Acta Otolaryngol (Stockh). 1999;119:1-5.
15. Vicini C, Agus G, De Vito A, et al. Atypical forms and differential diagnosis. Audiol Med. 2005;3:27-36.
16. Fife TD. Recognition and management of horizontal canal benign positional vertigo. Am J Otol. 1998;19:345-51.
17. Imai T, Ito M, Takeda N, et al. Natural course of the remission of vertigo in patients with benign paroxysmal positional vertigo. Neurology. 2005;64:920-1.
18. Cakir BO, Cakir ZA, Civelek S, et al. What is the true incidence of horizontal semicircular canal benign paroxysmal positional vertigo? Otolaryngol Head Neck Surg. 2006;134:451-4.
19. Saleh E. Diagnosis and management of lateral canal benign paroxysmal positional vertigo. Mediterr J Otol. 2006;3:103-11.
20. Riga M, Korres S, Korres G, et al. Apogeotropic variant of lateral semicircular canal benign paroxysmal positional vertigo: is there a correlation between clinical findings, underlying pathophysiologic mechanisms and the effectiveness of repositioning maneuvers? Otol Neurotol. 2013;34:1155-64.
21. Koo JW, Moon IJ, Shim WS, et al. Value of lying-down nystagmus in the lateralization of horizontal semicircular canal benign paroxysmal positional vertigo. Otol Neurotol. 2006;27:367-71.
22. Asprella-Libonati G. Pseudo-spontaneous nystagmus: a new sign to diagnose the affected side in lateral semicircular canal benign paroxysmal positional vertigo. Acta Otorhinolaryngol Ital. 2008;28:73-8.
23. Califano L, Melillo MG, Mazzone S, et al. Secondary signs of lateralization in apogeotropic lateral canalolithiasis. Acta Otorhinolaryngol Ital. 2010;30:78-86.
24. Oh SY, Kim JS, Jeong SH, et al. Treatment of apogeotropic benign positional vertigo: comparison of therapeutic head-shaking and modified Semont maneuver. J Neurol. 2009;256:1330-6.
25. Choi JY, Kim JS, Choi SY, et al. Apogeotropic central positional nystagmus: characteristics and mechanisms. Eur J Neurol. 2014;21(Suppl 1):275.
26. Lechner C, Taylor RL, Todd C, et al. Causes and characteristics of horizontal positional nystagmus. J Neurol. 2014;261:1009-17.
27. Taylor RL, Chen L, Lechner C, et al. Vestibular Schwannoma mimicking horizontal cupulolithiasis. J Clin Neurosci. 2013;20:1170-3.
28. Lempert T. Horizontal benign positional vertigo. Neurology. 1994;44:2213-4.
29. Baloh RW, Furman JMR, Halmagyi JM, et al. Recent advances in clinical neurotology. J Vest Res. 1995;5:231-52.
30. Tirelli G, Russolo M. 360-degree canalith repositioning procedure for the horizontal canal. Otolaryngol Head Neck Surg. 2004;131:740-6.

31. Asprella Libonati G, Gagliardi G, Cifarelli D, et al. "Step by step" treatment of lateral semicircular canal canalolithiasis under videonystagmoscopic examination. Acta Otorhinolaryngol Ital. 2003;23:10-5.
32. Vannucchi P, Giannoni B, Pagnini P. Treatment of horizontal semicircular canal benign paroxysmal positional vertigo. J Vestib Res. 1997;7:1-6.
33. Gufoni M, Mastrosimone L, di Nasso F. Repositioning maneuver in benign paroxysmal positional vertigo of the horizontal semicircular canal. Acta Otorhinolaryngol Ital. 1998;8:363-7.
34. Kim SH, Jo SW, Chung WK, et al. A cupulolith repositioning manoeuvre in the treatment of horizontal canal cupulolithiasis. Auris Nasus Larynx. 2012;39:163-8.

9B: SUBJECTIVE BENIGN PAROXYSMAL POSITIONAL VERTIGO

Dimitrios G Balatsouras

INTRODUCTION

Benign paroxysmal positional vertigo (BPPV) is one of the most common clinical entities encountered in a neurotology clinic.[1] Patients with this disorder complain of episodic vertigo of brief duration provoked by head movements and many of them can specify the exact movement that causes their symptoms. Benign paroxysmal positional vertigo is associated with a characteristic paroxysmal positional nystagmus, which is typically torsional-vertical or horizontal, depending on the semicircular canal involved, and is characterized by findings such as latency, crescendo and decrescendo, transience, reversibility, and fatigability. In most of the patients it occurs spontaneously, but it may be secondary to various other conditions, including head trauma, viral neurolabyrinthitis, vertebral-basilar ischemia, postsurgery, and prolonged bed rest as a result of unrelated diseases.[2] Diagnosis in most cases may be easily obtained using the Dix-Hallpike and the supine roll tests. Application of canalith repositioning procedures (CRPs) results in successful treatment of the disease, in most patients.[3]

A problem occasionally encountered in clinical practice is the presence of a positive history of BPPV with a negative diagnostic maneuver for positional nystagmus. Absence of vertigo and paroxysmal nystagmus during the Dix-Hallpike or the supine roll test usually may be attributed to fatigue due to previous motility, remission of the disease, or a different etiology. However, several patients experience a typical brief episode of vertigo with accompanying autonomic symptoms, but nystagmus is missing. This type of subclinical BPPV has been characterized as "subjective BPPV"[4] and, although not rare, has not been extensively studied in the vestibular literature. Although such cases have been quite often mentioned in several reviews and clinical studies on BPPV, in general the patients who did not have nystagmus during the Dix-Hallpike maneuvers have been excluded from the studies, to avoid confusion on the report of the results.[5]

LITERATURE REVIEW

Weider et al.[6] treated a group of 44 patients with BPPV, performing the Epley procedure for its treatment. Twenty-one patients (48%) did not have observable nystagmus in their provocative position during the authors' observation but all had subjective vertigo. However, some of these patients had nystagmus observed by their referring doctors and the authors hypothesized that the phenomenon of fatigue might probably account for these cases. Nine of the patients with subjective BPPV had at least 1-year duration of the disease, presenting the lower cure rate (55.6%). Patients with subjective BPPV in total were less responsive to CRP (76% cure rate) in comparison with patients with typical BPPV (94.7% cure rate), and the authors concluded that the underlying disorder might be another disease, such as vestibular atelectasis. They believed that the absence of observable nystagmus in several patients with typical episodes of brief vertigo during the maneuvers might be attributed to the long duration of the disease that interfered with ocular fixation, suppressing any existent nystagmus.

Norré[7] found 11 (11.5%) patients with no observable nystagmus out of 95 patients with BPPV and labeled them as having atypical paroxysmal vertigo. However, four patients had positional nystagmus in electronystagmography testing. The author treated his patients with vestibular habituation training and had less success in the atypical cases.

Tirelli et al.,[8] in the first study specific for subjective BPPV, found 43 patients fulfilling the criteria for this diagnosis, whereas 198 patients had objective BPPV. No patient was found with clinical findings of horizontal semicircular canal involvement. Treatment by CRP resulted in complete (60.5%) or partial (32.5%) recovery. In three (6.9%) patients the condition remained unchanged, with vertigo of the same intensity, whereas the condition did not worsen in any patient. The authors hypothesized that the lack of nystagmus was attributed to a small quantity of otoconia, leading to triggering of vertigo but not of nystagmus. They concluded that for the purpose of treatment of BPPV via CRPs, it is not essential to observe a positional/positioning nystagmus, but symptoms of vertigo connected to positional and positioning tests are sufficient. Accordingly, in all cases where positional and positioning vertigo is found, even without nystagmus, the patient should immediately undergo a CRP.

The term "subjective BPPV" was first coined by Haynes et al.[4] who noticed that a subset of patients with BPPV experienced positional vertigo on Dix-Hallpike testing, but did not demonstrate positional nystagmus observable to the examiner with the unaided eye. The vertigo in this subset of patients was described as similar to that of patients who had typical (objective) BPPV. The authors diagnosed and treated a group of 35 patients with subjective BPPV and compared it with a group of 127 patients with objective BPPV. Treatment with the Semont maneuver proved almost equally successful to both groups. The authors attributed the lack of nystagmus to fatigued nystagmus from previous testing or from attempts at habituation through provoking head positioning before referral to their setting. Another possibility was that subjective BPPV might be owing to less noxious form of cupulolithiasis or canalithiasis in which the neural signal is strong enough to elicit vertigo but not strong enough to reach the threshold necessary to stimulate the vestibulo-ocular pathway. They concluded that their study supported the use of the Semont maneuver in the treatment of BPPV of both the objective and the subjective type, because the procedure is well tolerated, noninvasive, without side effects and because none of the patients developed worsening symptoms.

Koga et al.[9] studied a group of 167 patients with vertigo/dizziness by means of vector-electronystagmography and the Dix-Hallpike test with the Frenzel goggles. Of the 167 patients, 68 (40.8%) presented with history and findings characterized as BPPV, even in the absence of nystagmus, but only seven (10.3%) of them had positional or positioning nystagmus visible with the Frenzel goggles. The authors characterized this condition as BPPV without nystagmus and attributed its pathogenesis to adaptation. Furthermore, Whitney et al.[10] studied the usefulness of a BPPV subscale developed from current Dizziness Handicap Inventory (DHI) items to determine whether the score could assist the practitioner in identifying individuals with BPPV. The subscale consisted of five items: (1) looking up, (2) difficulty getting out of bed, (3) quick head movements, (4) rolling over in bed, and (5) bending. The authors found that individuals with BPPV had significantly higher mean scores on the BPPV subscale of the DHI, which could serve as a predictor of the likelihood of having BPPV. However, they remarked that a positive Dix-Hallpike test result may depend on the time of day during which the test is performed. A negative result is possible, especially late in the day, because the otoconia may be dispersed throughout the semicircular canal, making it impossible to identify the characteristic nystagmus seen with BPPV. Also, if the patient has undergone vestibular testing immediately preceding the examination, the nystagmus may not be visualized because the nystagmus may have been fatigued from the head positions assumed during testing. Rescheduling the patient for testing early in the morning may be necessary under these circumstances.

In the Chinese literature, Zhang et al.[11] studied the clinical features and therapy of subjective BPPV in a retrospective clinical study. The authors compared a group of 12 patients with subjective BPPV with 24 patients with objective BPPV of the posterior semicircular canal. They found that patients with subjective BPPV had longer latency and shorter duration of the vertigo attacks, and responded more favorably to treatment than patients with objective BPPV.

Anagnostou et al.[12] studied retrospectively 70 patients complaining of dizziness. Thirty-seven (54.1%) of them had a typical history of BPPV with nystagmus and 33 (48.6%) had typical history without nystagmus, which was confirmed by the Dix-Hallpike test and the lateralization maneuver. Patients with typical BPPV were treated by CRPs and patients with subjective BPPV were asked to self-perform Brandt-Daroff exercises. Fifty percent of these patients followed the recommendation, which proved to be successful. All patients with either subjective or objective BPPV were found without vertigo, after 1-year of follow-up. The authors concluded that even in cases with normal neurotological examination, a typical medical history of BPPV, even without evident nystagmus upon positioning, diagnosis and treatment can be carried out, avoiding unnecessary complementary tests. A different aspect of subclinical BPPV was reported by Johkura et al.[13] These authors studied 155 patients complaining of dizziness who had an extremely weak, horizontal, direction changing apogeotropic positional nystagmus that had not been detected by conventional examination under Frenzel goggles, but could be detected only by a camera with infrared illumination and video-oculography. A group of 155 age-matched control subjects without dizziness was used as control. A subtle nystagmus matching that of horizontal semicircular canal BPPV was seen in 98 (49%) out of the 200 patients with chronic dizziness and in only 25 (16.1%) out of 155 patients in the control group. Additionally, a typical history of BPPV was present in 69 (34.5%) of the patients complaining of dizziness versus 18 (11.6%) in the control group. The authors assumed that the patient's weak horizontal positional nystagmus originated from BPPV and applied the Brandt-Daroff exercises as a treatment maneuver for subclinical horizontal canal BPPV. Forty-nine patients who accepted to perform the Brandt-Daroff exercise every day, had better symptom remission, as compared to the patients who did not. They concluded that the high prevalence of very weak horizontal positional nystagmus in patients with isolated chronic dizziness of otherwise unknown origin, together with the high proportion of patients with a history suggestive of BPPV, indicated that a very mild but chronic form of horizontal canal BPPV seems to be relatively common.

Munaro and Silveira[14] studied 86 patients with clinical history of positional vertigo, by positioning tests and vector-electronystagmography. Forty-five (49.45%) of them had typical BPPV and 41 (45.05%) had atypical form. Patients of the latter group presented with brief episodes of positional vertigo upon positional testing but had no nystagmus. The authors found that the two groups differed in associated pathologies, which were more common in atypical cases and in duration of disease, which was longer in patients with atypical BPPV. Also, Caldas et al.[15] analyzed the charts from 1,271 consecutive patients with BPPV examined in the past 6 years by means of the Dix-Hallpike maneuver and the Frenzel goggles. Typical BPPV with dizziness and positioning nystagmus occurred in

1,033 patients (81.3%), whereas BPPV with dizziness and no positioning nystagmus was present in 238 patients (18.7%). The authors applied CRPs and obtained cure or improvement in 77.9% of the patients. Recurrence rate was 21.8%, in 1 year of follow-up. Unfortunately, in this paper separate results of treatment success and recurrence rate for typical and atypical BPPV are not presented.

In a recent publication, Balatsouras and Korres[16] studied prospectively the demographic, clinical, pathogenetic, and nystagmographic features and treatment outcomes of subjective BPPV. They diagnosed during 3 years 63 patients with a positive history for BPPV, Dix-Hallpike or supine roll tests positive for vertigo, but negative for nystagmus. All patients underwent a complete audiologic and neurotologic examination, including videonystagmography. A group of 204 patients with typical BPPV was used for comparison. The authors obtained successful treatment by CRPs in 45 patients with subjective BPPV. Eighteen patients did not respond to treatment, but further diagnostic evaluation revealed transient vertebrobasilar ischemia (five cases), central positional vertigo (two cases), and vestibular paroxysmia (four cases), whereas the remaining seven patients remained undiagnosed. Comparison between patients with subjective and typical BPPV showed similar epidemiological and clinical features. Treatment failed in 13.5% of patients with subjective BPPV, after excluding patients with different causes of positional vertigo, as compared to 7.8% of patients with typical BPPV, which did not differ significantly. The authors concluded that subjective BPPV is quite common, accounting for more than one-fourth of patients with BPPV and sharing common features with objective BPPV, with the exception of nystagmus. Treatment by CRPs should be applied to patients of both groups, but in case of failure further diagnostic evaluation is needed, because another vestibular disease may be implicated.

More recently, Huebner et al.[17] studied patients with BPPV treated between 2003 and 2007. All patients underwent bilateral diagnostic Dix-Hallpike maneuver under Frenzel lenses and with the aid of videonystagmography, as a part of vestibular evaluation. The patients were asked to complete the 25-question DHI pre- and post-treatment by CRPs. The authors calculated DHI scores before and after treatment on both full-scale DHI and subscale DHI, the latter consisting of five items appropriate for the diagnosis of BPPV, as proposed by Whitney et al.[10] There were 36 participants with objective BPPV and 27 with subjective BPPV. The authors found a significant difference between pre- and post-treatment DHI scores for patients in both the subjective and objective groups when using the full-scale and BPPV-specific DHI. No significant difference was noted between groups for their initial or final full-scale and subscale DHI scores. Accordingly, they concluded that because of similar improvement in DHI full-scale and BPPV-specific subscale scores between the two groups following CRP, the presence or absence of nystagmus during Dix-Hallpike maneuvers is not related to the effectiveness of treatment using CRPs.

REVIEWS

The issue of subjective BPPV has also been reported in two reviews. The first one is by Ganança et al.,[18] who assessed 17 papers published between 1990 and 2002 dealing with the main diagnostic and treatment aspects associated with BPPV. The authors supported the use of Frenzel goggles or videonystagmography to study the type and direction of the nystagmus, which could be difficult upon simple observation. They also considered BPPV in the presence of vertigo without nystagmus detected in the Dix-Hallpike test and attributed the lack of nystagmus to habituation because of regular daily head movements. They also reported that the BPPV treatment in the absence of nystagmus is not different from the treatment with nystagmus, identifying the labyrinth involved by means of vertigo manifesting upon change in head position.

The second review was provided by Alvarenga et al.[5] The authors reviewed nine papers, published between 2001 and 2009, dealing with BPPV without nystagmus, whose diagnoses were based solely on clinical history and physical examination. The treatment of BPPV without nystagmus was carried out by means of CRPs or the Brandt-Daroff exercises. The authors reported that 50–97.1% of the patients (mean value of 67.64%) had remission of their symptoms. In several studies which compared treatment results from patients with and without nystagmus, symptom remission was by 17% greater among patients with nystagmus. On the other hand, in another study[4] a significant difference among patients with and without nystagmus was not found, and there was one study[11] in which patients without nystagmus had a significantly higher improvement when compared to the patients who had typical BPPV.

It should be also mentioned, that in the clinical practice guideline for BPPV, provided by the American Academy of Otolaryngology—Head and Neck Surgery Foundation,[19] the members of the panel remarked that several authors have loosened the historical criteria required for BPPV diagnosis with coinage of the term "subjective BPPV" without a positive Dix-Hallpike test. However, they proposed that history alone is insufficient to render an accurate diagnosis of BPPV and the majority of treatment trials and systematic reviews of BPPV require both episodic symptoms of positional vertigo noted in the patients' history and a positive for nystagmus Dix-Hallpike test.

SITTING-UP VERTIGO

A probably different variety of BPPV without nystagmus has been described by Büki et al.[20] These authors presented a group of patients who had typical complaints of BPPV and absence of nystagmus evoked by Dix-Hallpike and supine roll test, but manifested a short spell of vertigo while sitting up from either or both Dix-Hallpike positions. Among 200 consecutive patients with vertigo/dizziness examined in their setting the authors diagnosed 39 patients with typical BPPV and 86 patients with this type of vertigo, which has been named by the authors as "sitting-up vertigo". Twenty patients of the second group were submitted to posturography, and seven of them were found to present trunk oscillations during the act of sitting up and for a short time immediately afterward.

The authors attributed this type of BPPV to chronic short-arm canalolithiasis of the posterior canal on the involved side. According to them, in upright posture the posterior cupula is chronically deflected by the weight of the debris that lies on the utricular surface of the cupula, becoming adapted to the extreme position. During examination in the head hanging position, no nystagmus is evoked because the posterior canal cupula hangs vertically downward, so that it will not be deflected further. Moreover, in this head position the particles fall down from the cupula into the utriculus in the vestibulum. However, the chronically downward deflected cupula acts in an exaggerated fashion when sitting up, by losing its mechanical load, and because it had been adapted to an extreme deflected position. On this occasion, the endolymphatic flow pushes it toward the vestibulum and the patients receive the impression that they are falling forward, resulting in transient retropulsion. Trunk oscillation immediately after sitting up may be elicited by particles falling back onto the cupula in the upright position. The chronic dizziness experienced by patients with this type of disease may be attributed to the constantly changing mechanical load, which the debris exerts on the cupula during everyday activities.

For therapy, the authors suggested repetitive sit-ups from the Dix-Hallpike position at home, 20 times on both sides (with 4–5 seconds in each head-hanging position), once daily, in the morning. They proposed that the head hanging position during this maneuver should liberate the short arm of the posterior canal from otoliths and move them out from the constricted ampullar endolymphatic space.

As this author understands this is a quite common variety of BPPV, frequently encountered in daily clinical practice but it does not occur more frequently than objective BPPV and is probably less frequent than customary subjective BPPV. It may be successfully treated by the repetitive Dix-Hallpike maneuver. This type of disease represents a specific clinical entity with a different pathogenetic mechanism from the common type of subjective BPPV, because patients suffering from this disease experience vertigo only on sitting-up from the head-hanging position and not on lying down, which typically evokes a brief vertigo in patients with customary subjective BPPV.

TERMINOLOGY AND DIAGNOSTIC CRITERIA OF SUBJECTIVE BPPV

Various names have been used to describe BPPV without nystagmus, such as "atypical BPPV," "subclinical BPPV," and "subjective BPPV." It seems that the term "subjective BPPV," first used by Haynes et al.,[4] has prevailed in recent literature and this term has been used throughout this text. According to existing reports,[16] the following diagnostic criteria of subjective BPPV may be used:

1. History of repeated brief episodes of vertigo with changes in head position.
2. Vertigo provoked by the Dix-Hallpike or the supine roll test.
3. Absence of any detectable nystagmus, during and after the provoking maneuvers.
4. Presence of a latency period (usually a few seconds) between the completion of the diagnostic test and the onset of vertigo.
5. The provoked vertigo increases and then resolves within 1–2 minutes. However, in cases positive for involvement of the horizontal semicircular canal, the duration of the vertigo may be longer.
6. Absence of any clinical, laboratory, or imaging evidence for another peripheral or central vestibular disease.

When subjective BPPV is diagnosed, it is recommended to repeat the examination in the morning of the next day, using Frenzel goggles or videonystagmography, to confirm the diagnosis.

PATHOGENESIS

The main issue arising in cases with subjective BPPV is the explanation of the absence of nystagmus in patients with positional vertigo, during the provoking maneuver. Various explanations of this have been offered.

1. *Increased ocular fixation*: Weider et al.[6] hypothesized that the absence of open-eye nystagmus may be owing to excessive ocular fixation. This was attributed to the long duration of the disease that provides adequate time for the development of ocular fixation, to an extent that nystagmus with open eyes cannot be observed.
2. *Limited otoconia*: A more plausible explanation is the hypothesis of limited otoconia.[4,16] It is known that loose otoliths are quite common

in the lumens of all the semicircular canals, being most commonly found in the posterior canal, but their presence is asymptomatic.[21] Clinical manifestation of vertigo depends on the density, volume, and number of the suspending particles, which may vary in different patients. Thus, semicircular canal involvement may be subclinical and the neural signal is not strong enough to elicit symptoms. However, the patient may experience symptoms if a critical mass is surpassed.[22] Initially, vertigo may be the only manifestation if the neural signal is not strong enough to reach the threshold necessary to stimulate the vestibulo-ocular pathway. Apparently, with the increase of loose otoconia, the full picture of BPPV will become evident. It should be noticed that there is significant intersubject variability in the intensity of vertigo and its correlation with nystagmus. Cases of vertigo or dizziness without nystagmus is a common occurrence in clinical practice.[8] For example, during the final stage of caloric irrigations intense vertigo may be present, even in the absence of nystagmus. On the other hand, intense nystagmus may be present accompanied by minimal vertigo. Another example is the clinical evolution of vestibular neuritis in which disappearance of the nystagmus does not always correspond to disappearance of vertigo, which may persist for several days after the nystagmus has ceased. It may be thus concluded that the presence of a small quantity of loose otoconia is usually asymptomatic but may occasionally manifest as vertigo of varying intensity.

3. *Inadequate testing*: A mild positional nystagmus may get unnoticed with the naked eye, but may become evident on examination with Frenzel lenses or nystagmography. Accordingly, a prolonged search for nystagmus (2–3 minutes) should be conducted, using Frenzel glasses or a camera with infrared illumination, in cases with typical history of BPPV and vertigo but absence of nystagmus during positional testing. Another possibility is fatigability of the nystagmus due to dispersion of the loose otoliths during the day. Several patients may be negative for nystagmus on one occasion and on a repeat examination they may present with all the features of typical BPPV.[10] For this reason, in case of a negative test result, the patient should be re-examined early in the morning of the next day.[16]

4. *Disorders of the calcium metabolism*: Gans[23] presented another explanation based on some disorder of the metabolism of calcium. According to the author, the calcium carbonate needs to be in sufficient quantities for the excitation of the nerve endings. Although all humans have some amount of otoconia loose in the endolymph of the vestibular system, this otoconia gets absorbed and it never gets to

a point where it is heavy enough to cause dizziness. Difficulties with calcium absorption may result in the increase of otoliths within the semicircular canals, enabling thus the triggering of vertigo upon head movement.

5. *Posterior canal cupulolithiasis*: Büki[24] presented recently posterior canal cupulolithiasis as an appropriate explanation of subjective BPPV. According to this theory, the common canalolithiasis of the posterior canal occurs when the dislodged otoconia enters the common crus and the common opening of the vertical canals, in the supine position. However, on several circumstances the short arm and the upper surface of the cupula of the posterior canal may catch the debris, because it is located at the most inferior part of the vestibulum. It may be hypothesized that when the patient is in upright position, the debris adhering to the cupula of the posterior canal, should deflect it downward, away from the utricle. Over time, the cupula can adapt itself to this constant abnormal downward displacement. After positioning the patient from sitting to a Dix-Hallpike position, the cupula remains downward deflected and no nystagmus is seen. However, in patients with a more inferiorly attached ampulla and/or more inferiorly head hanging position, the cupula swings over and deflects upward, toward the utriculus, causing a slight, prolonged downbeat nystagmus.

FREQUENCY

In publications dealing with subjective BPPV, the reported data about its frequency are inconsistent. Its frequency may range from 10–12%[7] up to 90%[9] of the patients with BPPV, according to the relevant reports. The mean value of the existing studies (Table 9B.1) is 24.7%. Alvarenga et al.[5] found a mean value of 42% of the patients with BPPV, which was similar to the one found in the Ganança et al.[18] review, who reported that nystagmus was present in 50% of the patients with BPPV. Additionally, Büki et al.[20] found more than double patients with sitting-up vertigo than patients with typical BPPV. It is obvious that the issue of the frequency of subjective BPPV is not yet definitely set. This author is of the opinion that the frequency of subjective BPPV is <50%, and according to own data it approximates 20% of the patients with BPPV,[16] coming close to the mean value of the cumulative results of the previously reported papers.

DIFFERENTIAL DIAGNOSIS

Differential diagnosis between subjective BPPV and other causes of positional vertigo should be performed. There is a long list of such

Table 9B.1: Main pathogenetic theories of subjective BPPV.		
Authors	Theory	Explanation
Weider et al. (1994)[6]	Increased ocular fixation	Long duration of subjective BPPV provides adequate time for development of ocular fixation, so that nystagmus with open eyes cannot be observed
Haynes et al. (2002)[4]	Limited otoconia	Presence of a small quantity of loose otoconia within the canals may manifest as vertigo, but is not enough to provoke positional nystagmus
Tirelli et al. (2001)[8]	Inadequate testing	Fatigability of the positional nystagmus or difficulty in recording on naked-eye examination, without Frenzel lenses or camera with infrared illumination
Gans (2014)[23]	Disorders of the calcium metabolism	Difficulties with calcium absorption may result in the increase of otoliths within the canals, enabling the triggering of vertigo upon head movement
Büki (2014)[24]	Posterior canal cupulolithiasis	In upright position, the otoconia adhering to the cupula of the posterior canal deflects it downward, away from the utricle, but no nystagmus is seen, due to adaptation. In Dix-Hallpike test, the cupula remains downward deflected and no nystagmus is seen

(BPPV: Benign paroxysmal positional vertigo).

disorders, either central or peripheral.[25] The most significant central causes of positional vertigo include transient vertebrobasilar ischemia and central positional vertigo. Several central positional vertigo syndromes have been described, characterized mainly by prolonged nystagmus, usually downbeating, vertigo, and vomiting.[25,26] All patients who do not respond to treatment should be evaluated with magnetic resonance imaging to detect a central lesion. Less frequent causes of central positional vertigo[27] include cerebellar infarcts, small cerebellar hemorrhages, medulloblastoma, cerebellar degeneration, Arnold-Chiari malformation, and basilar invagination.

Peripheral causes of positional vertigo may include[25] perilymph fistulas, superior canal dehiscence syndrome, atypical Ménière disease, vestibular atelectasis, and positional vertigo with specific gravity differential between cupula and endolymph. In addition, vestibular paroxysmia attributed to neurovascular cross-compression may be implicated.[28]

TREATMENT

All authors proposed treatment using the same CRPs as those used for the typical BPPV. In various studies (Table 9B.2) the Epley (modified),

Table 9B.2: Frequency, type of treatment, and treatment outcome in subjective and objective BPPV.

Authors	No		% (sBPPV–oBPPV)	Outcome	
	sBPPV	oBPPV		sBPPV	oBPPV
Weider et al. (1994)[6]	21	23	48–52%	Epley	76%
Norré (1995)[7]	11	84	11.6–88.4%	Vestibular habituation training	
Tirelli et al. (2001)[8]	43	–	–	Epley	93%
Haynes et al. (2002)[4]	35	127	22–78%	Semont	86%
Koga et al. (2004)[9]	61	7	90–10%	–	–
Zhang et al. (2007)[11]	12	24	33–66%	CRP not specified	91.7%
Anagnostou et al. (2007)[12]	33	37	47–53%	Epley-Semont for oBPPV Brandt-Daroff for sBPPV	50% treated with Brandt-Daroff: remission after 1 year
Johkura et al. (2008)[13]	98 with weak, horizontal, positional nystagmus, and dizziness			Brandt-Daroff	
Munaro et al. (2009)[14]	41	45	47.7–52.3%	–	–
Caldas et al. (2009)[15]	238	1033	18.7–81.3%	CRPs not specified	
Balatsouras and Korres (2012)[16]	52	204	20.3–79.7%	Epley-Barbecue	86.5%
Huebner et al. (2013)[17]	27	36	42.9–57.1%	Epley Semont Appiani	

(BPPV: Benign paroxysmal positional vertigo; sBPPV: Subjective BPPV; oBPPV: Objective BPPV; CRP: Canalith repositioning procedures).

Semont, Appiani, and barbecue CRPs have been used. Occasionally, the Brandt-Daroff set of exercises has been administered.[12,13] In most studies, similar success rates were found in both groups of patients, those with subjective and those with objective disease.[4,16,17] Weider et al.[6] reported worse results for the subjective BPPV, whereas Zhang et al.[11] reported better treatment outcomes for the same group. In most studies, there is not adequate follow-up and report of recurrence rate, to extract valid conclusions, but the author's opinion is that this is similar to that of typical BPPV.

CONCLUSION

Subjective BPPV, defined as a positive history of BPPV with a positioning test positive for vertigo but negative for nystagmus, is a common occurrence, accounting probably for approximately one-fourth of patients with BPPV. Its demographic, clinical, pathogenetic, and nystagmographic features are similar to those of objective BPPV. Treatment is based on the application of the appropriate CRP, depending on the provoking positioning test. Similar success rates as those obtained in patients with objective BPPV are expected. In case of failure of treatment by CRP, further diagnostic workup is recommended, to detect possible central positional vertigo.

REFERENCES

1. Katsarkas A. Benign paroxysmal positional vertigo (BPPV): idiopathic versus post-traumatic. Acta Otolaryngol. 1999;119:745-9.
2. Korres SG, Balatsouras DG. Diagnostic, pathophysiologic, and therapeutic aspects of benign paroxysmal positional vertigo. Otolaryngol. Head Neck Surg. 2004;131:438-44.
3. Korres SG, Balatsouras DG, Papouliakos S, et al. Benign paroxysmal positional vertigo and its management. Med Sci Monit. 2007;13:CR275-282.
4. Haynes DS, Resser JR, Labadie RF, et al. Treatment of benign positional vertigo using the Semont maneuver: efficacy in patients presenting without nystagmus. Laryngoscope. 2002;112:796-801.
5. Alvarenga GA, Barbosa MA, Porto CC. Benign paroxysmal positional vertigo without nystagmus: diagnosis and treatment. Braz J Otorhinolaryngol. 2011;77:799-804.
6. Weider DJ, Ryder CJ, Stram JR. Benign paroxysmal positional vertigo: analysis of 44 cases treated by the canalith repositioning procedure of Epley. Am J Otol. 1994;15:321-6.
7. Norré ME. Reliability of examination data in the diagnosis of benign paroxysmal positional vertigo. Am J Otol. 1995;16:806-10.
8. Tirelli G, D'Orlando E, Giacomarra V, et al. Benign positional vertigo without detectable nystagmus. Laryngoscope. 2001;111:1053-6.
9. Koga KA, Resende BD, Mor R. Estudo da prevalência de tonturas/vertigens e das alterações vestibulares relacionadas à mudança de posição de cabeça por meio da vectoeletronistagmografia computadorizada. Rev. CEFAC. 2004;6:197-202.
10. Whitney SL, Marchetti GF, Morris LO. Usefulness of the dizziness handicap inventory in the screening for benign paroxysmal positional vertigo. Otol Neurotol. 2005;26:1027-33.
11. Zhang JH, Huang J, Zhao ZX, et al. Clinical features and therapy of subjective benign paroxysmal positional vertigo. Zhonghua Er Bi Yan Hou Tou Jing Wai Ke Za Zhi. 2007;42:177-80.

12. Anagnostou E, Mandellos D, Patelarou A, et al. Benign paroxysmal positional vertigo with and without manifest positional nystagmus: an 18-month follow-up study of 70 patients. HNO. 2007;55:190-4.
13. Johkura K, Momoo T, Kuroiwa Y. Positional nystagmus in patients with chronic dizziness. J Neurol Neurosurg Psychiatry. 2008;79:1324-46.
14. Munaro G, Silveira AF. Avaliação vestibular na vertigem posicional paroxística benigna típica e atípica. Rev. CEFAC. 2009;11:76-84.
15. Caldas MA, Ganança CF, Ganança FF, et al. Clinical features of benign paroxysmal positional vertigo. Braz J Otorhinolaryngol. 2009;75:502-6.
16. Balatsouras DG, Korres SG. Subjective benign paroxysmal positional vertigo. Otolaryngol Head Neck Surg. 2012;146:98-103.
17. Huebner AC, Lytle SR, Doettl SM, et al. Treatment of objective and subjective benign paroxysmal positional vertigo. J Am Acad Audiol. 2013;24:600-06.
18. Ganança MM, Caovilla HH, Munhoz MSL, et al. Lidando com a vertigem posicional paroxística benigna. Acta ORL. 2005;23:20-7.
19. Bhattacharyya N, Baugh RF, Orvidas L, et al.; American Academy of Otolaryngology—Head and Neck Surgery Foundation. Clinical practice guideline: benign paroxysmal positional vertigo. Otolaryngol Head Neck Surg. 2008;139 (Suppl 4):S47-S81.
20. Büki B, Simon L, Garab S, et al. Sitting-up vertigo and trunk retropulsion in patients with benign positional vertigo but without positional nystagmus. J Neurol Neurosurg Psychiatry. 2011;82:98-104.
21. Moriarty B, Rutka J, Hawke M. The incidence and distribution of cupulae deposits in the labyrinth. Laryngoscope. 1992;102:56-9.
22. Korres S, Balatsouras DG, Kaberos A, et al. Occurrence of semicircular canal involvement in benign paroxysmal positional vertigo. Otol. Neurotol. 2002;23:926-32.
23. Gans R. Benign paroxysmal positional vertigo: a common dizziness sensation. Audiology Online serial on the internet. 2002 Apr. Available from http://www.audiologyonline.com/articles/benign-paroxysmal-positional-vertigo-common-1150 [Assessed 16 Dec 2014].
24. Büki B. Benign paroxysmal positional vertigo-toward new definitions. Otol Neurotol. 2014;35:323-8.
25. Brandt T. Central positional vertigo. In: Brandt T, (Ed). Vertigo: its multisensory syndromes, 2nd edition. London: Springer; 2003. pp. 291-9.
26. Büttner U, Helmchen C, Brandt T. Diagnostic criteria for central versus peripheral positioning nystagmus and vertigo: a review. Acta Otolaryngol. 1999;119:1-5.
27. Bertholon P, Bronstein AM, Davies RA, et al. Positional down beating nystagmus in 50 patients: cerebellar disorders and possible anterior semicircular canalithiasis. J Neurol Neurosurg Psychiatry. 2002;72:366-72.
28. Hüfner K, Barresi D, Glaser M, et al. Vestibular paroxysmia: diagnostic features and medical treatment. Neurology. 2008;71:1006-14.

9C: CANAL SWITCH AND RE-ENTRY PHENOMENON IN BENIGN PAROXYSMAL POSITIONAL VERTIGO

Francesco Dispenza, Alessandro De Stefano, Maria Giglione, Rosetta Stagno, Sebastian Bianchini, Calogero Giancarlo Scarnà, Salvatore Maira, Ettore Bennici

Vertigo is a frequent and frustrating symptom for which patients seek help from an otolaryngologist, and benign paroxysmal positional vertigo (BPPV) accounts for ~20% of vestibular complaint,[1] becoming the most common cause of peripheral vertigo observed.[2] Diagnosis of BPPV is based mainly on history of onset of vertigo along with the elicitation of nystagmus during diagnostic maneuvers. This disease is generally underestimated by general practitioner and also by patients that wait some time before to refer an otologist. The most possible reason for this is the benign behavior of the disease and the fact that the pathology has a good probability to solve spontaneously.

The clinical features of BPPV are dominated by canal symptoms in acute condition (brief and intense spells of vertigo after hyperextension or hyperflexion of the head, lying down or standing up from lying position) and macular symptoms after acute condition (prolonged instability which persists even after that patient has recovered from canal symptoms).[3]

Being a mechanical disorder of the posterior labyrinth, the management consists of a "mechanical" repositioning of the otoconial debris detached from vestibular sensorineural epithelia. Posterior semicircular canal (PSC) is the most involved by BPPV with ~90% of cases, while horizontal semicircular canal (HSC) is the next most common.[4] Both theories canalithiasis and cupulolithiasis were accepted as pathophysiology of the BPPV, confirmed also by intraoperative findings of otoconial debris into canal.[5] The repositioning maneuvers to treat canalithiasis are well established and widespread used, with some variation recently reported in literature.[6-8]

The recurrence of the BPPV may be linked to some systemic diseases,[9,10] but the true recurrence should be differentiated from the persistence of the canalithiasis often due to a reflux of otoliths.

Although the repositioning maneuvers are free of major complications, a form of canalithiasis called "re-entry BPPV" may appear after therapeutic maneuvers.[11] Such kind of positional vertigo could also be called "canal switch BPPV" if the canal involved is different from the firstly affected canal,[12] before any repositioning session. These clinical entities arose when the maneuvers became common in clinical practice; hence, the clinician should consider a quick differential diagnosis distinguishing a re-entry form from a recurrent BPPV by an early verifying test.

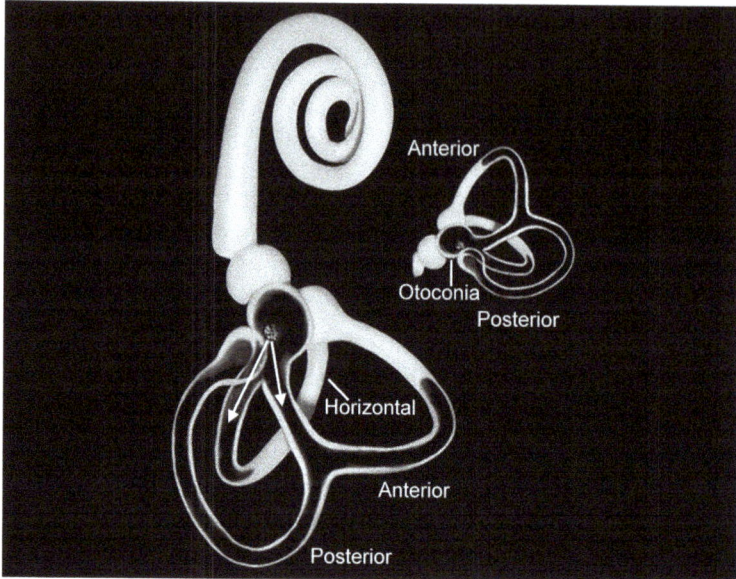

Fig. 9C.1: Right labyrinth with indication of possible otoconia reflux from vestibule to semicircular canals.

The treatment of BPPV is often simple and immediate, giving to the patient a prompt resolution of the symptoms. Sometimes, the neurotologists encounter patients with resistant BPPV requiring several maneuvers to reach the results, or patients that after an initial resolution of symptoms show again some delayed positional nystagmus, due to a canal re-entry of otoliths.

The reflux of otoliths into semicircular canals or them switching to other different canals is made possible by the casual position of otolith near the vestibular opening of the semicircular canal. Some head position gets after repositioning maneuver: early as a verify Dix-Hallpike test or after several days as supine position at home may cause the reflux of otoliths into canal, giving the patient a recurrence of symptoms (Fig. 9C.1).

We described two forms of canal re-entry and/or canal switch. The first is immediate, occurring some minutes after the repositioning session. The second is delayed, occurring after one or two days since maneuvers were done.[13]

The immediate reflux of otolith into PSC after a repositioning maneuver could be mistaken for a contralateral SSC BPPV, being the two form of nystagmus similar. As reported by Foster et al.[11] such form of nystagmus should be differentiated because in PSC reflux it is finest due to inhibiting endolymphatic flow. However, being that discrimination very difficultly detectable, the clinician should consider that it is highly unlikely that a contralateral disease, never diagnosed before, appears after a repositioning procedure.

The clinical experience in detect some canal conversion after reposition procedure was reported also by Babic et al. that described the transitional BPPV and the conversion occurred in a great number of cases after the final check to assess the freeing of the semicircular canal.[14] A great number of conversion in HSC cupulolithiasis is in our opinion not to be expected, because could be influenced by the consideration of all apogeotropic nystagmus in HSC as cupulolithiasis, rather than contemplate also the possibility of otolith in the ampullary arm of HSC, manageable with appropriate maneuver.[4]

The apogeotropic nystagmus in PSC during head-hanging position could be due to otolith into the nonampullary arm of PSC.[15] It could be possible that the apogeotropic nystagmus observed after retest could be caused by otolith mass stopped into ampullary arm, but if a liberatory nystagmus after first repositioning procedure is detected, the hypothesis of the otolith stopped into ampullary arm is less probably as cause of apogeotropic nystagmus.[13]

The BPPV patients may have a variable otoliths mass, ranging from fine particles unable to eliciting a clinical evident nystagmus,[16] to high mass particles visible with operating microscope.[5] The mass of otoliths in our opinion, supported by our results in clinical experience, have a role in determining not only the difficulty to obtain the particles repositioning, but also in the type of canal re-entry if presents.

We agree with the theory that the patients cleared with a single maneuver are likely to have some high mass or aggregated particles.[11] In those patients with an immediate reflux episode, the particles after the treatment procedure were probably located near the openings of the common crus and HSC, so the re-entry was more simple in case of high mass particles rather than dispersed otoliths.

The great portion of patients with BPPV requires a single maneuver to clean the canal. Those patients requiring more than three repositioning maneuvers to achieve the cleaning of the canal (negative Dix-Hallpike control test) have probably a large number of low-mass otoliths that are dispersed into utricle during the numerous maneuvers performed. Effectively, the patients with delayed re-entry/canal switch undergo generally more than two maneuvers in the same session and a negative final Dix-Hallpike/Roll test. The canal re-entry or switch could be evident after an average of 2–3 days; perhaps this time lapse is necessary in assembling the particles into utricle before a casual re-entry.

Certainly, to distinguish a delayed canal re-entry from a recurrence could be intriguing. The only consideration that leads us to believe that after 2–3 days a recurrence is effectively a re-entry phenomenon is the direction change of the nystagmus (i.e. a geotropic before the treatment becomes apogeotropic for PSC). For canal switch from PSC to LSC (lateral semicircular canal), BPPV the observation is different, because it is very likely that a new episode of BPPV after a few days since treatment affecting a different canal of the same side is due to re-entry of otoliths.

Foster et al. showed a relationship between timing of final test and canal re-entry.[11] These findings lead to couple the cause of re-entry BPPV or canal switch with the repetition of Dix-Hallpike test to assess the cleaning of the canal. We described the evidence that the minimum time that we should wait before doing a verification test, to reduce the risk of immediate re-entry/canal switch, was 10 minutes.[13] The delayed canal re-entry is not preventable increasing the time before performing the verification test, but it depends likely by a casual position/movements done by patients.

CONCLUSION

The canal re-entry or canal switch is a clinical entity that should be kept in mind of the neurotologist approaching the BPPV patients. It is important distinguishing it from recurrence when delayed and from maneuver failure when immediate. Probably, the mass of otoliths has a role in determining the type of canal re-entry. The timing of maneuver performing, in particular the final verification test after therapeutic sessions, is important to prevent the immediate reflux of particles into canals.

REFERENCES

1. De Stefano A, Dispenza F, Citraro L, et al. Are postural restrictions necessary for management of posterior canal benign paroxysmal positional vertigo? Ann Otol Rhinol Laryngol. 2011;120:460-64.
2. Dispenza F, De Stefano A, Mathur N, et al. Benign paroxysmal positional vertigo following whiplash injury: a myth or a reality? Am J Otolaryngol. 2011;32:376-80.
3. Marciano E, Marcelli V. Postural restrictions in labyrintholithiasis. Eur Arch Otorhinolaryngol. 2002;259:262-5.
4. Riggio F, Dispenza F, Gallina S, et al. Management of benign paroxysmal positional vertigo of lateral semicircular canal by Gufoni's manoeuvre. Am J Otolaryngol. 2009;30:106-11.
5. Parnes LS, Mc Clure JA. Free-floating endolymph particles: a new operative finding during posterior semicircular canal occlusion. Laryngoscope. 1992;102:988-92.
6. Dispenza F, Kulamarva G, De Stefano A. Comparison of repositioning maneuvers for benign paroxysmal positional vertigo of posterior semicircular canal: advantages of hybrid maneuver. Am J Otolaryngol. 2012;33:528-32.
7. Asprella Libonati G, Gagliardi G, Cifarelli D, et al. Step by step treatment of lateral semicircular canal canalolithiasis under videonystagmoscopic examination. Acta Otorhinolaryngol Ital. 2003;23:10-15.

8. Yacovino DA, Hain TC, Gualtieri F. New therapeutic maneuver for anterior canal benign paroxysmal positional vertigo. J Neurol. 2009;256:1851-5.
9. De Stefano A, Dispenza F, Suarez H, et al. A multicenter observational study on the role of comorbidities in the recurrent episodes of benign paroxysmal positional vertigo. Auris Nasus Larynx. 2014;41:31-6.
10. Talaat HS, Abuhadied G, Talaat AS, et al. Low bone mineral density and vitamin D deficiency in patients with benign positional paroxysmal vertigo. Eur Arch Otorhinolaryngol. 2015;272(9):2249-53.
11. Foster CA, Zaccaro K, Strong D. Canal conversion and reentry: a risk of Dix-Hallpike during canalith repositioning procedures. Otol Neurotol. 2012;33:199-203.
12. Lin GC, Basura GJ, Wong HT, et al. Canal switch after canalith repositioning procedure for benign paroxysmal positional vertigo. Laryngoscope. 2012;122:2076-8.
13. Dispenza F, De Stefano A, Costantino C, et al. Canal switch and re-entry phenomenon in benign paroxysmal positional vertigo: difference between immediate and delayed occurrence. Acta Otolaryngol Ital. 2015;35:116-20.
14. Babic BB, Jesic SD, Milovanovic JD, et al. Unintentional conversion of benign paroxysmal positional vertigo caused by repositioning procedures for canalithiasis: transitional BPPV. Eur Arch Otolaryngol. 2014;271:967-73.
15. Vannucchi P, Pecci R, Giannoni B, et al. Apogeotropic Posterior Semicircular Canal Benign Paroxysmal Positional Vertigo: Some Clinical and Therapeutic Considerations. Audiol Res. 2015; 5(1):130
16. Balatsouras DG, Koukoutsis G, Ganelis P, et al. Diagnosis of single- or multiple-canal benign paroxysmal positional vertigo according to the type of nystagmus. Otolaryngol. 2011;2011:48-3965.

9D: BPPV INVOLVING MULTIPLE CANALS

Alfarghal Mohamad, Essam Saleh

OVERVIEW

Benign paroxysmal positional vertigo (BPPV) is the most common cause of recurrent vertigo, with a lifetime prevalence of 2.4%. It is a condition that in most instances may be easily diagnosed and treated, with a simple office-based procedure.[1,2] Benign paroxysmal positional vertigo is characterized by brief periodic vertigo when the head is moved into certain positions. The most relevant etiology of this disorder is idiopathic (>50%) followed by post-traumatic (14-27%). Other causes include labyrinthitis, vertebrobasilar ischemia, Ménière's disease, chronic otitis, and ototoxicity.[3] The posterior canal is unilaterally affected in most cases, less commonly the problem is found in one of the horizontal canals and even more rarely in the anterior canal (AC), although it is uncommon for more than one canal in a single ear or bilaterally to be affected, it is not exceptional in the literature and such cases represent 6-20% of all patients with BPPV. Katsraks had defined bilateral disease as occurring only when both ears are simultaneously affected and reported that BPPV may present bilaterally in 7.5-15% of all cases.[4-9]

EPIDEMIOLOGY

Benign paroxysmal positional vertigo due to posterior canal involvement is the most common type of BPPV, accounting for up to 90% of the patients.[6] Benign paroxysmal positional vertigo originating from stimulation of the horizontal semicircular canal is the second most common type of BPPV, accounting for ~5-15% of the patients but its frequency has been occasionally reported up to 30%.[10-13] Unilateral anterior canal benign positional paroxysmal vertigo (AC-BPPV) is quite rare and its incidence has been reported to range from 1-2% to 15% of positional vertigo cases.[6,14] An apogeotropic variant of posterior BPPV (APC-BPPV) has recently been described in cases previously misdiagnosed as anterior canal BPPV, according to Vannucchi et al. It represents 2.5% of BPPV cases, and AC-BPPV represents only 1.2% of the cases.[15-17] Bilateral benign paroxysmal positional vertigo (biBPPV) is rather rare, accounting for 6-26% in the reported BPPV series. According to Pollack et al. 10% of BPPV cases showed positive Dix-Hallpike test in both sides, almost half of those cases were not true bilateral but rather unilateral mimicking bilateral cases of BPPV.[6,8,18]

ETIOLOGY

Despite the quite large amount of information about the mechanism of BPPV today, the cause of BPPV is known only in a small proportion of patients. Further studies for elucidation of the causes that lead to displacement of otoliths in cases of idiopathic BPPV are certainly justified.[8] Baloh et al. reported that head trauma in general is a well-recognized etiology, and has been documented in 17% of 240 patients presenting with BPPV. The etiology of head trauma was considered when it preceded symptoms by no more than 3 days, although they made no reference to the exact type and mechanism of trauma.[3] Patients with post-traumatic BPPV have a significantly higher incidence of bilateral involvement than do those with idiopathic BPPV. The incidence of biBPPV was significantly higher among post-trauma patients (14.3%) compared to those with idiopathic BPPV (6.3%).[19] Generally, the presence of bilateral disease has been reported to be often of traumatic origin.[5,20,21]

PATHOPHYSIOLOGY

Pollak et al. reported that more patients with biBPPV than unilateral BPPV were of traumatic origin (12.5% vs 0.9%), and they concluded that bilaterality of BPPV is probably a result of a mechanism mechanism that causes the debris dislodgment. The presence of bilateral disease has statistically significant influence on the number of treatment sessions necessary for the relief of symptoms. It is considered to have a less favorable prognosis than unilateral BPPV. Pollak et al. did not find differences in age, sex, duration of symptoms or treatment responsiveness between bilateral BPPV, unilateral mimicking bilateral BPPV and unilateral BPPV when compared separately.[8]

Pathophysiology of bilateral BPPV remains the same as unilateral cases based on the two main theories that explain BPPV, the more accepted theory that is canalolithiasis. Canalolithiasis is the implicated pathogenetic mechanism for this disorder, characterized by the presence of free floating debris within the posterior semicircular canal, detached from the otoconial layer by degeneration or head trauma. The otoconia gravitates into the posterior canal, where it forms a plug floating in its nonampullary branch. In the provoking Dix-Hallpike position, the endolymph pulls on the cupula, because the free-floating otoconia falls under the influence of gravity. In the vertical canals, ampullofugal deflection produces an excitatory response. This would cause an abrupt onset of vertigo and the typical nystagmus. Nystagmus latency is explained by inertia of the clot. The deflection of the cupula ends when the clot reaches its lowest position and accounts for the limited duration of the nystagmus.

Fatigue is due to dispersion of the clot particles and reactivation after bed rest is caused by renewed clot formation.[22-24]

An alternative pathogenetic theory, the cupulolithiasis of the posterior canal, may account for a small rate of cases with posterior canal BPPV. According to this theory, otoconia with a greater specific gravity than endolymph, originating from a degenerating utricular macula settle on the cupula of the posterior canal, rendering it sensitive to gravity. Certain head movements may then produce inappropriate endolymph cupula displacement, causing nystagmus and vertigo, which in this case is of longer duration. The latency before the onset of nystagmus reflects the inertia of the otoconial mass and the cupula, and the fatiguability is presumably due to dispersal of the debris attached to the cupula or even due to central vestibular adaptation.[23,25]

DIAGNOSIS

Benign paroxysmal positional vertigo is a common cause of vertigo and is characterized by episodes lasting for seconds. The diagnosis is established by inducing a rapid change from the sitting position to the left or right head-hanging position—the Dix-Hallpike maneuver. Typically, a torsional geotropic nystagmus is seen when the affected ear is downmost, accompanied with a sensation of vertigo. Other classic features of the nystagmus in posterior canal BPPV include a latency of several seconds, fatigability and reversal of the direction of nystagmus when the patient returns to the upright sitting position.[24] The Dix-Hallpike provoking maneuver is used to diagnose the disease by moving the patient rapidly from a sitting position to a position of head hanging with each ear alternately undermost. Posterior semicircular canal involvement is proved from the type of the visually observed paroxysmal positioning nystagmus, which is beating toward the undermost and affected ear, with a torsional component clockwise when following leftward movement, or counterclockwise, when following rightward movement.[25] Typically an upbeating nystagmus component is superimposed, resulting in a mixed torsional-vertical eye movement. Intense vertigo in conjunction with this pattern of nystagmus and the additional characteristics of a short latency, limited duration, intensity characterized by crescendo and decrescendo element, reversal on returning to the upright position, and fatiguability on repetitive provocation may easily establish the diagnosis of posterior canal BPPV.[23] The Dix-Hallpike maneuver is usually positive only when performed with the involved ear undermost and negative on the contralateral side, permitting thus easy localization of the side of the lesion. It should also be noticed that posterior canal paroxysmal positional nystagmus is dissociated, with the torsional component being more evident in the ipsilateral eye, and the vertical upbeating component is more evident in the contralateral eye, which can be explained by different angle of insertion of the oblique and rectus muscles.[26,27]

It should be noticed that the character of nystagmus changes with the direction of gaze, which is explained by contraction of the ipsilateral superior oblique and contralateral inferior rectus, following the stimulation of the posterior canal. When the patient lies in the lateral head hanging position, if he looks toward the uppermost unaffected ear, the axes of these two extraocular muscles nearly coincide, resulting in movement of the eyes in a vertical plane with predominance of the vertical component of the nystagmus, when looking toward the lower most involved ear, the axes of these two muscles are nearly at right angles with the direction of the gaze, and their contraction results in apogeotropic rolling of the upper pole of the eye (slow phase) and predominance of the torsional component of the nystagmus with geotropic fast phase.[28]

BILATERAL BPPV VERSUS BILATERALLY SYMPTOMATIZING BPPV

Clinicians should differentiate bilaterally symptomatizing BPPV cases from true bilaterally affected cases. Unilateral horizontal canal BPPV, unilateral anterior canal BPPV, and unilateral mimicking bilateral posterior canal BPPV all can provoke symptoms and nystagmus on both sides. Bilateral BPPV occurs when the disease is affecting same or different canals on either ear simultaneously. Cases where migration of otoconia from one canal to another occurs, as a complication of therapeutic maneuver is not considered multicanal BPPV. Horizontal canal BPPV patients complain that turning the head to either side in the supine position provokes intense vertigo, associated with a purely horizontal paroxysmal positional nystagmus. Vertigo may be more intense than in posterior canal involvement and is usually associated with severe autonomic symptoms. Two major types of horizontal canal BPPV may be distinguished according to the pathogenetic mechanism of canalolithiasis or cupulolithiasis. Canalolithiasis may manifest as BPPV with geotropic paroxysmal nystagmus, and less frequently with apogeotropic nystagmus, when the otoliths are located in the short arm of the horizontal semicircular canal near the ampulla. Cupulolithiasis manifests as apogeotropic persistent nystagmus commonly with absence of latency during the supine roll test (Table 9D.2 and 9D.5).[23]

It has been found that AC-BPPV produces bilaterally positive Dix-Hallpike maneuvers (Table 9D.4).[29] Bilateral posterior canal involvement is presumed when Dix-Hallpike maneuver is positive on both sides.

However, care should be taken to avoid the erroneous diagnosis of pseudobilateral posterior canal BPPV as true bilateral BPPV.[30]

The entity of unilateral mimicking bilateral BPPV was first described by Steddin and Brandt. According to these authors, inappropriate head positioning during testing of the unaffected ear causes displacement of the affected posterior canal from its perpendicular position. This makes the otolith debris move gravitationally toward the cupula, thus causing transient cupulolithiasis and evoking an inhibitory nystagmus. This nystagmus is directed toward the lower unaffected ear and this situation may be erroneously diagnosed as bilateral posterior canal BPPV. The inhibitory nystagmus usually has a lower amplitude and frequency than the excitatory nystagmus of the affected ear, and patients report less symptoms when the unaffected ear is tested.[23,30,31] They have postulated that quite often unilateral BPPV may mimic biBPPV. Their observations are based on performing a body tilt from the sitting position similar to Semont's maneuver and not the Dix-Hallpike maneuver. In their testing, when the head of the patient is parallel to the plane of the body tilt, a tortional geotropic nystagmus may be elicited with the unaffected ear downmost. According to their theory, when the patient is positioned with the unaffected side downmost, without tilting the head on the affected side, the posterior canal becomes uppermost and may also be stimulated by the debris, as it settles on the cupula, ampullopetally. This mechanism of cupulolithiasis on the unaffected side mimics a contralateral BPPV, but the nystagmus is characterized by low amplitude, low frequency, and a longer duration.[23,30,31] It should be taken into consideration that when performing the provoking maneuver, the semicircular canal plane does not always lie in the ideal position.[32] This is due to the fact that the head is put into the required plane by the examiner only approximately by eye judgment. Moreover, the head positioning can be influenced by limitation of the patient's neck movement, his skull form, or hairstyle.[33] The lack of optimal positioning of the semicircular canals is also the cause in cases when horizontal canalithiasis mimics a uni- or bilaterally positive Dix-Hallpike test. However, here, the nystagmus has a clearly horizontal component and should be easily recognized by the examiner.[8]

Differential diagnosis between true bilateral and pseudobilateral posterior canal BPPV may be obtained based on the following. (i) The presence of asymmetric nystagmus and symptoms of different intensity between right and left Dix-Hallpike maneuvers should arouse the suspicion of pseudobilateral posterior BPPV. The side with more intense nystagmus and symptoms may probably be the affected side. (ii) Performance of a head-down test, extending the head of the patient directly backward from the sitting to the supine straight head hanging position, might be helpful, during this test, both posterior canals get irritated, resulting in the appearance of nystagmus. This nystagmus has only a vertical upbeating component, because the torsional components having opposite directions are cancelled. True bilateral BPPV may be concluded in this case, whereas in case that the nystagmus retains its torsional component, pseudobilateral BPPV is probable. The true side of the disease may be found, observing the direction of this component, which beats clockwise on left posterior canal BPPV and counterclockwise on right posterior canal involvement. Pollak et al. reported that for this strategy to be valid patients's eyes should be kept in midposition during examination. (iii) The criterion of responsiveness to treatment is quite helpful. Successful treatment of the patient after performing the appropriate canalith repositioning procedure on the side with more intense manifestations is proof of previously pseudobilateral BPPV.[31,8,30] When it is necessary to repeat the CRP contralaterally to obtain remission of the symptoms, this may be proof of bilateral posterior BPPV.[23]

Pollack et al. studied 232 patients treated for BPPV; they found 28 with bilaterally positive Dix-Hallpike maneuver. Sixteen patients (6%) were diagnosed with biBPPV and 12 (5%) with unilateral mimicking biBPPV.[8] Correct diagnosis of unilateral versus biBPPV may be important when surgical intervention such as a posterior canal occlusion is considered. Parnes and McClure performed a posterior semicircular canal occlusion on an 82-year-old woman diagnosed with biBPPV. Surgery was performed unilaterally, on the more symptomatic side and the patient was free of symptoms on long-term follow-up[34] (Table 9D.1 and Flowchart 9D.1).

ANTERIOR CANAL BPPV

Anterior canal involvement is rare for anatomic considerations, because it is higher in position than the other canals, and its posterior arm descends directly into the common crus and the vestibule, which should lead to continuous self-clearance of otolith from the canal. AC-BPPV is believed to be more frequent in post-traumatic cases.[15,29] The common clinical picture of AC-BPPV is characterized by vertical down-beating paroxysmal nystagmus in the Dix-Hallpike test, as well as in the straight head hanging position, with clockwise torsional component when left canal is involved and counter-clockwise torsional component when right canal is involved, without inversion of the nystagmus when coming back to the sitting position.[15, 39,40] This typical nystagmus is coherent with Flourens-Ewald's law, because it respects the plane of the interested canal, whereas according to Zapala, a unilateral form of AC-BPPV can be presented by a purely vertical down-beating nystagmus due to the orientation of

Flowchart 9D.1: Algorithm for management of bilateral posterior canal BPPV based on work of Pollak et al. and author's experience.

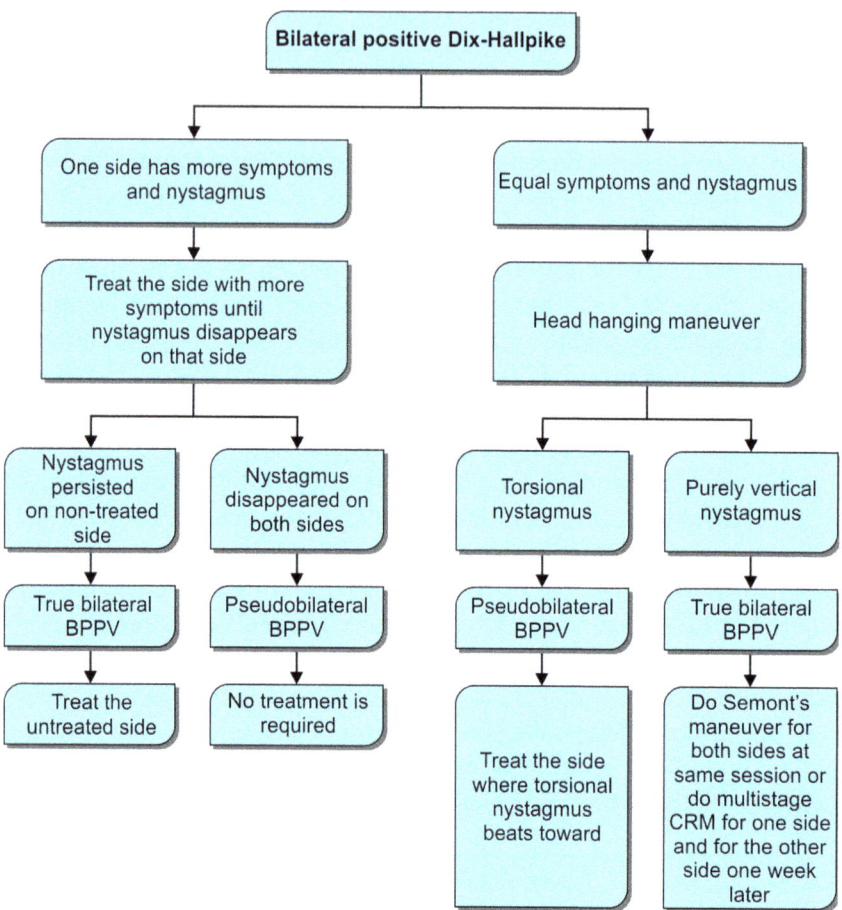

(BPPV: Benign paroxysmal positional vertigo; CRM: Canalith reposition maneuver).

the anterior canal which is closer to the sagittal plane ,and the fact that torsional vestibulo-oculomotor reflex gain is smaller than horizontal and vertical components gain[15, 35] Cambi et al reported that AC-BPPV is a very probable cause of peripheral down beating nystagmus.[36]

To explain AC-BPPV, changes in the diameter of the common crus, stenosis of membranous duct and changes in the position of the canal have been proposed.[37] Downbeating nystagmus syndrome can be associated with cerebellar diseases, and in such cases, it is mandatory to exclude these from peripheral downbeating nystagmus syndrome. Bertholon et al.[29] reported 50 consecutive cases of positional downbeating nystagmus, 12 of which presented without central neurological symptoms or signs and a clinical picture of an AC-BPPV. Cambi et al.

recently showed that the natural course of most cases of downbeating nystagmus syndrome is toward a spontaneous resolution and that it is sometimes associated with BPPV, so that the frequency of peripheral downbeating nystagmus syndrome appears to be more frequent than previously suggested. Cerebral MRI is required in cases of downbeating nystagmus if there are associated neurological signs or symptoms or in case of failure of therapeutic maneuvers (Tables 9D.1 and 9D.4)[36]

APOGEOTROPIC POSTERIOR SEMICIRCULAR CANAL BPPV

Recently, Vannucchi et al. described a new form of BPPV that he called "apogeotropic posterior canal BPPV" that is characterized by a torsional downbeating nystagmus clockwise for the right posterior canal and counterclockwise for the left posterior canal.[15-17] They explained the oculomotor pattern of Apogeotropic Posterior Canal BPPV (APC-BPPV) is caused by ampullopetal stimulation of the posterior semicircular canal due to free-floating otoconial debris in the nonampullary arm, perhaps because putative alterations of posterior canal morphology which can cause otolith entrapment in that zone. The less severe paroxysm could be due to the reduced movement of the otoconial mass and to the weaker inhibitory ampullopetal endolymphatic flow (III Ewald's law) caused by otoliths on diagnostic positioning tests. Differential diagnosis between APC-BPPV and Anterior Canal BPPV is possible due to the prevalence of the torsional component compared with the vertical one in APC-BPPV, whereas differential diagnosis between APC-BPPV and traditional Posterior canal BPPV is possible because of the inverted characteristics of the nystagmus, in APC-BPPV nystagmus is downbeating, clockwise in the right Dix-Hallpike position and counterclockwise in the left Dix-Hallpike position. Anterior canal appears to be rarer than reported in the literature if APC cases identified and no more labeled as AC-BPPV.[15-17]

As reported by Giannoni and Korres, sometimes nystagmus reversed its direction with higher intensity in returning to the sitting position, probably because of the stronger excitatory ampullofugal endolymphatic flow (III Ewald's law).[38-40] APC-BPPV was treated through Quick Liberatory Repositioning maneuver usually used in typical posterior canal BPPV; the efficacy of therapeutic maneuvers in the form of canal conversion or direct resolution of the disease confirmed that oculomotor patterns reported in the literature allow correct identification of both AC-BPPV and APC-BPPV; analysis of positioning-evoked nystagmus through infrared videonystagmography permits differential diagnosis between AC-BPPV, characterized by a prevalent vertical downbeating nystagmus and APC-BPPV in which the torsional component is prevalent and reverted

Table 9D.1: Differentiation between traditional posterior canal, anterior canal, and apogeotropic posterior canal BPPV based on our clinical experience and the above-mentioned references.

	AC-BPPV	APC-BPPV	TPC–BPPV
Tortional component	Less prevalent clockwise left, counterclockwise right	Prevalent tortional component clockwise for the right posterior canal and counterclockwise for the left posterior canal	Prevalent clockwise for left, counterclockwise for right
Vertical component	Downbeating	Downbeating	Upbeating
Reversal of nystagmus	No reversal of nystagmus	Weak reversed nystagmus on sitting from supine position	Weak reversed nystagmus on sitting from supine position
Severity of vertigo and nystagmus	No enough reports, in our experience strong nystagmus but less vertigo	Less severe	Severe
Response to CRP	Respond to Yacovino or reversed Epley's maneuver	Quick Liberatory Maneuver	Respond to Epley's maneuver or Quick Liberatory Maneuver

(AC-BPPV: Anterior canal BPPV; APC-BPPV: Anterior posterior canal BPPV; TPC-BPPV: Traditional posterior canal BPPV).

compared to TPC-BPPV.[15,39,40] A new maneuver proposed for treatment of AC-BPPV is the Yacovino maneuver.[41] Correct differential diagnosis is of significant importance to identify the affected ear and to adopt the most appropriate therapeutic maneuver to obtain a good therapeutic outcome in these rare and atypical forms of BPPV.[15] This variant of APC-BPPV could support the previously mentioned mechanism of unilateral mimicking biBPPV (Tables 9D.1 and 9D.4).

BILATERAL HORIZONTAL CANAL BPPV

Bilateral horizontal canal BPPV is quite difficult to diagnose. The critical point in this case is that during the supine roll test, unilateral horizontal canal BPPV elicits horizontal nystagmus on both sides, either geotropic (canalolithiasis mechanism) or apogeotropic (cupulolithiasis and canalolithiasis mechanism). In a theoretical case of bilateral horizontal BPPV with geotropic nystagmus, supine roll test on either side would result in excitation of the horizontal canal of the lowermost ear due to ampullopetal endolymph flow and at the same time inhibition of the horizontal canal of the uppermost ear due to ampullofugal endolymph flow vectorial summation would result in an intense, symmetric geotropic nystagmus. It may be assumed that the nystagmus would be more intense in apogeotropic bilateral horizontal canal BPPV because of a dual pathogenetic mechanism: inhibition of the horizontal canal of the lower ear and, concurrently, excitation of the horizontal canal of the upper ear. In comparison, in cases with unilateral involvement of the horizontal canal, only one mechanism contributes to the produced apogeotropic nystagmus: either inhibition of the affected ear on turning toward its direction or excitation of the affected ear on turning toward the healthy ear. The same mechanism is valid in cases with canalolithiasis of the ampullary arm of the horizontal canal.[23] It has been reported that 10% of the cases with unilateral horizontal BPPV may present with symmetrical nystagmus.[32]

In cases of bilateral symmetrical nystagmus, owed to bilateral involvement, neither pseudospontaneous nystagmus nor nystagmus during the head down test should be present most of the time. However, if some type of nystagmus could be observed, its direction should not be stable, but changing according to the prevailing movement of otoconia in each horizontal canal. It should be further noticed that the criterion of symmetry of the nystagmus to diagnose bilateral horizontal canal BPPV is not a solid one, because asymmetric involvement of the two horizontal canals may occur as well. Combination of canalolithiasis-cupulolithiasis, either on the same or on different horizontal canals, would complicate the matter further. It has been reported that reversal of the geotropic nystagmus to apogeotropic, while the subject remains in the same lateral position during the supine roll test, may be explained from concomitant canalolithiasis—cupulolithiasis in the horizontal canal of the lower ear.[42] It may be thus concluded that although patients with bilateral disease of the horizontal canal may exist, difficulty in diagnosis may explain why cases with this type of vertigo have been scarcely reported. Horii et al. described such an interesting case of bilateral horizontal BPPV treated successfully by canal plugging of the horizontal canal on one side and the Lempert's maneuver on the other side[43] (Tables 9D.2 and 9D.5).

BILATERAL AC-BPPV

Bilateral AC-BPPV is also very difficult to diagnose. Theoretically, the Dix-Hallpike maneuver on the right side would cause paroxysmal nystagmus with a vertical downbeating component and a torsional component with the upper pole of the eye beating clockwise (at opposite direction of the posterior canal BPPV). This type of nystagmus is attributed to excitation of the contralateral anterior canal. However, the ipsilateral anterior canal would also be excited, resulting in a downbeating vertical component and a torsional component in the opposite direction, but probably of a smaller intensity.[40] The vectorial summation of all the components would result in an intense vertical downbeating component

Table 9D.2: Comparison between unilateral and bilateral horizontal canal BPPV based on above references and author's clinical experience.

	Unilateral HC-BPPV	Bilateral HC-BPPV
Intensity of vertigo and nystagmus	Less intense	More intense
Symmetry of nystagmus	Usually asymmetrical	Theoretically symmetrical
Pseudospontaneous nystagmus	Commonly present	Theoretically rare
Response to unilateral therapeutic maneuver	Symptoms and nystagmus disappear	Symptoms and nystagmus persist

(HC-BPPV: Horizontal canal BPPV).

and a weak torsional component toward the upper ear. In conclusion, the Dix-Hallpike maneuvers on both sides would produce a mixed nystagmus, with an intense vertical and a weak torsional component on both occasions opposite to those of posterior canal involvement. Differential diagnosis would be difficult because in unilateral anterior BPPV, the torsional nystagmus vector may be quite often absent. Furthermore, in a head down test, performed in a similar way as in the case of bilateral posterior canal BPPV, both ACs would get irritated again, resulting in the appearance of nystagmus. This nystagmus should be characterized by only an intense purely vertical downbeating component, because the torsional components would cancel each other, as having opposite directions, a unilateral form of AC can also cause a vertical downbeating nystagmus, due to the orientation of the AC that is closer to the sagittal plane (usually by a 41° angle) than the posterior canal (usually by a 56° angle); these considerations are enough to justify the frequent occurrence of a purely vertical downbeating nystagmus on both sides even in unilateral forms.[29,44] Differential diagnosis on these grounds would not be safe, because unilateral AC involvement, as previously mentioned, may manifest as purely vertical as well. Finally, the criterion of responsiveness to treatment is not helpful in this case, as there is no established therapeutic maneuver for treatment of the AC-BPPV, and both standard Epley and reversed Epley's maneuvers have been used, as well as various specifically designed maneuvers.[41,45] To conclude, although the entity of bilateral anterior BPPV has been previously reported, details concerning its diagnosis and treatment are missing. That makes us believe that this diagnosis is presently highly hypothetical[9,14,23] (Tables 9D.1, 9D.3 and 9D.4).

HORIZONTAL AND POSTERIOR CANAL BPPV

This is the most common case of mixed canal BPPV. The involved canals may be either on the same side or on both sides. Diagnosis may be easily obtained, considering the features of the nystagmus on either maneuver.

Table 9D.3: Comparison between unilateral and bilateral anterior canal BPPV based on above references and author's experience.

	Unilateral AC-BPPV	Bilateral AC-BPPV
Torsional component of nystagmus on head hanging test	Present but can be absent	Absent but can be present
Reponses to unilateral treatment with reversed Epley's maneuver	Symptoms and nystagmus disappear	Symptoms and nystagmus persist

(AC-BPPV: Anterior canal BPPV).

Mixed torsional geotropic-vertical upbeating nystagmus in Dix-Hallpike maneuvers reveals involvement of the posterior canal, additionally geotropic or apogeotropic horizontal nystagmus during the supine roll test will be evidence of horizontal canal BPPV. In most mixed cases, the horizontal nystagmus is geotropic due to canalolithiasis, although cupulolithiasis has been occasionally reported. It should be noticed, however, that during the Dix-Hallpike tests, the horizontal canal is also, at least, partially stimulated, and a horizontal component of nystagmus may be evident in conjunction with the torsional-upbeating nystagmus of posterior canal origin. Additionally, it has been shown that horizontal nystagmus, provoked during the supine roll test, exhibits also a vertical and a torsional component.[20,44-47]

HORIZONTAL AND ANTERIOR CANAL BPPV

Occurrence of this combination is quite unusual, due to rare involvement of the AC. Diagnosis of horizontal canal involvement is evident, according to previously described characteristics of the nystagmus. Anterior canal BPPV may be also diagnosed by an experienced clinician, as already described. The main feature for differential diagnosis from the posterior canal BPPV is the downbeating vertical component of the nystagmus. Additionally, the direction of the torsional component will show if either the ipsilateral or the contralateral canal is involved.[23]

POSTERIOR AND ANTERIOR CANAL BPPV

This combination has also been reported, but its diagnosis presents difficulties. Two categories of involvement should be distinguished on the same side and on different sides.[9,14] If the involved posterior and anterior canal are on the same side, then Dix-Hallpike on this side would cause theoretically a torsional component with the upper eye pole moving geotropically and a vertical upbeating component due to posterior canal disease; a torsional component with the same direction and a vertical downbeating component due to anterior canal disease. The net result would be only a strong torsional component, because the two torsional components would be added and the two vertical components would be cancelled, as having opposite directions. Dix-Hallpike on the none affected ear would cause a torsional component with the upper eye pole moving apogeotropically and a vertical downbeating component, due to anterior canal disease. If the involved posterior and anterior canals are on different sides, then Dix-Hallpike on the side where the posterior canal is involved, theoretically would cause a torsional component with the upper eye pole moving geotropically and a vertical upbeating component due to posterior canal disease; a torsional component with opposite direction and a vertical downbeating component due to AC disease of the contralateral side. The net result will be absence of nystagmus due to vectorial subtraction of the partial components. However, some asymmetry of canal involvement may manifest as mild nystagmus, either torsional, or vertical, or mixed, depending on the intensity of the partial components. Dix-Hallpike on the side of the involved anterior canal would cause a mixed nystagmus, with a torsional component with the upper eye pole moving geotropically and a vertical downbeating component, due to ipsilateral anterior canal disease. Mixed posterior-anterior canal is so difficult to be diagnosed with certainty. In case of suspicion, separate Canalith Repositioning Procedures for the posterior canal (mainly the Epley's Canalith Repositioning Procedure) and a specific therapeutic procedure for the Anterior Canal could support the diagnosis, if treatment could be obtained. However, it should be noticed that an Epley's maneuver for posterior canal BPPV is also a reverse Epley (and probably therapeutical) for the contralateral Anterior Canal, thus complicating this issue further (Tables 9D.4).[40]

TREATMENT

Treatment of Bilateral Posterior Canal BPPV

The management of biBPPV remains unclear. The studies reviewed by Katsarkas, Longridge, and Barber did not report on management or outcome of their patient.[5,19] In keeping with the two theories of BPPV (cupulolithiasis and canalithiasis), single treatment approaches such as the Epley's maneuver are aimed at moving debris into the vestibule or into the crus commune by the force of gravity. Performing Epley's maneuver on both sides at the same session may be counterproductive as the side first treated may become restimulated, while the maneuver is being performed on the contralateral side. A staged strategy of initially treating the side with more symptoms and with a higher magnitude of

Table 9D.4: Summary of type of nystagmus with different vertical canal involvement.

Involved canal	Diagnostic maneuver	Vertical component of nystagmus	Torsional component of nystgmus
Right posterior	Dix-Hallpike Rt (+) Dix-Hallpike Lt (–)	Upbeating No nystagmus	Counter-clockwise No nystagmus
Left posterior	Dix-Hallpike Rt (–) Dix-Hallpike Lt (+)	No nystagmus Upbeating	No nystagmus Clockwise
Right anterior	Dix-Hallpike Rt (+) Dix-Hallpike Lt (+)	Downbeating Downbeating	Counter-clockwise Counter-clockwise
Left anterior	Dix-Hallpike Rt (+)	Downbeating	Clockwise
	Dix-Hallpike Lt (+)	Downbeating	Clockwise

Table 9D.5: Horizontal canal BPPV nystagmus.

Involved SCC	Diagnostic maneuver	Direction of nystagmus	Intensity of nystagmus	Pathogenetic mechanisms
H-BPPV right ear	Supine roll test R (+) Supine roll test L (+)	Geotropic Geotropic	More intense Less intense	Canalithiasis
H-BPPV left ear	Supine roll test R (+) Supine roll test L (+)	Geotropic Geotropic	Less intense More intense	Canalithiasis
H-BPPV right ear	Supine roll test R (+) Supine roll test L (+)	Apogeotropic Apogeotropic	Less intense More intense	Cupulolithiasis or canalithiasis of short arm of H-SCC
H-BPPV left ear	Supine roll test R (+) Supine roll test L (+)	Apogeotropic Apogeotropic	More intense Less intense	Cupulolithiasis or canalithiasis of short arm of H-SCC

(BPPV: Benign paroxysmal positional vertigo; SCC: Semicircular canal).

nystagmus and only when an improvement in the patient's symptoms on the Dix-Hallpike maneuver are seen, does the patient can undergo treatment on the contralateral side. Semont's maneuver, which does not restimulate the side treated first, could be used as an alternative to Epley's maneuver, and may be more suitable for a single-stage bilateral treatment of bilateral posterior canal BPPV.[48] BiBPPV usually requires greater number of treatment sessions and relatively longer time than typical BPPV for patients to be symptom free. In our experience, staged Epley's maneuver gives better results than one-stage Semont's maneuver (*see* Table 9D.1 and Flowchart 9D.1).

Treatment of Multi-canal BPPV

Treatment of multi-canal BPPV should depend on the clinician's judgment either to start treatment of the most symptomatic canal or to start by treating posterior canal if involved, as being the most dependent canal it could be the primary source of otoconial debris, beside the fact that, successful treatment of the posterior canal BPPV is often achievable with one repositioning maneuver Table 9D.1.

CONCLUSION

Typical posterior canal BPPV and horizontal canal BPPV are usually easy to diagnose, using the standard Dix-Hallpike and supine roll maneuvers, respectively. Anterior canal BPPV presents difficulties in diagnosis, because it may demonstrate mixed vertical-torsional nystagmus on both right and left Dix-Hallpike maneuvers. Additionally, the torsional nystagmic component may be missing. It is difficult to differentiate AC-BPPV from recently described apogeotropic posterior canal BPPV. Benign paroxysmal positional vertigo involving both posterior canals may be easily detected; true bilateral involvement can be distinguished from unilateral mimicking biBPPV by applying certain criteria. The diagnosis of bilateral horizontal or anterior canals involvement is almost theoretical; BPPV involving two different canals, either on the same or on different sides, may be quite safely diagnosed in typical cases of posterior-horizontal and anterior-horizontal involvement. However, the combination of posterior-anterior canal involvement is more difficult to diagnose with certainty. Appropriately diagnosing bilateral or multicanal involvement in cases of BPPV and appropriately choosing the type and sequence of therapeutic maneuvers are the bases for proper management of such relatively complicated cases.[8,23]

REFERENCES

1. Korres S, Balatsouras D. Diagnostic, pathophysiologic, and therapeutic aspects of benign paroxysmal positional vertigo. Otolaryngol Head Neck Surg. 2004;131(4):438-44.
2. Von Brevern M, Radtke A, Lezius F, et al. Epidemiology of benign paroxysmal positional vertigo: a population based study. J Neurol Neurosurg Psychiatr. 2007;78:710-15.
3. Baloh RW, Honrubia V, Jacobson K. Benign positional vertigo: clinical and oculographic features in 240 cases. Neurology. 1987;37:371-8.
4. Balatsouras DG. Benign paroxysmal positional vertigo with multiple canal involvement. Am J Otolaryngol. 2012;33(2):250-8.
5. Katsarkas A. Benign paroxysmal positional vertigo (BPPV): idiopathic versus post-traumatic. Acta Otolaryngol. 1999;119:745-9.
6. Korres S, Balatsouras DG, Kaberos A, et al. Occurrence of semicircular canal involvement in benign paroxysmal positional vertigo. Otol Neurotol. 2002;23(6):926-32.
7. Lopez-Escamez J, Molina M, Gamiz M, et al. Multiple positional nystagmus suggests multiple canal involvement in benign paroxysmal vertigo. Acta Otolaryngol. 2005;125(9):954-61.

8. Pollak L, Stryjer R, Kushnir M, et al. Approach to bilateral benign paroxysmal positioning vertigo. Am J Otolaryngol. 2006;27(2):91-5.
9. Tomaz A, Gananc MM, Gananc CF, et al. Benign paroxysmal positional vertigo: concomitant involvement of different semicircular canals. Ann Otol Rhinol Laryngol. 2009;118(2):113-7.
10. Uno A, Moriwaki K, Kato T, et al. Clinical features of benign paroxysmal positional vertigo. Nippon Jibiinkoka Gakkai Kaiho. 2001;104:9-16.
11. Bhattacharyya N, Baugh R, Orvidas L, et al. American Academy of Otolaryngology Head and Neck Surgery Foundation. Clinical practice guideline: benign paroxysmal positional vertigo. Otolaryngol Head Neck Surg. 2008;139(5) (Suppl 4):s47-81.
12. Fife TD. Benign paroxysmal positional vertigo. Semin Neurol. 2009;29(5): 500-08.
13. Parnes L, Agrawal S, Atlas J. Diagnosis and management of benign paroxysmal positional vertigo (BPPV). Can Med Assoc J. 2003;169(7):681-93.
14. Lopez-Escamez J, Molina M, Gamiz M. Anterior semicircular canal benign paroxysmal positional vertigo and positional downbeating nystagmus. Am J Otolaryngol. 2006;27(3):173-8.
15. Califano L, Salafia F, Mazzone S, et al. Anterior canal BPPV and apogeotropic posterior canal BPPV: two rare forms of vertical canalolithiasis. Acta Otorhinolaryngol Ital. 2014;34(3):189-97.
16. Vannucchi P, Pecci R, Giannoni B, et al. Apogeotropic posterior semicircular canal benign parosysmal positional vertigo: some clinical and therapeutic considerations. Audiol Res. 2015 Mar 31;5(1):130.
17. Vannucchi P, Pecci R, Giannoni B. Posterior semicircular canal benign paroxysmal positional vertigo presenting with torsional downbeating nystagmus: an apogeotropic variant. Int J Otolaryngol. 2012;2012:1-9.
18. Gacek RR. Technique and results of singular neurectomy for the management of benign paroxysmal positional vertigo. Acta Otolaryngol. 1995;115:154-7.
19. Longridge NS, Barber HO. Bilateral paroxysmal positioning nystagmus. J Otolaryngol. 1978;5:395-9.
20. Macias J, Lambert M, Massingale S, et al. Variables affecting treatment in benign paroxysmal positional vertigo. Laryngoscope. 2000;110(11):1921-4.
21. McClure JA, Parnes LS. A cure for benign positional vertigo. Baillieres Clin Neurol. 1994;3(3):537-45.
22. Boniver R. Benign paroxysmal positional vertigo: an overview. Int Tinnitus J. 2008;14(2):159-67.
23. Balatsouras DG, Koukoutsis G, Ganelis P, et al. Diagnosis of single- or multiple-canal benign paroxysmal positional vertigo according to the type of nystagmus. Int J Otolaryngol. 2011;2011:483965.
24. Hal SF, Ruby RR, McClure JA. The mechanics of benign paroxysmal vertigo. J Otolaryngol. 1979;8:151-8.
25. Korres S, Balatsouras D, Papouliakos S, et al. Benign paroxysmal positional vertigo and its management. Med Sci Monit. 2007;13(6):CR275-CR282.
26. Brandt T. Positional and positioning vertigo and nystagmus. J Neurol Sci. 1990;95(1):3-28.
27. Honrubia V, Baloh R, Harris M, et al. Paroxysmal positional vertigo syndrome. Am J Otol. 1999;20(4):465-70.
28. Harbert F. Benign paroxysmal positional nystagmus. Arch Ophthalmol. 1970;84(3):298-302.

29. Bertholon P, Bronstein A, Davies R, et al. Positional down beating nystagmus in 50 patients: cerebellar disorders and possible anterior semicircular canalithiasis. J Neurol Neurosurg Psychiatry. 2002;72(3):366-72.
30. Steddin S, Brandt T. Unilateral mimicking bilateral benign paroxysmal positioning vertigo. Arch Otolaryngol Head Neck Surg. 1994;120:1339-41.
31. Imai T, Takeda N, Sato G, et al. Differential diagnosis of true and pseudo-bilateral benign positional nystagmus. Acta Otolaryngologica. 2008;128(2):151-8.
32. Epley JM. Human experience with canalith repositioning maneuvers. Ann N Y Acad Sci. 2001;942:179-91.
33. Blanks RHI, Curthoys IS, Markham CH. Planar relationships of the semicircular canals in man. Acta Otolaryngol. 1975;80:185-96.
34. Parnes LS, McClure JA. Free floating endolymph particles: a new operative finding during posterior semicircular canal occlusion. Laryngoscope. 1992;102:988-92.
35. Zapala DA. Down-beating nystagmus in anterior canal benign paroxysmal positional vertigo. J Am Acad Audiol. 2008;19:257-66.
36. Cambi J, Astore S, Mandala M, et al. Natural course of positional down-beating nystagmus of peripheral origin. J Neurol. 2013;260:1489-96.
37. Crevits L. Treatment of anterior canal benign paroxysmal positional vertigo by a prolonged forced position procedure. J Neurol Neurosurg Psychiatry. 2004;75:779-81.
38. Ichijo H. Asymmetry of positioning nystagmus in posterior canalolithiasis. Acta Otolaryngol. 2013;133:159-64.
39. Giannoni B. Vertical canal lithiasis. In: Guidetti VG, Pagnini P (Eds). Labyrintholithiasis-Related Paroxysmal Positional. Excerpta Medica; 2002. pp. 157-70.
40. Korres S, Riga M, Sandris V, et al. Canalithiasis of the anterior semicircular canal (ASC): treatment options based on the possible underlying pathogenetic mechanisms. Int J Audiol. 2010;49(8):606-12.
41. Yacovino D, Hain T, Gualtieri F. New therapeutic maneuver for anterior canal benign paroxysmal positional vertigo. J Neurol. 2009;256:1851-5.
42. Lee S, Kim M, Cho K, et al. Reversal of initial positioning nystagmus in benign paroxysmal positional vertigo involving the horizontal canal. Ann N Y Acad Sci. 2009;1164:406-8.
43. Horii A, Imai T, Mishiro Y, et al. Horizontal canal type BPPV: bilaterally affected case treated with canal plugging and Lempert's maneuver. J Otorhinolaryngol. 2003;65(6):366-9.
44. Aw S, Todd M, Aw G, et al. Benign positional nystagmus: a study of its three-dimensional spatio-temporal characteristics. Neurology. 2005;64(11):1897-905.
45. Leopardi G, Chiarella G, Serafini G, et al. Paroxysmal positional vertigo: short- and long-term clinical and methodological analyses of 794 patients. Acta Otorhinolaryngol Italica. 2003;23(3):155-60.
46. Imai T, Takeda N, Ito M, et al. Benign paroxysmal positional vertigo due to a simultaneous involvement of both horizontal and posterior semicircular canals. Audiol Neurotol. 2006;11:198-205.
47. Ichijo H. Positional nystagmus of horizontal canalolithiasis. Acta Otolaryngol. 2011;131(1):46-51.
48. Kaplan DM, Uriel Attal, Mordechai Kraus. Bilateral benign paroxysmal positional vertigo following a tooth implantation. J Laryngol Otol. 2003;117:312-13.

Chapter 10

Secondary Benign Paroxysmal Positional Vertigo

Maria Riga

DEFINITIONS AND PITFALLS

Benign paroxysmal positional vertigo (BPPV) is characterized as either idiopathic or secondary. A disease is characterized as idiopathic when it is of unknown pathogenesis or apparently spontaneous origin. On the contrary, a condition that follows and results from an earlier disease, injury, or event is characterized as secondary. Secondary BPPV is, by definition, the direct consequence of an ipsilateral disease process affecting the labyrinth and causing the detachment of otoconia without totally destroying semicircular canal (SCC) function.

Benign paroxysmal positional vertigo is generally considered as a disorder in which otoconia exceeding a critical mass, is displaced into one or more SCCs and is capable of dislodging the cupula, either by being directly attached to it (cupulolithiasis), or by sedimenting freely through the canals and exerting transcupular pressure (canalithiasis). Recently, the theory of light cupula, which indicates cupula with lower specific gravity than the surrounding endolymph, as well as new pathophysiological data on the afferent and efferent innervation of the vestibular organs, has been introduced. The etiology underlying these disorders (both otoconial detachment and light cupula) is currently obscure. This may explain the discrepancies regarding the perception of "secondary" BPPV by various researchers.

Epidemiological observations have established an association between BPPV and other inner ear diseases such as endolymphatic hydrops, vestibular neuritis, and sudden sensorineural hearing loss (SSNHL). In this respect, BPPV is characterized as secondary when additional inner ear disease is diagnosed. An issue that may need to be clarified is the time period between the onset of the primary-causative condition and the diagnosis of secondary BPPV. Most authors do not specify the time period between the two events, while others extend it to several months or years. Furthermore, there is no consensus, regarding the lateralization of the two lesions. For some authors contralateral inner ear disease is a sufficient condition for the characterization of BPPV as secondary,[1] while others refer strictly to ipsilateral lesions.² Laterality issues do not obviously apply for inner ear pathologies with obvious bilaterality such as head trauma (contrecoup injuries) or bilateral Ménière's disease (MD). In other cases, however, where the bilaterality of the disease is doubtful or the time interval between the two events is long, the characterization of BPPV as secondary becomes questionable. Some researchers regard these cases of BPPV as an incidental unrelated finding, while others inquire into additional common underlying pathophysiological factors. Related theories are described in further detail in the pathophysiology section of this chapter.

INCIDENCE AND EPIDEMIOLOGICAL CHARACTERISTICS

Cross-sectional and case-control studies have indicated that the incidence of BPPV is higher among patients with a number of inner ear diseases and vice versa the diagnosis of certain inner ear diseases is more frequent among BPPV patients. Endolymphatic hydrops, vestibular neuritis, head trauma, SSNHL and migraine are the most common conditions related to secondary BPPV. A wide variation of incidence of secondary BPPV (3–66%) is observed across studies.³ This may reflect differences in patient cohorts, referral patterns, and diagnostic protocols. Prospective studies tend to attribute higher incidence rates than retrospective ones. In the literature review that follows, only incidence rates coming from studies with strictly mentioned ipsilateral criteria are included, at least in cases where no apparent pathophysiological mechanism can justify contralateral involvement (such as vestibular neuritis, SSNHL, and endolymphatic hydrops). In order to flatten the discrepancies among patient populations and referral patterns, each one of the different inner ear diseases that have been associated with BPPV is assessed separately.

Vestibular Neuritis

Vestibular neuritis seems to represent the inner ear disease that is most commonly associated with secondary BPPV.² The incidence of vestibular neuritis among BPPV patients has also been reported within the wide range of 0.8–24.1%.[2,4-7] In patients with vestibular neuritis the incidence of BPPV appears to be more frequent (9.8–20%) than in the general population.[8-12] These incidence differences seem to reflect further discrepancies among the respective studies, especially regarding their referral patterns. The main methodological issue, however, that may need to be clarified is the time window between the diagnoses of vestibular neuritis and secondary BPPV. Balatsouras et al.⁶ (2014) adopted the criterion of a 12-week time interval to ensure the causative relationship between vestibular neuritis and BPPV and found that the prevalence of vestibular neuritis among BPPV patients was 5.2%. In studies where this time period is extended up to a few years[5,8] the causative relationship between the two inner ear diseases might be questionable. On the other hand, the prospective study of Mandalà et al.[8] (2010) reported that during the 6-year-long follow up of the study, the incidence of BPPV in a vestibular neuritis cohort was found to be 9.8%, significantly higher than in the general population and significantly higher than expected if the two events had been independent. Further prospective multicentered studies are needed in order to comment on the chronological association between vestibular neuritis and BPPV.

The involved SCC is typically the posterior one, while no clear reports on lateral or anterior SCC BPPV secondary to vestibular neuritis have been presented so far. This is to be expected considering that the typical vestibular nerve lesion regards the superior vestibular nerve sparing the inferior division of the nerve, due to the anatomic differences between the respective bony canals.[13] The bony canal of the superior vestibular nerve is longer and presents more spicules than that of the singular and inferior vestibular nerve, thus rendering the former more susceptible to ischemia and neuritis.[14] As a result of this preferential insult of the superior vestibular nerve, potential otoconial displacement toward the lateral and anterior SCCs is bound to remain asymptomatic, since these SCCs are innervated by the affected superior-division of the vestibular nerve. Any clinical signs and symptoms are expected to originate from the healthy inferior-division of the vestibular nerve that innervates the crista of the posterior SCC and the macula of the saccule. Secondary BPPV in inferior vestibular neuritis cases has not been reported so far.

Benign paroxysmal positional vertigo secondary to vestibular neuritis has mainly been reported in the context of larger studies investigating secondary BPPV in general. There are only a few studies focusing on this particular subtype of secondary BPPV, which seems to be both highly heterogeneous and underdiagnosed. Evaluation of the degree of involvement of each vestibular end-organ through detailed neurotological examination is usually not provided. Consequently the incidence, epidemiological characteristics, underlying pathophysiological mechanisms, and any particular issues regarding its diagnostic and therapeutical assessment actually remain unclear. Further studies are needed in order to gain a clear insight in the particularities of BPPV secondary to vestibular neuritis.

Ménière's Disease

Significant differences in the incidence of cupular and free-floating deposits in the posterior and lateral SCCs between temporal bones with and without MD were found in a temporal bone research, thus verifying the association between BPPV and MD supported by observational studies.[15] An important conclusion of the same study is that the incidence of these deposits was associated with the duration of disease rather than with aging.

The incidence of ipsilateral MD among BPPV patients has been reported within a wide range (5-30%), which seems to reflect further methodological differences among the respective retrospective studies.[16,17] Authors seeking a strictly causative relationship between MD and secondary BPPV, refer only to preceding ipsilateral definite MD diagnoses, while others may disconnect the clinical diagnosis of a definite MD from the ongoing underlying pathophysiological processes and refer to "associated" MD. It is of note, that MD patients are a heterogeneous population involving patients in different stages of the disease. Most authors do not offer a detailed staging of the patients included in their cohorts. The time-window of a retrospective study, the patients' referral, and follow-up patterns as well as the inclusion of subjective BPPV cases may also have an impact on the estimated incidence rates. Vice versa, in a study involving 500 patients with MD, Paparella et al. (2008) estimated that approximately 65-70% of patients experience BPPV between attacks of the disease.[18]

There is not enough epidemiological data to comment on the chronological relationship between BPPV and MD. The existing studies referring to this detail, present substantial differences regarding their referral patterns and diagnostic protocols. Limited data suggest that simultaneous onset is not common. Onset is usually noted one week to several months after the stabilization and successful control of MD.[4,19,20] There are also few references on patients with BPPV dating before MD. These cases seem to have better prognosis probably because underlying pathophysiological mechanisms are different.[21]

The reported time window between the onset of BPPV symptoms and their diagnosis and treatment is unexpectedly long (mean 7.3 months, range 1-36 months).[16] This might be an indicator of the low suspicion index of a second inner ear disease in known vertiginous patients, which may apply for both the treating physicians and the patients themselves. Difficulties in treatment, as discussed below, may be another explanation for the long duration of BPPV symptoms. Female predominance seems to be in accordance with the current epidemiology of MD.[20,22] Most authors agree that the posterior SCC is the most frequently affected, followed by the horizontal SCC, which seems to be involved in 15-24% of the patients.[15,16,22] In the population of Lee et al.[4] (2010), however, the lateral SCC seems to be the most susceptible to secondary BPPV by 65%. The incidence of horizontal SCC BPPV has been reported to be highly dependent upon the duration of symptoms, with percentages being substantially reduced with time progression due to spontaneous resolution.[23] Differences in patient referral patterns and diagnostic protocols may account for these discrepancies among studies.

Sudden Sensorineural Hearing Loss

Sudden sensorineural hearing loss is encountered in 0.2-5% of BPPV patients. The diagnosis of BPPV has been reported for 5-19% of patients with SSNHL.[12,24] The time window between the two events is usually very short (<12 hours) and most authors refer to the two conditions as synchronous. The posterior and the lateral SCC seem to be the most frequently involved with relevant studies on small populations presenting controversial results.[12,24]

Head Trauma

Head trauma seems to be the most common and best studied cause of secondary BPPV, with the relevant literature being substantially more extended than that regarding BPPV secondary to inner ear conditions and migraine. The incidence of head trauma among BPPV patients has been reported to be significantly higher than in the general population, ranging between 7% and 27%.[25,26] The nature and severity of the traumas causing trauma-BPPV are diverse, ranging from minor head injuries to more severe head and neck trauma with brief loss of consciousness.

The most commonly affected SCCs are the posterior and the lateral.[27] Noteworthy clinical characteristics of traumatic BPPV are bilaterality in 14-20% of the patients and multiple SCC involvement.[25,28]

Postsurgical

All surgeries involving drilling and/or osteotomes are potentially capable of developing secondary BPPV. The incidence of secondary BPPV after surgical drilling of the temporal bone for various indications has been reported to be around 1%, while in otosclerotic patients it is significantly higher, ranging between 6.3% and 8.5%.[29,30] Cochlear implantation has been extensively reported as a cause of secondary BPPV with incidence rates ranging between 0% and 28%.[31,32] The incidence of secondary BPPV among patients undergoing maxillofacial and dental surgery including placement of dental implants with or without sinus floor elevation has been reported to be around 3%.[33,34]

In nonotologic and otologic surgeries where the inner ear is not directly involved in the surgical intervention, secondary BPPV tends to present immediately or shortly after the procedure. Regarding cochlear implantation, on the other hand, a considerably heterogeneous and long-time interval has been reported between surgery and initiation of BPPV symptoms (ranging from a few hours to several months).[31,32] Similarly, for patients undergoing stapes surgery (where utricular trauma may be involved), the time-interval till the development of secondary BPPV seems to extend to the first 3 weeks after surgery.[29]

In correspondence to post-traumatic vertigo, contralateral, bilateral and multiple SCC involvement are to be expected.[30] The most commonly affected SCCs are the posterior and the lateral.

Migraine

The association between migraine and BPPV has been reported both as a high prevalence of migraine in patients with BPPV (twice as high as that in age- and sex-matched controls) and as a high prevalence of BPPV in patients with migraine (more than twice as high as that in patients with other forms of headache).[35,36] Patients with migraine seem to experience BPPV at earlier age (at early forties versus mid-fifties for patients with other headache causes) and seem to be more likely to develop recurrent BPPV.[36] The relevant literature is quite limited. Benign paroxysmal positional vertigo secondary to migraine should be distinguished from migrainous positional vertigo, which is characterized by migrainous symptoms during episodes with positional vertigo and atypical positional nystagmus.

PATHOPHYSIOLOGY

Most theories regarding underlying pathophysiological mechanisms seek to explain respective clinical observations. There are only a limited number of temporal bone studies and a few promising studies exploiting advanced imaging techniques. Further studies on the pathophysiology of secondary BPPV are needed, in order to offer insight to the underlying mechanisms that may be useful for the effective diagnosis, treatment, and counseling of patients diagnosed with a specific subtype of secondary BPPV.

Vestibular Neuritis

The etiology and pathogenesis of vestibular neuritis remain unknown. Proposed theories include viral infections, vascular occlusion, and immunomediated mechanisms. Otoconial detachment in vestibular neuritis could be considered as a result of the degeneration in the utricular neuroepithelium, usually following viral infection or vascular compromise and ischemic necrosis.[6] It could be hypothesized that more extended utricle damage might be more likely to induce detachment of otoconia. The utricle has been considered as the most possible source of otoconia in BPPV, since otoconial debris of saccular origin would have to transverse the utricular-saccular duct before reaching the vestibule and the SCCs. The typical superior vestibular nerve lesion sparing the inferior division of the nerve seems to be the main pathogenetic mechanism explaining the typical posterior SSC involvement in BPPV secondary to vestibular neuritis (more detailed analysis is provided in the "Incidence and Epidemiology" section). Both the macula of the saccule and the crista of the posterior canal are innervated by the inferior vestibular nerve. The presence of secondary posterior SCC BPPV in vestibular neuritis patients implies that at least some function in the inferior vestibular nerve remains, as it is also supported by the preserved vestibular evoked myogenic potentials, most likely of saccular origin, in postneurolabyrinthitis patients.[10]

It should be noted that vestibular neuritis patients comprise a highly heterogeneous population. Detailed neurotological examination of such populations has revealed that patients actually present different degrees of vestibular involvement considering the evaluation of each single vestibular end-organ.[37] This clinical fact is quite far from any simplistic inferior and/or superior vestibular neuritis analysis. In any case, otolith organs seem to have a role in the pathogenesis of BPPV that has been underestimated. Three-dimensional analyses of the nystagmus properties, off-vertical axis rotation, and subjective visual vertical studies have confirmed otolith dysfunction in BPPV patients.[38] Although further research on the field is definitely needed, it seems that otolith organs may serve a double mission. Apart from their sensory role, otolith organs might exert an inhibitory effect on the responsiveness of SCC(s) of the same vestibular nerve division. Thus, the saccule inhibits the excitatory responsiveness of the posterior SCC and the utricle that of the lateral and the anterior SCCs. Experimental studies in cats have demonstrated that selective denervation of the utricle can produce horizontal nystagmus if the innervation of the lateral canal crista remains intact. Because of their double assignment, which presumably divides into two halves the afferent innervation of the macula, otolith organs have been hypothesized to be more vulnerable to vestibular deafferentiation (as it is the case in vestibular neuritis). According to Gacek (2008), this loss of the inhibitory effect of otolith organs on SCCs, may itself generate BPPV symptoms.[39] Although otoconial displacement remains the main pathophysiological basis for BPPV secondary to vestibular neuritis since in a large percentage of patients BPPV symptoms and signs subside through canalith repositioning maneuvers, there seems to be a role for those new pathophysiological data in the understanding of BPPV/vestibular neuritis cases that need more time to recover or complain of residual dizziness after repositioning maneuvers. The study of the efferent vestibular system is another promising field, which may attribute important clinical implications. Further well designed and diagnostically integrated studies are definitely needed. Vestibular neuritis patients with secondary BPPV seem to be an ideal population for the study of the pathophysiology of BPPV in general, due to their variability in vestibular end-organ involvement.

Endolymphatic Hydrops and Ménière's Disease

Experimental animal models of endolymphatic hydrops have demonstrated that the endolymph becomes abnormally rich in calcium ions. This change in the ionic environment of the endolymph may also facilitate the detachment of otoconia.[21] Paparella et al.[18] on the other hand, proposed that not only may BPPV originate from endolymphatic hydrops, but the opposite might apply as well. Dislocated otoconia could secondarily induce a decrease in endolymphatic absorption that could provoke endolymphatic hydrops. There is, however, limited clinical data to support this theory, since BPPV is usually reported to follow the diagnosis of endolymphatic hydrops.

Periodic hydropic distension, as seen in the natural course of MD, and vascular compromise seem to account for the fibrosis and destruction of the maculae of the utricle and saccule that may in turn enhance detachment of otoliths and induce secondary BPPV in MD. Furthermore, repeated hydrolabyrinth might reduce the elasticity of the membranous labyrinth thus inducing partial collapse of SCCs and complicating otoconial sedimentation within the SCCs and toward the vestibule.[15,20,22] Paparella et al. (1984) also suggested that positional vertigo in MD could be attributed to saccular distension up to the SCCs.[40]

Apart from offering explanation regarding the association between MD and BPPV, these hypotheses may explain why incidence rate increases as the course of MD is prolonged and why BPPV may exist independently after effective control of endolymphatic hydrops. According to clinical observations, most patients (80-90%) presenting with secondary BPPV have been diagnosed with MD >6 years earlier and are classified as stage 2 or 3.[16,22] Additionally they also interpret why BPPV secondary to MD requires for repositioning maneuvers to be repeated more than twice before effective treatment can be achieved and for close patient follow up due to high BPPV recurrence rates (further relevant information are discussed in the "Treatment implications" section). However, they also suggest that, vice versa, the effective treatment of endolymphatic hydrops may be a prerequisite for the avoidance of repeated BPPV episodes and for the successful repositioning of otoconial debris.[15,20,22]

Sudden Sensorineural Hearing Loss

Concurrent BPPV in SSNHL might indicate extension of the labyrinth damage to otolith organs and detachment of otoconia, which is subsequently displaced toward a SCC. The utricle has been considered as the most possible source of otoconia in BPPV, since the utricular-saccular duct seems to severely suspend the accessibility of the vestibule and the SCCs to otoconial debris of saccular origin. On the other hand, simultaneous involvement of the saccule and the cochlea is more plausible to be explained on the basis of the theory of vascular compromise. Vascular compromise, usually in the form of transient ischemia rather than that of arterial occlusion, has been one of the proposed theories regarding the pathophysiology of SSNHL and BPPV. Occlusion of the common cochlear artery after the branching of the anterior vestibular artery could account for the simultaneous involvement of the saccule and the basal turn of the cochlea (supplied by the vestibulocochlear artery) and the middle and apical turn of the cochlea (supplied by the posterior cochlear artery). Saccular involvement has been investigated through cervical vestibular evoked myogenic potentials (cVEMPs), which are thought to be of saccular origin. Vestibular evoked myogenic potentials were found to be abnormal in 14/26 patients with SSNHL and BPPV tested by Song et al.[24] (2012), while caloric testing revealed ipsilesional canal paresis in four patients. In the absence, however, of a similar noninvasive method that may provide information on the condition of the utricle, this finding hardly represents any proof that the displaced otoconia is of saccular rather than utricular origin.

On the other hand, damage of the utricle and the cochlea may not be plausibly explained on a strict vascular supply basis. A suggestion that could still validate the vascular theory is that the different structures of the inner ear may present different susceptibility to ischemia (perhaps reinforced by other comorbidities). In this respect, vascular compromise might actually refer to additional inner ear structures, which due to their resistance to ischemia may not produce relevant clinical signs.[41] The validity of this suggestion, as well as that of the vascular theory on the whole, remains to be seen, probably through relevant and efficient temporal bone studies.

Loss of inner ear function that does not follow a consistent vascular distribution has been attributed to viral labyrinthitis, in the form of either infection or reactivation[42] and, less likely, to transient inner ear ischemia. Finally, Kim et al.[42] expressed the hypothesis that BPPV in SSNHL patients may result from inner ear hemorrhage within the endolymphatic space. Since specific gravity of the whole blood is higher than that of the endolymph, the former may settle into the SCC acting as an analog to otoconia.

The mechanism underlying the association between SSNHL and BPPV remains actually unknown.

Head Trauma

Mechanical detachment of otoconia during head trauma seems to be a well-recognized pathophysiological mechanism. Long bed resting seems to favor the gravitation of the dislocated otoconia from the utricle toward the lumen or the ampulla of the posterior and the lateral SCC. The mechanism of contrecoup injuries may justify otoconial detachment from the contralateral otolith organs and explain the causative association between head trauma and contralateral BPPV.

Postsurgical

Any dental, craniofacial, otosurgical, neurosurgical procedure involving drilling or preparation of implant beds with osteotome and mallet transmits percussive and vibratory forces, which are thought to propagate through the bony structures of the head toward the posterior labyrinth, both the ipsilateral and the contralateral. Based on epidemiological studies these forces are apparently capable of detaching otoconia mechanically. The patient is positioned with the contralateral ear down during both surgery (usually supine with head over-extension) and postoperative bed-rest or sleeping (usually side-lying on the healthy side). Thus, dislocated otoconia in the contralateral ear, where the utricle is placed at a higher level, is more likely to gravitate toward an SCC. This may explain the high incidence of contralateral involvement in postsurgical BPPV.[30] The patient's head position also seems to favor the displacement of otoconia toward the posterior SCC.

Regarding surgical procedures involving the inner ear, additional pathophysiological mechanisms have been hypothesized. When performing cochlear implantation surgery, disruption of endolymph mechanics during cochleostomy and implant insertion might induce movement of dislocated otoconia toward one or more SCCs. Furthermore, direct falling of bone dust particles into the cochlea during cochleostomy has also been suggested to trigger BPPV.[31] After falling into the cochlea, bone dust particles might through a microrupture of the basilar membrane, travel into the endolymphatic compartment of the scala media and into the lumen usually of the posterior SCC, thereby producing canalolithiasis and subsequent delayed-onset BPPV.[32] The hypothesis of the dislodging of otoconia because of electrical stimulation is also possible for patients who experience BPPV symptoms after implant activation, although this theory has been considered as less likely by most authors.[32,33] Benign positional paroxysmal vertigo in patients undergoing cochlear implantation has not been associated with any anatomic variants or intra/postoperative complications. In otosclerotic patients on the other hand, secondary BPPV has been attributed to utricular trauma probably following incorrect measurement of the distance between the incus and the stapes footplate[29] and pneumolabyrinth after stapedectomy.[43]

Migraine

The underlying pathophysiological mechanism remains obscure. Presumably, patients with migraine suffer recurrent damage to the utricle (due to vasospasm or other unknown mechanism) that may account for detachment of otoconial debris and BPPV.

Other Hypotheses and Related Comorbidities

In 2008, Manzari reported the hypothesis that an excessive secretion or/ and a defect in the elimination of the osmotically active components of the endolymph reflected in the form of a dilated vestibular aqueduct (yet not clinically expressed as endolymphatic hydrops) might account for recurrent vertigo in some patients. Volumetric abnormalities documented with computed tomography scan were found in 63 out of the 108 patients with recurrent BPPV (yet not expressing audiological signs of enlarged vestibular aqueduct syndrome) who comprised the study cohort. This proportion was significantly higher than in control group. Since the evaluation of the vestibular aqueduct is hardly a common examination in current neurotology, further prospective controlled studies are needed in order to evaluate this hypothesis. A few years later, Song et al.[24] reported an association between radiologically confirmed enlarged vestibular aqueduct syndrome and BPPV attacks (in some cases recurrent), which usually accompanied sensorineural hearing loss in a pediatric population. This type of secondary BPPV seemed to respond well to canalith repositioning maneuvers.

Although not specified as etiological factors, a variety of other comorbidities seem to affect the onset and relapse of BPPV episodes according to recent data. Common conditions such as hypertension, diabetes, atherosclerosis, and osteoporosis frequently combined with each other and with old age, all seem to promote otoconial detachment as well as dysfunction of both maculae and crista. These factors should probably be taken into consideration when estimating incidence or recurrence rates in various populations. Further studies are needed in order to clarify the degree and mechanisms by which these factors may interact with each other and may contribute to the onset and the course of BPPV.[44] A detailed analysis of this subject is offered in the respective chapter.

DIAGNOSTIC IMPLICATIONS

The aforementioned association of a number of conditions and inner ear pathologies with BPPV seems to encourage the application of a simple clinical examination, such as the Dix-Hallpike examination, even in cases where a typical history of BPPV attacks is not present. However, the diagnosis of secondary BPPV in the acute phase of MD or vestibular neuritis may be quite difficult. The co-existence of two pathologies that are typically associated with dizziness (and nystagmus) inevitably modifies the clinical findings and symptoms. Consequently, the clinical findings in secondary BPPV are in several cases atypical and substantially different from those of idiopathic BPPV. The performance of the Dix-Hallpike examination with video-Frenzel glasses may be indicated in order to reinforce diagnostic sensitivity. Although problematic in the acute phase, the Dix-Hallpike examination seems to be strongly recommended in cases of vestibular neuritis and MD that do not respond to the indicated treatment, or vice versa, in cases of BPPV that recurs or does not respond as expected to canalith repositioning maneuvers. Depending on the symptoms and clinical findings that are most prominent, those of the causative inner ear disease or those of secondary BPPV, either one might escape diagnosis or account for the unsatisfactory response to treatment. Especially in chronic diseases such as MD, secondary BPPV might be underdiagnosed, because dizziness is attributed to the primary pathology, by both the patient and the treating physician. The performance of a detailed clinical and laboratory neurotological testing seems to reveal the unexpected coexistence of another underlying pathological condition in a considerable number of cases (as it has been analyzed in the "Incidence and Epidemiological characteristics" section).

In cases of SSNHL and migraine, on the other hand, the performance of a Dix-Hallpike examination is expected to attribute typical findings. The implementation of this simple and nontime consuming examination to the typical diagnostic protocol of these patients may prevent underdiagnosis of secondary BPPV. On the other hand, the indications of a Dix-Hallpike examination for patients with head trauma are to be set with caution, even though this is the most common cause of secondary BPPV. Any injury of the spinal cord, frequently present in patients with head trauma, must be accordingly evaluated by the respective experts before investigating the possible diagnosis of secondary BPPV.

Some authors have pointed out that in a considerable number of BPPV patients, additional inner ear diseases that do not seem to have any causative role (e.g. because they refer to the contralateral ear), may be revealed after performing a detailed neurotological examination.[1] Any additional inner ear disease may potentially interfere with the patients' symptoms and signs during both the diagnostic and the therapeutical procedure, even though not in concept of secondary BPPV. In fact, the application of nystagmography in idiopathic BPPV patients has been reported to reveal ipsilateral canal paresis at a percentage of 13–47%.[45,46] Furthermore, the percentage of abnormal VEMP and subjective visual vertigo in idiopathic BPPV patients has been reported to be statistically higher than in controls.[38,47] Therefore, a thorough neurotological examination seems to be indicated in all BPPV patients who remain symptomatic after repositioning maneuvers or recur frequently.

TREATMENT IMPLICATIONS

The outcome of repositioning maneuvers between the several types of secondary and idiopathic BPPV seems to differ, thus requiring different diagnostic, counseling, treatment, and follow-up strategies. Several studies have highlighted the fact that secondary BPPV seems to be more debilitating, more difficult to treat, and more prone to recurrences than idiopathic.[3,21,36] Incomplete resolution of symptoms in patients with secondary BPPV seems to be more often and it can be attributed to an additional SCC and/or otolithic dysfunction. On the other hand, the prognostic role of secondary BPPV in the recovery or rehabilitation of the primary inner ear disease has not been adequately addressed in literature. The same seems to apply for the therapeutical outcome of repositioning maneuvers in postsurgical BPPV patients.

Vestibular Neuritis

Although the relevant literature is quite limited, authors apparently agree that the treatment of patients with BPPV secondary to vestibular neuritis seems to be significantly more time-consuming and less effective than that of idiopathic.[4,6] Success rates for the first application of canalith repositioning maneuver have been reported to be only 13.6%, while overall treatment failure (despite the performance of multiple maneuvers) has been reported as high as 40.9%.[6] The potentially late emergence of BPPV after vestibular neuritis may highlight the necessity for the repentance of the Dix-Hallpike examination at the follow-up sessions, especially in patients who present a slow recovery. Benign paroxysmal positional vertigo seems to be in these cases a negative prognostic index, since it seems to present predominantly in patients who did not fully recover from the disease.[8] Treatment strategies and results are obviously affected by the time window between the onset of the two conditions as well as the course (full, partial, or no recovery) and extent (division and degree of vestibular nerve lesion, degree of otolith organ participation) of the primary inner ear disease. The current literature lacks relevant studies.

Another important issue is a possible tendency for recurrences. Recurrence rates (referring to the same ear) have been reported to be as high as 67–71% within the following 12 months.[6,11] Substantially lower recurrence rates (8%) have been reported by other authors.[8] Most of these patients presented with multiple (more than three) recurrent episodes of BPPV. Discrepancies among recurrence rates might be attributed to different follow-up patterns, e.g. telephone interviews versus clinical examination, which may result in biased conclusions due to spontaneous resolution of BPPV recurrences. Further prospective studies are needed in this field in order to clarify the clinical characteristics and pathophysiology of recurrences in BPPV secondary to vestibular neuritis. Future studies might assess the association between BPPV recurrences and recovery from vestibular neuritis and the hypothesis that continuous deafferentiation due to partial recovery might be more likely to be related to higher recurrence rates than complete recovery and stabilization of a normal vestibular nerve function. The prognostic role of BPPV in patients with vestibular neuritis, also, has not been investigated yet.

Ménière's Disease

Before attempting any comparisons among studies and during patient consultation, one should bear in mind that MD patients are a heterogeneous population involving patients in different stages of the disease and consequently patients with substantially different pathophysiology profiles (as it has been analyzed in the "Pathophysiology" section). As it is the case in all secondary BPPV patients, those with MD also seem to need more than one therapeutical sessions in order to become asymptomatic (as opposed to the excellent results reported for idiopathic BPPV patients). However, the overall cure rate (after the performance of the required number of canalith repositioning maneuvers) does not seem to differ significantly between patients with and without endolymphatic hydrops.[16,17,19,20,22]

The particular characteristic of this subcategory of secondary BPPV seems to be the higher probability of recurrence. Endolymphatic hydrops has been associated with BPPV recurrence rates as high as 20–75% within the next 12 months.[16,17,48] At this point laterality issues seem to come along for once more. There is no consensus on whether the appearance of a BBPV episode on the contralateral ear should be considered as a recurrence, since there is no explanation to justify the involvement of the contralateral ear. Another notable observation reported in a study of 162 patients with MD is that 5.5% of these patients, mostly females, seem to develop intractable BPPV.[20] An interesting study by Perez et al.[21] investigated the effect of gentamycin intratympanic injections on patients with definite MD and secondary BPPV. The study was based on the hypothesis that gentamycin intratympanic injections might affect the prognosis of BPPV through ototoxic damage of the hair cells of the corresponding crista that might be expected due to the proximity of the ampulla of the posterior SCC to the round window. However, the hypothesis was not verified and treatment of secondary BPPV was also achieved through a number of canalith repositioning maneuvers.

Sudden Sensorineural Hearing Loss

Although several studies have debated the prognostic value of vertigo in idiopathic SSNHL, little is known concerning the role of BPPV as a prognostic factor for SSNHL. The prognostic value of the presence of BPPV for the recovery of hearing is a matter of controversy, having been reported as both unfavorable and irrelevant.[4,12] The same seems to apply for the recurrence of BPPV secondary to SSNHL. The number of canalith repositioning maneuvers required for successful treatment seems to be also larger than those required in idiopathic BPPV, as it seems to be the case for all forms of secondary BPPV.

Head Trauma

Benign paroxysmal positional vertigo secondary to head trauma seems to require more canalith repositioning maneuvers than idiopathic BPPV to be performed before achieving successful treatment.[27] This might in part be attributed to the fact that in traumatic BPPV multiple canal involvement or bilaterality is more often.

Regarding the tendency of traumatic BPPV to recur, the relevant literature is quite controversial. In the series studied by Kansu et al.[49] (2010), history of head trauma was one of the factors contributing to recurrence. Conversely, idiopathic and traumatic BPPV presented similar recurrence rates in the population studied by Ahn et al.[27] Recurrences may refer to different side and canal.[21]

Postsurgical

In postsurgical BPPV, contralateral, bilateral, and multiple SCC involvement are expected to render treatment through canalith repositioning maneuvers more difficult and more time-consuming requiring multiple sessions and/or maneuver performances. However, no tendency to recur has been reported.[30]

Migraine

Canalith repositioning maneuvers in patients with BPPV and migraine seem to attribute success rates similar to those reported for idiopathic BPPV, although in migraineurs, BPPV seems to have a tendency to recur.[36,50]

GENERAL CONSIDERATIONS

Secondary BPPV seems to be an underdiagnosed entity among patients with another known inner ear disease especially when the latter produces more alerting and/or chronic symptoms such as MD, vestibular neuritis, and idiopathic SSNHL. The reverse also seems to apply. Physicians treating patients with intractable BPPV may misinterpret the symptoms of another inner ear disease as incomplete resolution of BPPV. A higher suspicion index promptly investigated by a comprehensive clinical, audiological, and neurotological evaluation are essential in order to reach an integrated diagnosis. In most cases, the two inner ear diseases do not seem to present concomitantly. This might mean that an integrated diagnosis may require multiple sessions before being reached and that the symptoms and signs of the patient with intractable vertigo should probably be de novo evaluated at each session.

A precise diagnosis seems to be essential in order to offer patients with intractable vertigo an optimal and efficient treatment. Most studies agree that secondary BPPV is more difficult to treat than idiopathic and patients require longer time intervals and more canalith repositioning maneuvers before becoming free from clinical symptoms. In chronic inner ear diseases, such as MD and vestibular neuritis with partial or no recovery, secondary BPPV seems to have a tendency to recur. Further clinical studies are needed in order to establish generally accepted diagnostic and therapeutical protocols for secondary BPPV.

REFERENCES

1. Pollak L, Davies RA, Luxon LL. Effectiveness of the particle repositioning maneuver in benign paroxysmal positional vertigo with and without additional vestibular pathology. Otol Neurotol. 2002;23(1):79-83.
2. Karlberg M, Hall K, Quickert N, et al. What inner ear diseases cause benign paroxysmal positional vertigo? Acta Otolaryngol. 2000;120(3):380-5.
3. Riga M, Bibas A, Xenellis J, et al. Inner ear disease and benign paroxysmal positional vertigo: a critical review of incidence, clinical characteristics, and management. Int J Otolaryngol. 2011;2011:709469.
4. Lee NH, Ban JH, Lee KC, et al. Benign paroxysmal positional vertigo secondary to inner ear disease. Otolaryngol Head Neck Surg. 2010;143(3):413-7.
5. Caldas MA, Ganança CF, Ganança FF, et al. Clinical features of benign paroxysmal positional vertigo. Braz J Otorhinolaryngol. 2009;75(4):502-6.
6. Balatsouras DG, Koukoutsis G, Ganelis P, et al. Benign paroxysmal positional vertigo secondary to vestibular neuritis. Eur Arch Otorhinolaryngol. 2014;271(5):919-24.
7. Roberts RA, Gans RE, Kastner AH, et al. Prevalence of vestibulopathy in benign paroxysmal positional vertigo patients with and without prior otologic history. Int J Audiol. 2005;44(4):191-6.

8. Mandalà M, Santoro GP, Awrey J, et al. Vestibular neuritis: recurrence and incidence of secondary benign paroxysmal positional vertigo. Acta Otolaryngol. 2010;130(5):565-7.
9. Halmagyi GM, Cremer PD, Curthoys IS. Peripheral vestibular disorders and disease in adults. In: Linda L (ed). Textbook of audiological medicine. Clinical aspects of hearing and balance. Martin Dunitz: London; 2003. p. 805.
10. Murofushi T, Halmagyi GM, Yavor RA, et al. Absent vestibular evoked myogenic potentials in vestibular neurolabyrinthitis. An indicator of inferior vestibular nerve involvement? Arch Otolaryngol Head Neck Surg. 1996;122(8):845-8.
11. Huppert D, Strupp M, Theil D, et al. Low recurrence rate of vestibular neuritis: a long-term follow-up. Neurology. 2006;67(10):1870-1.
12. Kim YH, Kim KS, Choi H, et al. Benign paroxysmal positional vertigo is not a prognostic factor in sudden sensorineural hearing loss. Otolaryngol Head Neck Surg. 2012;146(2):279-82.
13. Fetter M, Dichgans J. Vestibular neuritis spares the inferior division of the vestibular nerve. Brain. 1996;119:755-63.
14. Gianoli G, Goebel J, Mowry S, et al. Anatomic differences in the lateral vestibular nerve channels and their implications in vestibular neuritis. Otol Neurotol. 2005;26(3):489-94.
15. Morita N, Cureoglu S, Nomiya S, et al. Potential cause of positional vertigo in Ménière's disease. Otol Neurotol. 2009;30(7):956-60.
16. Balatsouras DG, Ganelis P, Aspris A, et al. Benign paroxysmal positional vertigo associated with Meniere's disease: epidemiological, pathophysiologic, clinical, and therapeutic aspects. Ann Otol Rhinol Laryngol. 2012;121(10):682-8.
17. Rossi Izquierdo M, Soto Varela A, Santos Pérez S, et al. Association between endolymphatic hydrops and benign paroxysmal positional vertigo: coincidence or causality?. Acta Otorrinolaringol Esp. 2009;60(4):234-7.
18. Paparella MM. Benign paroxysmal positional vertigo and other vestibular symptoms in Ménière disease. Ear Nose Throat J. 2008;87(10):562.
19. Ganança CF, Caovilla HH, Gazzola JM, et al. Epley's maneuver in benign paroxysmal positional vertigo associated with Meniere's disease. Braz J Otorhinolaryngol. 2007;73(4):506-12.
20. Gross EM, Ress BD, Viirre ES, et al. Intractable benign paroxysmal positional vertigo in patients with Meniere's disease. Laryngoscope. 2000;110(4):655-9.
21. Perez N, Martin E, Zubieta JL, et al. Benign paroxysmal positional vertigo in patients with Ménière's disease treated with intratympanic gentamycin. Laryngoscope. 2002;112(6):1104-9.
22. Li P, Zeng X, Li Y, et al. Clinical analysis of benign paroxysmal positional vertigo secondary to Meniere's disease. Sci Res Essays. 2010;5(23):3672-5.
23. Chung WH, Chung KW, Kim JH, et al. Effects of a single intratympanic gentamicin injection on Meniere's disease. Acta Otolaryngol Suppl. 2007;(558):61-6.
24. Song JJ, Yoo YT, An YH, et al. Comorbid benign paroxysmal positional vertigo in idiopathic sudden sensorineural hearing loss: an ominous sign for hearing recovery. Otol Neurotol. 2012;33(2):137-41.
25. Katsarkas A. Benign paroxysmal positional vertigo (BPPV): idiopathic versus post-traumatic. Acta Otolaryngol. 1999;119(7):745-9.

26. Motin M, Keren O, Groswasser Z, et al. Benign paroxysmal positional vertigo as the cause of dizziness in patients after severe traumatic brain injury: diagnosis and treatment. Brain Inj. 2005;19(9):693-7.
27. Ahn SK, Jeon SY, Kim JP, et al. Clinical characteristics and treatment of benign paroxysmal positional vertigo after traumatic brain injury. J Trauma. 2011;70:442-6.
28. Suarez H, Alonso R, Arocena M, et al. Clinical characteristics of positional vertigo after mild head trauma. Acta Otolaryngol. 2011;131(4):377-81.
29. Magliulo G, Gagliardi M, Cuiuli G, et al. Stapedotomy and post-operative benign paroxysmal positional vertigo. J Vestib Res. 2005;15(3):169-72.
30. Park SK, Kim SY, Han KH, et al. Benign paroxysmal positional vertigo after surgical drilling of the temporal bone. Otol Neurotol. 2013;34(8):1448-55.
31. Viccaro M, Mancini P, La Gamma R, et al. Positional vertigo and cochlear implantation. Otol Neurotol. 2007;28(6):764-7.
32. Limb CJ, Francis HF, Lusting LR, et al. Benign positional vertigo after cochlear implantation. Otolaryngol Head Neck Surg. 2005;132:741-5.
33. Chiarella G, Leopardi G, De Fazio L, et al. Iatrogenic benign paroxysmal positional vertigo: review and personal experience in dental and maxillo-facial surgery. Acta Otorhinolaryngol Ital. 2007;27(3):126-8.
34. Sammartino G, Mariniello M, Scaravilli MS. Benign paroxysmal positional vertigo following closed sinus floor elevation procedure: mallet osteotomes vs. screwable osteotomes. A triple blind randomized controlled trial. Clin Oral Implants Res. 2011;22(6):669-72.
35. Lempert T, Leopold M, von Brevern M. Migraine and benign positional vertigo. Ann Otol Rhinol Laryngol. 2000;109:1176.
36. Faralli M, Cipriani L, Del Zompo MR, et al. Benign paroxysmal positional vertigo and migraine: analysis of 186 cases. B-ENT. 2014;10(2):133-9.
37. Magliulo G, Gagliardi S, Ciniglio Appiani M, et al. Vestibular neurolabyrinthitis: a follow-up study with cervical and ocular vestibular evoked myogenic potentials and the video head impulse test. Ann Otol Rhinol Laryngol. 2014;123(3):162-73.
38. Marom T, Oron Y, Watad W, et al. Revisiting benign paroxysmal positional vertigo pathophysiology. Am J Otolaryngol. 2009;30(4):250-5.
39. Gacek RR. A place principle for vertigo. Auris Nasus Larynx. 2008;35(1):1-10.
40. Paparella MM. Pathogenesis of Meniere's disease and Meniere's syndrome. Acta Otolaryngol Suppl. 1984;406:10-25.
41. El-Saied S, Joshua BZ, Segal N, et al. Sudden hearing loss with simultaneous posterior semicircular canal BPPV: possible etiology and clinical implications. Am J Otolaryngol. 2014;35(2):180-5.
42. Kim CH, Shin JE, Park HJ, et al. Concurrent posterior semicircular canal benign paroxysmal positional vertigo in patients with ipsilateral sudden sensorineural hearing loss: is it caused by otolith particles? Med Hypotheses. 2014;82(4):424-7.
43. Mandalà M, Colletti L, Carner M, et al. Pneumolabyrinth and positional vertigo after stapedectomy. Auris Nasus Larynx. 2011;38(4):547-50.
44. De Stefano A, Dispenza F, Suarez H, et al. A multicenter observational study on the role of comorbidities in the recurrent episodes of benign paroxysmal positional vertigo. Auris Nasus Larynx. 2014;41(1):31-6.

45. Blessing R, Strutz J, Beck C. Epidemiology of benign paroxysmal positional vertigo (in German). Laryngol Rhinol Otol (Stuttg). 1986;65:455-8.
46. Korres SG, Balatsouras DG, Ferekidis E. Electronystagmographic findings in benign paroxysmal positional vertigo. Ann Otol Rhinol Laryngol. 2004;113(4): 313-8.
47. Korres S, Gkoritsa E, Giannakakou-Razelou D, et al. Vestibular evoked myogenic potentials in patients with BPPV. Med Sci Monit. 2011;17(1):CR42-7.
48. Tanimoto H, Doi K, Nishikawa T, et al. Risk factors for recurrence of benign paroxysmal positional vertigo. J Otolaryngol Head Neck Surg. 2008;37(6):832-5.
49. Kansu L, Avci S, Yilmaz I, et al. Long-term follow-up of patients with posterior canal benign paroxysmal positional vertigo. Acta Otolaryngol. 2010;130:1009-12.
50. Uneri A. Migraine and benign paroxysmal positional vertigo: an outcome study of 476 patients. Ear Nose Throat J. 2004;83(12):814-5.

Chapter 11

Benign Paroxysmal Positional Vertigo and Migraine-Associated Vertigo

Terry D Fife, Kristen Steenerson

OVERVIEW

Benign paroxysmal positional vertigo (BPPV) is a disorder of the inner ear related to calcium carbonate material that becomes dislodged from otoconia of the macula of the utricle, which moves within the lumen of one of the semicircular canals during certain head movements by the effect of gravity. The movement of these particles causes endolymph movement that inappropriately stimulates the ampullary nerve of the affected semicircular canal resulting in a burst of positional vertigo and nystagmus.

The pathophysiology of BPPV and that of migraine seem to have little in common. However, an association between BPPV and migraine has been recognized in the literature. Furthermore, there are important features of each condition that are noteworthy in distinguishing BPPV from migrainous vertigo, which can, sometimes, also have positional features.

VESTIBULAR MIGRAINE

Migraine is a common condition associated with episodic moderate to severe headaches often associated with nausea and sensitivity to light, sound and odors.[1] However, in some people, periodic vertigo, sensations of motion, and sensitivity to movement occur without accompanying headache. When such vestibular features dominate the symptom complex, we refer to it as vestibular migraine.[2] In the past few years, diagnostic criteria have been set forth by a subcommittee of the International Headache Society (IHS) and a committee of the Barany Society.[3] Table 11.1 outlines the criteria for classifying vestibular migraine.

The cause of migraine is not well understood. There is evidence in the case of migraine headache that brainstem nuclei become hypersensitized to ordinary sensory stimulation. In particular, the nucleus caudalis and, possibly, the raphe nuclei become activated. The susceptibility of persons for this kind of activation appears to be influenced by both genetic and environmental factors. A similar hypersensitization may occur in the vestibular nuclei rendering prone to spontaneous

Table 11.1: Diagnostic criteria for vestibular migraine.[3]	
A	At least five episodes of vestibular symptoms (spontaneous or positional vertigo, visual vertigo, head motion-related dizziness, or motion sickness) of moderate-to-severe intensity lasting 5 minutes to 72 hours
B	Current or prior history of migraine by IHS criteria
C	One or more of the following: throbbing or unilateral headache, photophobia or phonophobia, migraine visual aura
D	Not better explained by another vestibular or headache disorder

(IHS: International Headache Society).

illusions of motion and also especially sensitive to head motion and optokinetic stimuli.[4] The underlying pathophysiology may relate to derangements in the communications between neurons such as ion channels. Thus, vestibular migraine is probably due to a multitude of genetic factors leading to varying degrees of susceptibility to environmental stimuli. Although migraine is commonly familial, a rat model for migraine-related neurogenic inflammation and cortical spreading depression assume no family predisposition.[45] This suggests that all humans may be hard-wired for migraine and what is inherited is our degree of susceptibility to innate and external environmental factors. Thus, unlike the mechanical and the anatomic basis of BPPV, migraine is more closely tied to actual nerve-to-nerve physiological interactions carried out by the brain on a daily and continuing basis.[5]

ASSOCIATION BETWEEN BPPV AND MIGRAINE

Benign paroxysmal positional vertigo is the most common cause of episodic recurrent vertigo. Although historically incidence has been estimated between 0.01%[6] and 0.06%,[7] these data were based on recorded clinical cases, thus likely were an underestimation of the true incidence. In a German population-based survey, the lifetime prevalence of BPPV was 2.4%.[8] The 1-year prevalence of BPPV increased with age being seven times higher in those older than age 60 years than in those 18 to 39 years. Benign paroxysmal positional vertigo was more common in women than men in all age groups. Approximately 18% of patients seen in dizziness clinics[9] and 25% of patients sent for vestibular testing have BPPV.[10] This also accounts for about 20% of pediatric referrals.[11]

Meanwhile, vestibular migraine accounts for a large proportion of dizziness and is the second most common cause of recurrent vertigo.[8] In the general population, lifetime prevalence of migraine is 14%[12] and 7% in vertigo.[8] The lifetime prevalence of definite vestibular migraine is ~1%.[8] However, if one considers probable vestibular migraine and benign recurrent vertigo, vestibular migraine may be much more common than previously appreciated.[13]

The co-occurrence of BPPV and migraine in the same individual occurs more often than would be predicted by pure change.[14] The expected co-occurrence of both BPPV and vestibular migraine is about 1%. However, the population prevalence of both conditions is 3.2%, which is three times greater than anticipated.[8,15] In a study of 476 patients with posterior canal BPPV, 54.8% had a history of migraine by IHS criteria, and two-thirds of the 476 BPPV patients had motion hypersensitivity, which is much higher than the baseline population.[16] Another study found that of 247 patients with BPPV, a history of migraine was threefold greater among those who developed idiopathic BPPV versus those who had BPPV following head trauma or surgery.[17] In a population-based study, prevalence of lifetime vestibular vertigo (not purely BPPV but substantially so) without migraine is of 7.4%, whereas the lifetime prevalence of having both vestibular vertigo and migraine is 3.2%, suggesting a stronger-than-expected prevalence of the two conditions together.[15]

POSSIBLE MECHANISTIC RELATIONSHIP BETWEEN BPPV AND MIGRAINE

In general, BPPV and vestibular migraine have been described as two separate conditions with some overlapping symptomatology. Indeed, BPPV may occur with headache and likewise vestibular migraine may have a positional component, which may appear similar to BPPV.[5,18,19]

One possible explanation for the association between migraine and BPPV is that vertigo itself may be a trigger for a migraine event, particularly, headaches.[20] This would explain why migraine is more common in BPPV patients but not so much why BPPV is seen more among migraineurs. In addition, patients with vestibular migraine are more affected by visual commotion and also by head movement than by the general population.[4,21,22] This increased sensitivity to visual and actual motions renders them more symptomatic to vertigo of any cause when they develop vertigo from any cause.[4,23] Vestibular migraine patients have a reduced perceptual tolerance for dynamic head movements[24] and they tend to be particularly prone to motion sickness.[25] Thus, the occurrence of BPPV symptoms is more disabling and alarming and is more apt to bring them into medical attention, possibly explaining why those with vestibular migraine or migraine headaches are found to have BPPV more often than the general population.

Increasing evidence supports the likelihood that degeneration of otoconia[26] may be related to aging, osteopenia, vitamin D deficiency, and female gender.[27,28,44] Since migraine generally has a 3:1 female-to-male predominance[29] and BPPV has a 2:1 female-to-male predominance,[30] the presence of the association might be tied more to gender susceptibility than to a direct mechanism.

Some have proposed other more direct mechanisms by which migraine may predispose to BPPV. It has been proposed that migraine may cause vasospasm-related ischemia within the labyrinth that over time may promote or hasten the breakdown of otoconia.[13] Alternatively, calcitonin gene-related peptide, serotonin, norepinephrine, and dopamine modulate the neuronal activity of both centrally and peripherally vestibular neurons.[46] It is conceivable that the effects of modulation of peripheral vestibular function could have indirect effects on the integrity of otoconia though at present there is no direct evidence of this.

Recently, a form of BPPV that seems to run in families was localized to chromosome 15[31] so there could also genes predisposing to recurrent BPPV could cosegregate with a gene or genes that influence the propensity for migraine.

DISTINGUISHING MIGRAINE POSITIONAL VERTIGO FROM BPPV

Clinical Features

Vestibular migraine is associated with varying sensations of dizziness ranging from floating to rocking to spinning to simply motion sensitivity.[2,32-34] One of the ways that migraine-related vertigo can present is with a positional element,[5,14,19] which can make it, in some cases, similar to the history of BPPV. Table 11.2 describes some of the clinical and nystagmus features that help distinguish vestibular migraine with positional vertigo from BPPV.

Vestibular migraine has been more often associated with a history of long-standing symptoms since childhood.[19] This might include recurrent dizziness or motion sickness. Spells of dizziness related to migraine may at times be short-lived and may thus be confused with BPPV. One should enquire about other more characteristic migraine features including general sensitivity to motion, aversion to bright lights (photophobia), and loud sounds (phonophobia), migraine headaches, and migraine visual phenomena all of which may occur temporally not related to the vertigo or dizziness. That is, fairly, commonly, the dizziness occurs independently of any migraine headaches, and migraine headaches may actually be infrequent or rare.[2,32,35]

Nystagmus of Migraine Positional Vertigo and of BPPV

The forms of positional nystagmus that may occur due to migraine include: static positional upbeating nystagmus, low velocity direction changing static positional nystagmus[32, 33, 36-38] The nystagmus may resolve as dizziness improves but in some cases persists even between spells of dizziness.[38, 39]

Table 11.2: Features of benign paroxysmal positional vertigo (BPPV) versus migraine positional vertigo.

	BPPV	Migraine positional vertigo	Benign paroxysmal vertigo of childhood
Age of peak incidence	40–60 years	25–55 years	3–10 years
Duration of vertigo	10–30 seconds	1 minute to hours	15 minutes to hours
Positional trigger	Turning in bed, rolling in bed, tilting head back, bending over	Lying on one side for a period of at least 1 minute	None
Response to Dix-Hallpike maneuver	Burst of intense spinning vertigo	Little or no dizziness except that associated with general head movement	None
Latency	2–6 seconds	1–15 minutes	None
Nystagmus	With Dix-Hallpike maneuver, there is paroxysmal upbeating and torsional nystagmus with top pole rotating toward downward ear; in horizontal canal variant: direction changing paroxysmal horizontal positional nystagmus	Little or no nystagmus or low-velocity static positional upbeating, horizontal or direction changing positional nystagmus (less commonly)	Little or no nystagmus or low-velocity static positional upbeating, horizontal or direction changing positional nystagmus (less commonly).
Treatment	Canalith repositioning maneuvers; Semont's liberatory maneuver	Migraine prophylactic medications when severe	Migraine prophylactic medications when severe

It has been observed that noxious stimulation of trigeminal dermatomes in patients with vestibular migraine induced nystagmus compared to no nystagmus in healthy controls.[40] Compensatory mechanisms also seem to be decreased as one study described decreased suppression of otoacoustic emissions in patients with vestibular migraine compared to controls.[20] Toglia et al.[41] described labyrinthine abnormalities in 80% of patients with migraine with aura using quantitative vestibular testing.

Benign paroxysmal vertigo of childhood is a syndrome of recurrent spontaneous spells of vertigo, occasionally with nystagmus and imbalance that occur in young children.[42] It can occasionally be confused with BPPV but is widely believed to be a form of vestibular migraine in children.[43]

Finally, it should be remembered that both BPPV and vestibular migraine may be present in the same person at the same time in some cases. The nystagmus that is characteristic of BPPV and the history of a clear positional trigger are good clues to the presence of BPPV but other features more related to vestibular migraine may confuse the clinical history and occasionally low-velocity static positional nystagmus may be observed.

TREATMENT OF VESTIBULAR MIGRAINE

Prophylactic migraine pharmacotherapy is indicated when vestibular migraine is causing symptoms frequently and reducing the patient's quality of life. There are no good randomized controlled trials to guide therapy at present, but several are underway looking at verapamil, metoprolol, and rizatriptan. Pending the results, we rely on randomized trials for the treatment of migraine headaches. Tricyclic amines (e.g. nortriptyline, imipramine, and amitriptyline) may be used in dosages from 25 to 100 mg, especially if there are concomitant problems with anxiety or insomnia. Verapamil usually at dosages of 180–240 mg daily is generally well tolerated and perhaps surprisingly, only occasionally, causes hypotension but more often is associated with constipation. Selective serotonin norepinephrine reuptake inhibitors such as venlafaxine or duloxetine may be helpful with slow titration schedules to 75 mg of venlafaxine or 60 mg of duloxetine daily. Topiramate at dosages of 50–200 mg daily may also provide relief of symptoms. Patients should be advised that most migraine prophylactic medications take several weeks to noticeably reduce symptoms.

The treatment of BPPV is described elsewhere. It is important to treat the BPPV early on[36] and not let symptoms linger and continue, as they may be a recurring trigger for migraine symptoms and may also cause increased anxiety and thus complicate recovery.

CONCLUSION

Together, vestibular migraine and BPPV account for many cases of recurrent vertigo. These two conditions occur together more often than one would expect on the basis of prevalence alone raising the possibility that vestibular migraine may predispose to BPPV or that BPPV makes it more likely for patients to seek medical attention. Vestibular migraine may cause chronic positional dizziness and low-velocity static positional nystagmus but does not cause the classical nystagmus of BPPV. The positional nystagmus of vestibular migraine is more likely to build up over a period of minutes whereas BPPV is paroxysmal and results in a burst of nystagmus and vertigo upon lying back or turning in bed. Benign paroxysmal positional vertigo is effectively treated with canalith repositioning maneuvers whereas vestibular migraine-related positional vertigo does not. Vestibular migraine, when severe enough to warrant it, requires migraine preventative drugs.

REFERENCES

1. Olesen J, Steiner TJ. The international classification of headache disorders, 2nd edition. Oxford: International Headache Society; 2004.
2. Lempert T. Vestibular migraine. Semin Neurol. 2013;33:212-8.
3. Lempert T, Olesen J, Furman J, et al. Vestibular migraine: diagnostic criteria. J Vestib Res. 2012;22;167-72.
4. Bronstein AM, Golding JF, Gresty MA. Vertigo and dizziness from environmental motion: visual vertigo, motion sickness and drivers' disorientation. Semin Neurol. 2013;33:219-30.
5. Furman JM, Balaban CD. Vestibular migraine. Ann N Y Acad Sci. 2015;1343:90-6.
6. Mizukoshi K, Watanabe Y, Shojaku H, et al. Epidemiological studies on benign paroxysmal positional vertigo in Japan. Acta Otolaryngol Suppl. 1988;447:67-72.
7. Froehling DA, Silverstein MD, Mohr DN, et al. Benign positional vertigo: incidence and prognosis in population-based study in Olmsted County, Minnesota. Mayo Clin Proc. 1991;66(6):596-601.
8. Neuhauser HK, Lempert T. Vertigo: epidemiologic aspects. Semin Neurol. 2009;29(5);473-81.
9. Nedzelski JM, Barber HO, McIlmoyl L. Diagnoses in a dizziness unit. J Otolaryngol. 1986;15:101-4.
10. Hughes CA, Proctor L. Benign paroxysmal positional vertigo. Laryngoscope. 1997;107:607-13.
11. Wiener-Vacher SR. Vestibular disorders in children. Int J Audiol. 2008;47:578-83.
12. Jensen R, Stovner LJ. Epidemiology and comorbidity of headache. Lancet Neurol. 2008;7(4):354-61.
13. Cha YH, Lee H, Santell LS, et al. Association of benign recurrent vertigo and migraine in 208 patients. Cephalalgia. 2009;29(5):550-5.
14. Lempert T, Leopold M, von Brevern M, et al. Comment on migraine and benign positional vertigo. Ann Otorhinolaryngol. 2000;109(12 Pt 1):1176.
15. Neuhauser HK, Radtke A, von Brevern M, et al. Migrainous vertigo: prevalence and impact on quality of life. Neurology. 2006;67(6):1028-33.
16. Uneri A. Migraine and benign paroxysmal positional vertigo: an outcome study of 476 patients. Ear Nose Throat J. 2004;83(12):814-5.
17. Ishiyama A, Jacobson KM, Baloh RW. Migraine and benign positional vertigo. Ann Otorhinolaryngol. 2000;109(4):377-80.
18. Stolte B, Holle D, Naegel S, et al. Vestibular migraine. Cephalalgia. 2015;35(3):262-70.
19. von Brevern M, Radtke A, Clarke AH, et al. Migrainous vertigo presenting as episodic positional vertigo. Neurology. 2004;62(3):469-72.
20. Murdin L, Davies RA, Bronstein AM. Vertigo as a migraine trigger. Neurology. 2009;73(8):638-42.
21. Page NG, Gresty MA. Motorist's vestibular disorientation syndrome. J Neurol Neurosurg Psychiatry. 1985;48:729-35.

22. Bronstein AM. Visual vertigo syndrome: clinical and posturography findings. J Neurol Neurosurg Psychiatry. 1995;59:572-6.
23. Golding JF. Motion sickness susceptibility questionnaire revised and its relationship to other forms of sickness. Brain Res Bull. 1998;47:507-16.
24. Lewis RF, Priesol AJ, Nicoucar K, et al. Dynamic tilt thresholds are reduced in vestibular migraine. J Vestib Res. 2011;21(6):323-30.
25. Jeong SH, Oh SY, Kim HJ, et al. Vestibular dysfunction in migraine: effects of associated vertigo and motion sickness. J Neurol. 2010;257(6):905-12.
26. Jang YS, Hwang CH, Shin JY, et al. Age-related changes on the morphology of the otoconia. Laryngoscope. 2006;116:996-1001.
27. Jeong SH, Choi SH, Kim JY, et al. Osteopenia and osteoporosis in idiopathic benign positional vertigo. Neurology. 2009;72(12):1069-76.
28. Yu S, Liu F, Cheng Z, et al. Association between osteoporosis and benign paroxysmal positional vertigo: a systematic review. BMC Neurol. 2014;14:110.
29. Van Ombergen A, Van Rompaey V, Van de Heyning P, et al. Vestibular migraine in an otolaryngology clinic: prevalence, associated symptoms and prophylactic medication effectiveness. Otol Neurotol. 2015;36:133-8.
30. Ogun OA, Janky KL, Cohn ES, et al. Gender-based comorbidity in benign paroxysmal positional vertigo. PLoS One. 2014;9:e105546.
31. Gizzi MS, Peddareddygari LR, Grewal RP. A familial form of benign paroxysmal positional vertigo maps to chromosome 15. Int J Neurosci. 2015;125(8):593-6.
32. Cutrer F, Baloh RW. Migraine-associated dizziness. Headache. 1992;32:300-4.
33. Cass SP, Furman JM, Ankerstjerne K, et al. Migraine-related vestibulopathy. Ann Oto Rhinol Laryngol. 1997;106(3):182-9.
34. Neuhauser H, Lempert T. Vertigo and dizziness related to migraine: a diagnostic challenge. Cephalalgia. 2004;24(2):83-91.
35. Neff BA, Staab JP, Eggers SD, et al. Auditory and vestibular symptoms and chronic subjective dizziness in patients with Meniere's disease, vestibular migraine, and Meniere's disease with concomitant vestibular migraine. Otol Neurotol. 2012;33(7):1235-44.
36. Roberts RA, Gans RE, Kastner AH. Differentiation of migrainous positional vertigo (MPV) from horizontal canal benign paroxysmal positional vertigo (HC-BPPV). Internat J Audiol. 2006;45(4):224-6.
37. Kuritzky A, Toglia UJ, Thomas D. Vestibular function in migraine. Headache. 1981;21(3):110-2.
38. Polanesk SH, Tusa RJ. Nystagmus during attacks of vestibular migraine: an aid in diagnosis. Audiol Neurootol. 2010;15(4):241-6.
39. Kayan A, Hood HD. Neuro-otological manifestations of migraine. Brain. 1984;107:1123-42.
40. Marano E, Marcelli V, Di Stasio E, et al. Trigeminal stimulation elicits a peripheral vestibular imbalance in migraine patients. Headache. 2005;45(4):325-31.
41. Toglia JU, Thomas D, Kuritzky A. Common migraine and vestibular function. Electronystagmographic study and pathogenesis. Ann Otorhinolaryngol. 1981;90(3 Pt 1):267-71.
42. Watson P, Steele JC. Paroxysmal dysequilibrium in the migraine syndrome of childhood. Arch Otolaryngol. 1974;99(3):177-9.

43. Koehler B. Benign paroxysmal vertigo of childhood: a migraine equivalent. Eur J Pediatr. 1980;134(2):149-51.
44. Whitman GT, Baloh RW. Seasonality of benign paroxysmal positional vertigo. JAMA Otolaryngol Head Neck Surg. 2015;141:188-9.
45. Bolay H, Reuter U, Dunn AK, et al. Intrinsic brain activity triggers trigeminal meningeal afferents in a migraine model. Nat Med. 2002;8(2):136-142.
46. Babalian A, Vibert N, Assie G, et al. Central vestibular networks in the guinea-pig: functional characterization in the isolated whole brain in vitro. Neuroscience 1997;81:405-426.

Chapter 12

Benign Paroxysmal Postural Vertigo in the Childhood

Hamlet Suarez

INTRODUCTION

Vestibular organs provide sensory information about motion and spatial orientation, along with the visual and somatosensory information, and are essential for postural control and gait. Therefore the normal function of these three sensory inputs (Visual, vestibular and somatosensory) is crucial in a child development. Specifically, vestibular receptors have the role of stabilizing the image on the retina during head movements. Vestibular receptor lesions in children affect the ability of learning to read and write and in fine and gross skills.

Benign paroxysmal positional vertigo (BPPV) is the most common cause of vertigo and is related to the displacement of fragments of otolith organs (otoconia debris) into semicircular canals, mainly in the posterior semicircular canal. Although BPPV occurs in all age groups,[1] it has less incidence in children, reported only 3% of 3,341 patients with BPPV who were studied.[2] Basser related the BPPV in childhood as a clinical presentation of the vestibular neuronitis.[3] Baloh and Honrubia reported three members of the same family who developed BPPV before the age of 13. All three had migraine headaches and two of them had spontaneous episodes of vertigo. Their hypothesis about the mechanisms of macule disorders is related to ischemic damage due to vasospasm because all three patients had a vestibular migraine syndrome.[4] Such approaches of positional vertigo during childhood must, perhaps, be considered in order to assess factors that can be related to the etiology of the pathology of vestibular maculae.

CLINICAL PRESENTATION OF BPPV IN CHILDREN

Many times vertigo is clearly linked with body movements, such as getting up from the bed or tilting to a side. In other times, the positional vertigo is not reported accurately by the child who feels dizzy and cannot define exactly if the symptoms start with the head or body movement.

Besides the positional vertigo, the child at other times can report chronic dizziness, which may be associated with nausea or vomiting. This

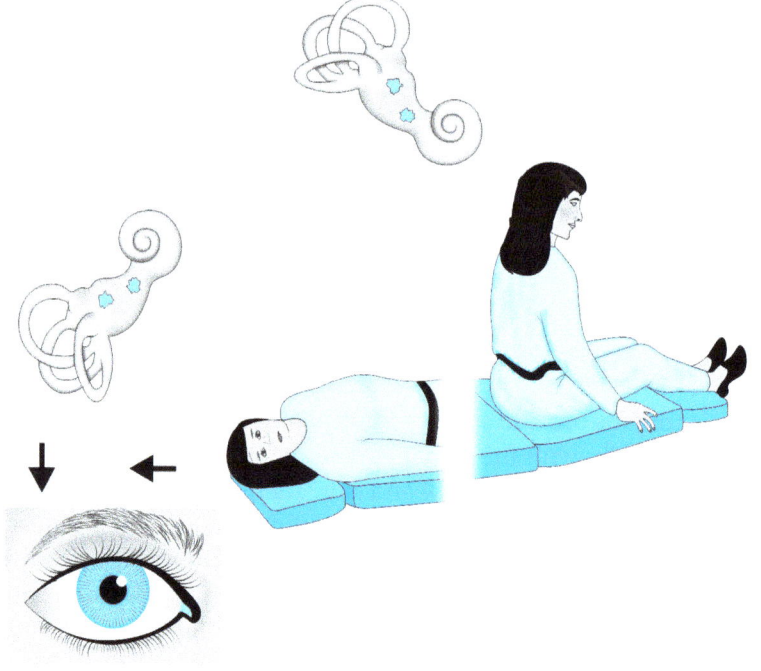

Fig. 12.1: Dix-Hallpike test.

kind of clinical presentation mainly occurs after head trauma, and the exploration by means of electronystagmography (ENG) or videonystagmography (VNG) usually shows a unilateral vestibular hypofunction.

The history of vertigo in children may be confused with an onset of symptoms of vestibular migraine and, therefore—obtaining a detailed description of the characteristics of the symptomatology—it will be necessary to find the typical presentation of BPPV positional nystagmus.

CHARACTERISTIC OF THE POSITIONAL NYSTAGMUS

The Dix-Hallpike maneuver is a suitable clinical test for BPPV, generating a rotatory nystagmus with latency and limited duration. Sometimes a negative test can indicate that active canalithiasis is not present at that moment because the reposition of the debris from the canal can occur spontaneously, although it is usually recurrent. Posterior canal BPPV produces geotropic rotatory nystagmus when the affected ear is positioned downward during the Dix-Hallpike maneuver (Fig. 12.1). Horizontal nystagmus indicates the presence of canalithiasis in horizontal canal. Canalithiasis in the anterior canal is least frequent in BPPV and is diagnosed when the positional nystagmus is downbeating and sometimes with torsional movements in the Dix-Hallpike position. Occasionally, anterior canal canalithiasis occurs as a complication of the repositioning maneuver. Nonfatiguing nystagmus may indicate cupulolithiasis rather than canalithiasis.

FREQUENT ETIOLOGY OF BPPV IN THE CHILDHOOD

Head Trauma

Many mechanisms of head trauma, such as domestic or car accidents and sports trauma, have been described related to BPPV. They can be divided into those producing severe neurological disorders and those with mild head trauma. A patient with mild traumatic brain injury has typically had a head trauma without any period of loss of consciousness or significant loss of memory of events immediately before or after the accident, or focal neurological disorders.[5] Mild head trauma can generate utricular or saccular macula lesions and even damage the semicircular canal receptor with different clinical features.[6] The symptoms can appear immediately after trauma or deferred in time, even months later. The clinical presentation of positional vertigo after mild head trauma is most frequently bilateral canalithiasis and multicanal BPPV when compared to BPPV not related to trauma. However, no significant differences had been found in a sample that shows the index of recurrence between BPPV after trauma and "idiopathic" BPPV.[7] Benign paroxismal positional vertigo after trauma can be associated with unilateral or bilateral vestibular receptor hypofunction, which is related to the concussion and assessed by ENG or VNG, and it must be considered in order to design a vestibular rehabilitation program. Another association, which is evidenced, is with cognitive disorders, mainly if the head trauma included loss of consciousness or related to neurosurgical procedures.

A special clinical situation arises when BPPV occurs as an associated lesion in a patient with diffuse axonal injury, which represents a very complex challenge in order to achieve vestibular as well as neurological rehabilitation.

As mentioned above, BPPV after trauma can be manifested in three main clinical presentations:
1. Isolated BPPV, appearing immediately or delayed, related to mild head trauma
2. Associated with cognitive disorders
3. Associated with diffuse axonal injury.

All of these clinical presentations can be related to vestibular receptor hypofunction, involving partial or total loss of utricular and saccular macula and semicircular canal functions. These situations will need different approaches for designing an adequate rehabilitation program, performing repositioning maneuvers when the BPPV is exclusively due to vestibular disturbance, and adding training of the vestibulo-ocular reflex when the BPPV is associated with vestibular receptor hypofunction and the patient complains of chronic dizziness. A multidisciplinary team will be necessary to work on rehabilitation when the BPPV is present along with major neurological lesions with cognitive alterations or diffuse axonal injury.

BPPV and Genetic

The clinical expertise shows that if a child has BPPV it is frequent for some other members of his or her family to have the history of positional vertigo. Gizzi et al.[8] reported a study in which they performed a genome-wide scan on a three-generation family in which multiple family members developed BPPV. They studied the whole genome mapping with 400 microsatellite repeat markers and analyzed the autosomal dominant and recessive models of inheritance. They found two-point linkage analysis that showed LOD (logarithm of the odds) scores of one or greater than one on chromosomes 7, 15, 16, and 20. Independent of the model of inheritance, the highest two-point LOD scores localized the same marker on chromosome 15. Logarithm of the odds is a test used to compare the likelihood if two loci are linked versus that of the two loci if they are unlinked. The formula for the calculation is as follows:

$$LOD = \log10 \frac{\text{likelihood if the loci are linked}}{\text{likelihood if the loci are unlinked}}$$

This involvement of chromosome 15 in this studied family is a significant finding and opens a new way for the study and understanding of the role of genes in the pathology of the otolith organs, mainly when the clinical disorders have an expression during childhood.

Metabolism of the Otoconia

The metabolism of the otoconia can suffer alterations with demineralization, decreasing the anchoring of the fibrils interconnecting the otoconia and causing weakening of this matrix with an increase in the chance of otolith detachment and movement toward the endolymphatic space, generating the mechanism of the BPPV. These findings have been reproduced in 2-year-old mice and these alterations can also be related to genetic disorders[9] and to modifications in the autophagy, which is a catabolic process where cells degrade their constituents to dispose of unwanted cytoplasmic elements recycling nutrients which have a important role in the process to remodeling the cells. Recent studies showed that in mice with lack of autophagin-1 evidenced alterations in the development of the otoconia.[10] Metabolic disorders that had been described experimentally can be involved in the generation of BPPV in the early stages of life.

BPPV LINKED WITH OTOLOGIC DISEASE

Positional vertigo can appear as a delayed symptom in the evolution of vestibular neuritis. Although Ménière's disease is rare during childhood, after a crisis, a positional nystagmus with clinical characteristic of BPPV related to otolith organ lesions by endolymphatic hydrops can be observed. Also, chronic otitis media can generate alterations on the otolith receptors due to a nearby inflammatory process, causing debris to be released from the otoconia to the endolymphatic space eliciting BPPV.[11]

TESTING

ENG-VNG

In addition to the bedside examination, ENG-VNG can provide relevant information indicating if BPPV is associated with a semicircular canal hypofunction. The patients who have BPPV and vestibular receptor hypofunction feel chronic dizziness as well as positional vertigo. This is a significant fact to know if the BPPV is an isolated disorder or can be a secondary symptom of a major lesion on the inner ear.

A vestibular hypofunction evidenced in the ENG-VNG must be taken into account in order to design a vestibular rehabilitation program, which must include repositioning maneuvers as well as vestibular ocular reflex training to compensate the deficit.

The registry of vestibular responses during caloric or rotatory stimulation and the behavior of the ocular movements (smooth pursuit and saccadic) and optokinetic nystagmus give the possibility of knowing the function of the vestibular system as a whole. All these data are significant in cases in which BPPV is recurrent or the response to the repositioning maneuver is poor.

Vestibular Evoked Myogenic Potentials

Vestibular evoked myogenic potentials (VEMPs) can be useful in cases in which BPPV patients complain of a nonspecific symptom of chronic dizziness even after the disappearance of the positional nystagmus with the repositioning maneuvers. With the ocular and cervical VEMPs, it is possible to know about the utricular and saccular functions, which can be useful in BPPV posthead concussion or BPPV postvestibular neuritis.

Audiological Testing

The audiometry is a suitable procedure to perform an easy assessment of the cochlear function while the impedanciometry, otoacoustic emissions, or auditory evoked potentials must be explored when BPPV is a symptom of a more complex disturbance, such as head trauma or BPPV in a chronic otitis media.

Image Exploration

When a lesion of the temporal bone or the posterior fossa is presumed, with associated symptoms of a positional nystagmus, the computed tomography scanning or magnetic resonance imaging can be accurate for the diagnosis. It can provide relevant information, especially in children with a head trauma.

Treatment

The BPPV treatment is mainly addressed to improve the patient´s clinical condition by means of repositioning maneuvers. Maneuvers of Epley, Semont, Vanucci, and others are described in the corresponding chapters and each of them is more suitable when the canalithiasis is placed in the posterior, horizontal, or anterior semicircular canal. These procedures follow the same rules in children as they do with adults.

When BPPV is associated with chronic dizziness due to hypofunction of a vestibular receptor, it will be necessary, in addition to the repositioning maneuvers, to design a vestibular rehabilitation program in order to achieve a vestibular compensation.

Norré[12] described habituation training, which is a classic approach where the treatment of vestibular deficit and different kinds of exercises have been proposed,[13] including the use of virtual reality techniques,[14] with a goal of compensating the vestibular deficit. These procedures are sometimes carried out for weeks, being the psychological support of the children essential for therapeutic success.

REFERENCES

1. von Brevern M, Radtke A, Lezius F, et al. Epidemiology of benign paroxysmal positional vertigo: a population based study. J Neurol Neurosurg Psychiatry. 2007;78(7):710-5.
2. Saka N, Imai T, Seo T, Ohta S, et al. Analysis of benign paroxysmal positional nystagmus in children. Int J Pediatr Otorhinolaryngol. 2013;77(2):233-6.
3. Basser LS, Benign paroxismal vertigo of childhood. (A variety of vestibular neuritis). Brain. 1964;87:141-52.
4. Baloh RW, Honrubia V. Childhood onset of benign positional vertigo. Neurology. 1998;50(5):1494-6.
5. Vanderploeg RD, Belanger HG, Curtiss G. Mild traumatic 273 brain injury and posttraumatic stress disorder and their 274 associations with health symptoms. Arch Phys Med Rehabil. 2009;90:1084-93.

6. Rabbitt RD, Breneman KD, King C, et al. Dynamic displacement of normal and detached semicircular canal cupula. J Assoc Res Otolaryngol. 2009;10:497-509.
7. Suarez H, Alonso R, Arocena M, et al. Clinical characteristics of positional vertigo after mild head trauma. Acta Otolaryngol. 2011;131(4):377-81.
8. Gizzi MS, Peddareddygari LR, Grewal RP. A familial form of benign paroxysmal positional vertigo maps to chromosome 15. Int J Neurosci. 2015;125(8):593-6.
9. Andrade LR, Lins U, Farina M, et al. Immunogold TEM of otoconin 90 and otolin—relevance to mineralization of otoconia, and pathogenesis of benign positional vertigo. Hear Res. 2012;292(1-2):14-25.
10. Mariño G, Fernández AF, Cabrera S, et al. Autophagy is essential for mouse sense of balance. J Clin Invest. 2010;120(7):2331-44.
11. Babić B, Arsović N. [Assessment of senses of hearing and balance in chronic suppurative otitis media]. Srp Arh Celok Lek. 2008;136(5-6):307-12. (Article in Serbian)
12. Norré ME, Beckers A. Vestibular habituation training: exercise treatment for vertigo based upon the habituation effect. Otolaryngol Head Neck Surg. 1989;101(1):14-9.
13. Herdman SJ, Whitney SL. Interventions for the patient with vestibular hypofunction. In: Herdman SJ (Ed). Vestibular rehabilitation. Philadelphia, PA: FA Davis; 2007. pp. 309-37.
14. Suarez H, Arocena M, Geisinger D, et al. Virtual reality in the assessment and rehabilitation of vestibular disorders. In: Vincent M, Moreau M (Eds). Accidental falls: causes, prevention and intervention, Chapter 5. New York: Nova-publisher; 2008. pp. 766-3.

Chapter 13

Medical Management of Benign Paroxysmal Positional Vertigo

Kourosh Parham

INTRODUCTION

Benign paroxysmal positional vertigo (BPPV) is believed to arise from displacement of particulate matter, likely fragments of otoconia from the utricle, into the semicircular canals. This idea was initially put forth by Schucknecht[1,2] based on intricate insight into vestibular structure and function, and histopathologic observations of basophilic staining masses of granular or homogeneous material found attached to the cupula of the posterior semicircular canal on the affected side. In a subsequent report, Schuknecht and Ruby reported finding copular deposits in 37% of temporal bone specimens and that 58% of these were located in the posterior canal.[3] Although the mechanisms leading to BPPV symptoms were a matter of long-standing debate,[4] today, there is little doubt about the role of particulate matter. The involvement of particulate matter within the posterior semicircular canal has been established intraoperatively in patients with BPPV.[5,6] Welling et al. prospectively examined the posterior semicircular canal of patients with and without a clinical history of BPPV for the presence of particulate matter. No particles were observed intraoperatively in any of the 73 patients undergoing labyrinthine surgery (vestibular schwannoma excision or labyrinthectomy) without a history of BPPV.[7] Particulate matter was observed in 8 of 26 patients with intractable BPPV at the time of the posterior semicircular canal occlusion procedure. Similarly, Beyea et al. reported 20% incidence of free floating particles in the posterior semicircular canal of patients undergoing transmastoid posterior canal plugging for intractable BPPV.[8]

Based on clinical and experimental evidence,[9-14] displaced fragments of otoconia into the semicircular canals are now widely accepted as the cause of BPPV symptoms. Depending on the location of the displaced fragments, BPPV can arise from either canalolithiasis (particles in one or more semicircular canals) or cupulolithiasis (particles adherent to the cupula of one or more semicircular canals). It is important to realize that mere presence of fragments within the semicircular canal is not always sufficient to induce a change in vestibular nerve activity and that a critical mass is needed to evoke clinical symptoms.[15]

TREATMENT

Canalith Repositioning

Historically, as the proposed mechanism involving cupulolithiasis and canalolithiasis became more widely accepted, the idea of using head positioning maneuvers to relieve symptoms of BPPV evolved as an alternative to conservative management (i.e. avoidance of provocative head positions and changes) and surgical procedures. Brandt and Daroff used a physical therapy approach involving repeated maneuvers to loosen and disperse the degenerated otolithic material from the cupula.[16] These efforts were followed by liberatory maneuver of Semont[17] and subsequently canalith repositioning procedure (CRP) of Eply.[18,19] Given that the dominant view at that time was that BPPV arose from the involvement of the posterior semicircular canal, these repositioning procedures were mainly directed at providing relief of posterior canal BPPV. However, several varieties of BPPV can be experienced depending on the semicircular canal involved, whether or not cupula is involved, single or multiple canal involvement, and sidedness of the affected structures. In fact, the effectiveness of the repositioning maneuvers varies depending on the correct identification of the affected canal.

To assess the effectiveness of the Epley maneuver in treatment of posterior semicircular canal BPPV, a Cochrane review compared Epley maneuver versus placebo Epley maneuver versus untreated controls[20] and concluded that the Epley maneuver is a safe effective treatment for posterior canal BPPV. A more recent review[21] arrived at the same conclusion, noting that based on a systematic review of all relevant randomized controlled trials (level I evidence) there is strong evidence of efficacy of the Epley maneuver in treatment of posterior canal BPPV, with no serious adverse effects.

There are currently two practice guidelines available for diagnosis and management of BPPV, one by the American Academy of Neurology[22] and another by American Academy of Otolaryngology—Head and Neck Surgery.[23] They both offer through reviews of the available evidence and validate the effectiveness of the Epley maneuver in management of posterior semicircular canal BPPV, and elsewhere in this book detailed rationale and description are provided.

Pharmacotherapy

Given that primary treatment for BPPV is canalith repositioning, then the question becomes as follows: is there any role for pharmacotherapy in management of BPPV? In fact, current clinical practice guideline from the American Academy of Otolaryngology—Head and Neck Surgery recommends against the use of vestibular suppressants or antianxiety

Table 13.1: Medications commonly used for relief of severe benign paroxysmal positional vertigo associated symptoms in the acute setting.

Drug name	Class	Dose and route
Meclizine	Antihistamine	12.5–25 mg PO Q6–8 h
Betahistine	Antihistamine	8–24 mg PO QD or BID
Dimenhydrinate	Antihistamine	25–100 mg PO Q4–6 h
Hydroxyzine	Antihistamine	25–100 mg PO Q6 h
Promethazine	Antihistamine/Antiemetic	12.5–50 mg PO or PR Q4–12 h
Prochlorperazine	Antiemetic	5–10 mg PO Q6–8 h or 25 mg PR Q12 h
Metoclopramide	Antiemetic	10–20 mg PO Q6 h
Ondansetron	Antiemetic	4–8 mg PO/ODT Q6–8 h
Diazepam	Benzodiazepine	2–10 mg PO Q4–8 h
Lorazepam	Benzodiazepine	0.5–2 mg PO Q4–8 h
Scopolamine	Anticholinergic	1 transdermal patch Q72 h

(PO: Per oral; PR: Per rectum; ODT: Oral disintegrating tablet; Q: Every; QD: Every day; BID: Twice daily).

medications for primary treatment of BPPV.[23] Practice parameter published by the American Academy of Neurology does not comment on pharmaceutical management of BPPV.[22] In general, long-term use of drugs in treatment of vertigo is believed to prolong or prevent central compensation of vestibular tone imbalance. There are however several situations in which pharmaceutical management of BPPV as a supplement or an alternative to canalith repositioning is desired. For example, when the patient refuses to do the treatment due to excessive vertigo and nausea,[24] he or she is physically unable to or is not fully responsive to canalith repositioning (e.g. cupulolithiasis). In addition, even though management of BPPV is primarily through canalith repositioning, it should be kept in mind that initial care for patients with acute vertigo is either provided by the primary care or by the emergency room provider. Benign paroxysmal positional vertigo has notoriously poor recognition rate in the primary care setting[25] and therapeutic maneuvers are underutilized in the emergency room.[26] Presentation with vertigo in these settings commonly elicits an attempt to control symptoms with medication (Table 13.1). The "motion sickness" associated with vertigo includes autonomic responses such as nausea and vomiting. Thus, medications are often utilized to (1) reduce the spinning sensations of vertigo specifically and/or (2) to reduce the accompanying motion sickness symptoms.[23] Treatment commonly consists of one or more vestibular suppressants.

Antihistamines are one class of medications often utilized. A popular antihistamine choice in management of acute vertigo is meclizine, a first-generation antihistamine (i.e. H_1 receptor antagonist). H_1 receptor antagonism also induces anticholinergic effects, as well as, central nervous system suppression commonly manifesting as dry mouth and drowsiness, respectively. Dry mouth from meclizine appears to be less severe than other first-generation antihistamines. Motion sickness relief comes through peripheral action, i.e. reduced labyrinthine excitability and central action in the brainstem. Other members of the first-generation antihistamines of the piperazine class with longer half-life than meclizine (e.g. 20 hours for hydroxyzine vs 6 hours for meclizine) can provide prolonged relief. Benefits of antihistamines can be enhanced by combining with opioids.

Betahistine dihydrochloride is a medication whose structure closely resembles that of antihistamines and commonly used in Europe to manage Ménière's disease.[27] Betahistine is believed to have beneficial antivertigo effects through both vascular and neural mechanisms. It has been reported to increase vestibular blood flow.[28] Dilation of peripheral vasculature is likely mediated by action at H_1 receptors on blood vessels of the inner ear. Furthermore, betahistine produces postsynaptic inhibition of the vestibular afferents in response to hair cell neurotransmitters of the vestibular endorgans.[29] Betahistine may also produce its beneficial effects, in part, through action on the histamine H_3 receptor in the brain.[30] Betahistine metabolites, aminoethylpyridine, and hydroxyethylpyridine have also been shown to increase cochlear blood flow; thus, they may represent additional therapeutic approaches in management of vertigo.[31]

Anticholinergic agents have also been found to be beneficial in relieving nausea and motion sickness. One example is scopolamine, a belladonna alkaloid, which can be applied as a transdermal patch for continuous effect over 3 days. Scopolamine exerts its effects by acting as a competitive antagonist at muscarinic (M1) acetylcholine receptors.

Benzodiazepines, such as diazepam, clonazepam, lorazepam, and alprazolam, have anxiolytic, sedative, muscle relaxant, and anticonvulsant properties derived from potentiating the inhibitory effect of the γ-aminobutyric acid system.[23] This system is a major inhibitory neurotransmitter in the central vestibular pathways. In small dosages, they are extremely useful in management of acute vertigo[32] and motion sickness.[33] Benzodiazepines are commonly classified according to their half-lives into long acting (diazepam), intermediate acting (clonazepam, lorazepam, and alprazolam), and short acting (midazolam). In clinical practice, however, duration of action is determined by lipid solubility that determines the rate at which medication leaves the bloodstream and crosses the blood-brain barrier. In severe BPPV, associated with nausea and vomiting, benzodiazepine can provide much needed symptom relief.

In particular, owning to their rapid absorption, dosing half an hour before liberatory maneuvers[34] can make the canalith repositioning maneuvers more tolerable.

Other medications that are often used for motion sickness include promethazine, which is a phenothiazine with antihistamine properties, and serotonin-5-hydroxytryptamine-3 antagonists[23] such as ondansetron.

Population studies consistently show "loose crystals," i.e. BPPV, is the most common cause of dizziness, especially among geriatric patients.[35,36] In a large registry that includes data collected from 4,294 patients with vertigo in 13 countries generated over a 28-month period, nearly one third were diagnosed to have BPPV.[37] The 1-year prevalence of individuals with BPPV attacks rises steeply with age: from 0.5% in 18–39-year-old to 3.4% in individuals over 60 years of age and the cumulative (lifetime) incidence of BPPV reaches almost 10% by the age of 80.[35] These statistics are very reproducible, e.g. 11% of a large population of 75-year-olds manifested BPPV symptoms.[38] As noted above, prolonged use of medication in management of vertigo is generally discourages because of interference with central compensation in peripheral vestibular conditions.[23] However, given that the majority of BPPV patients are over age 60, caution in use of pharmacotherapy and polypharmacy is essential population. For example, use of benzodiazepines bears increased risk of amnesia or confusion (i.e. delirium) in geriatric patients. Furthermore, anticholinergic medications place older patients at higher risk for developing drug-induced urinary retention, because of existing comorbidities such as benign prostatic hyperplasia and the use of other concomitant medication that could reinforce the impairing effect on micturition.[39] In the geriatric setting, management of vertigo is complicated by the inherent difficulties in assessment as there are often multiple vestibular and nonvestibular causes contributing to patient symptoms (*see* also the "Prevention" section).[40]

Combination Therapy

Canalith repositioning procedures are the most effective treatment for BPPV; however, after repositioning maneuver, there can exist either persistent or residual symptoms. Failure to relieve symptoms after canalith repositioning could be because of adherent particles to the cupula, incomplete transfer of the canaliths into the utricle, incorrect diagnosis of the canal involved, multicanal involvement, or bilateral disease. Canal switching is a common complication of CRPs[41] and may contribute to persistence of symptoms. Even when successful in relieving vertigo, residual symptoms can persist. In a prospective investigation of 135 BPPV patients in whom CRP was performed until nystagmus and vertigo disappeared, dizziness handicap inventory

(DHI) was completed 5–7 days later.[42] Although post-CRP DHI scores were improved, this improvement was incomplete, particularly, in the emotional scale. Residual symptoms such as lightheadedness or floating sensation 1 week after successful repositioning maneuver and resolution of positional nystagmus are present in up to 57% of patients.[43] Other symptoms included ear fullness, general weakness, and vertigo. Some of these residual symptoms have been attributed to small fragments of otoconia, which may persist in the affected semicircular canals. An alternative source is autonomic dysfunction. In a prospective study of 58 consecutive patients with BPPV who had successful CRPs with resolution of nystagmus or positional vertigo, standardized autonomic function tests were carried out.[44] About 43% of patients had residual dizziness, characterized as postural lightheadedness when righting from sitting, or short-lasting nonspecific dizziness that occurred during head movement or walking. Orthostatic hypotension occurred in 19% of patients with the incidence being significantly higher in patients with residual dizziness at the next follow-up than those without residual dizziness (40% and 3%, respectively). When compared to patients without residual dizziness, patients with residual dizziness had larger falls in systolic blood pressure during the Valsalva maneuver and head-up tilt test. However, cardiovagal parasympathetic function was not different in the patients with or without residual dizziness.

Thus, another area where pharmacotherapy may be applicable to management of BPPV is residual symptoms after CRP. A recent study investigated Danhong injection in management of residual dizziness after successful CRP.[45] Danhong is a traditional Chinese medicine that can dilate blood vessels and improve microcirculation and had previously been proven to be effective in improving cervical vertigo and posterior circulation ischemic vertigo. Danhong significantly improved the residual dizziness after successful repositioning treatment in patients with BPPV.

In another study, BPPV patients who underwent successful treatment with CRPs were randomized into two groups: benzodiazepine (low-dose anxiolytic etizolam 0.5 mg qhs) for 2 weeks or no medication.[46] Subjective symptoms before and after CRP were measured using the DHI. The benzodiazepine group had significantly decreased total, functional, and emotional DHI scores suggesting that the patients with BPPV had a benefit from adjuvant medication after CRP with respect to their anxieties and daily activities.

In a controlled, randomized trial, it was demonstrated that the vestibular suppressant antihistamine, dimenhydrinate 50 mg daily, administered after canalith repositioning produced significantly improved control of residuals symptoms compared to nonmedically treated control and placebo groups.[43]

Finally, in a prospective, randomized, controlled study, BPPV subjects who were treated with Cawthorne-Cooksey exercises six times per day for 4 weeks had significantly better outcomes than those treated with betahistine alone.[47] However, there is evidence that as an adjunct to positional maneuvers, betahistine provides improved outcomes. In a double-blind, randomized, controlled trial, BPPV subjects who underwent the Epley maneuver and followed by betahistine for 1 week showed significantly improved symptoms in a subset of BPPV patients.[48] Specifically, those with duration of BPPV of <60 days show improved postural stability when treated with betahistine after Epley maneuver.[49]

PREVENTION

As we gain better understanding of pathophysiological conditions that may influence BPPV, other avenues in management of BPPV become available. Given that BPPV affects a substantial proportion of the population and that there remain significant limitations in our ability to fully control its symptoms and recurrences, over the past decade effort has been directed at identification of medical factors that may predispose a patient to development of idiopathic BPPV. Associations have been reported between BPPV and diabetes.[50] In a case–control histopathologic human temporal bone study, temporal bones from patients with type 1 diabetes mellitus and normal temporal bones from age-matched individuals were histopathologically examined.[51] It was found that the prevalence of cupular and free-floating deposits in the lateral and posterior semicircular canals was significantly higher in type 1 diabetes mellitus patients compared with normals. Another systemic link was described recently where the lipid profiles and serum uric acid levels were found to be higher in patients with BPPV than in controls.[52] Curiously, serum uric acid levels decreased 1 month after the BPPV attack; however, the mechanisms behind these observations have not yet been elucidated. Other conditions that have been associated with BPPV include chronic thyroiditis,[53] hypertension, hyperlipidemia, and stroke.[35]

To find a statistical link between common comorbidities affecting the elderly population (hypertension, diabetes, osteoarthrosis,[54] and depression) and recurrent episodes of BPPV data from over 1,000 BPPV patients in 11 centers across 7 countries were examined.[55] The results showed the presence of at least one comorbid disorder in 20% of subjects and two or more in 37% of subjects. Furthermore, it was noted that >50% of subjects had at least one recurrence and that the higher the number of comorbidities, the greater the number of recurrences.

Above findings imply that optimal management of comorbid conditions may somewhat influence BPPV occurrence/recurrences. However, among the comorbidities, the association between BPPV and osteoporosis[54,56-59] has raised much interest, in part, because it implies abnormal bone turnover may underlie BPPV. As the link between the two disorders appears to be strong, then a paradigm shift in management of BPPV away from management of individual BPPV episodes with canalith reposition to treatment of the acute episode plus prevention of both initial and recurrent episodes may occur in near future. Such a proactive management of BPPV will lead to a substantial reduction in fall and fracture risk particularly in the geriatric population where the association of BPPV (increased fall risk) with osteopenia/osteoporosis (reduced bone mass) substantially increases fracture risk. Some support for this approach exists in the literature. Mikulec et al. conducted a retrospective chart review to assess the prevalence of "treated osteoporosis" (on antiresorptive therapy) in 260 women with and without BPPV between 51 and 80 years of age.[60] They observed a statistically significant negative association between BPPV and "treated osteoporosis" in women aged 51-60 years but not in the older group. Another supporting evidence comes from studies showing a high prevalence of vitamin D deficiency among BPPV patients.[61,62] A recent pilot study showed that in a small group patients with BPPV recurrence, vitamin D levels were lower than those without recurrence and recurrences were relieved with vitamin D supplementation.[63]

CONCLUSION

Benign paroxysmal positional vertigo is caused by displacement of otoconia fragments from utricle into the semicircular canals. It follows that the principal management of BPPV is canalith repositioning. However, there are a number situations in which canalith repositioning is not utilized, practical, effective, or leaves residual symptoms. In such scenarios, vestibular suppressants such as antihistamines, anticholinergics, and benzodiazepines can be effective in symptom relief. Better understanding of comorbid conditions associated with BPPV provides an opportunity to proactively treat BPPV and prevent recurrences. These conditions include osteoporosis and vitamin D deficiency, which typically prompt treatment with bisphosphonates and vitamin D supplements, respectively.

REFERENCES

1. Schuknecht HF. Positional vertigo: clinical and experimental observations. Trans Am Acad Ophthalmol Otolaryngol. 1962;66:319-32.
2. Schuknecht HF. Further observations on the pathology of presbycusis. Arch Otolaryngol. 1964;80:369-82.
3. Schuknecht HF, Ruby RR. Cupulolithiasis. Adv Otorhinolaryngol. 1973;20:434-43.

4. Lanska DJ, Remler B. Benign paroxysmal positioning vertigo: classic descriptions, origins of the provocative positioning technique, and conceptual developments. Neurology. 1997;48(5):1167-77.
5. Schuknecht HF. Destructive labyrinthine surgery. Arch Otolaryngol. 1973;97(2):150-1.
6. Parnes LS, McClure JA. Free-floating endolymph particles: a new operative finding during posterior semicircular canal occlusion. Laryngoscope. 1992;102(9):988-92.
7. Welling DB, Parnes LS, O'Brien B, et al. Particulate matter in the posterior semicircular canal. Laryngoscope. 1997;107(1):90-4.
8. Beyea JA, Agrawal SK, Parnes LS. Transmastoid semicircular canal occlusion: a safe and highly effective treatment for benign paroxysmal positional vertigo and superior canal dehiscence. Laryngoscope. 2012;122(8):1862-6.
9. Furuya M, Suzuki M, Sato H. Experimental study of speed-dependent positional nystagmus in benign paroxysmal positional vertigo. Acta Otolaryngol. 2003;123(6):709-12.
10. Rajguru SM, Rabbitt RD. Afferent responses during experimentally induced semicircular canalithiasis. J Neurophysiol. 2007;97(3):2355-63.
11. Squires TM, Weidman MS, Hain TC, et al. A mathematical model for top-shelf vertigo: the role of sedimenting otoconia in BPPV. J Biomech. 2004;37(8):1137-46.
12. Rajguru SM, Ifediba MA, Rabbitt RD. Biomechanics of horizontal canal benign paroxysmal positional vertigo. J Vestib Res. 2005;15(4):203-14.
13. Obrist D, Hegemann S, Kronenberg D, et al. In vitro model of a semicircular canal: design and validation of the model and its use for the study of canalithiasis. J Biomech. 2010;43(6):1208-14.
14. Zucca G, Valli S, Valli P, et al. Why do benign paroxysmal positional vertigo episodes recover spontaneously? J Vestib Res. 1998;8(4):325-9.
15. Kveton JF, Kashgarian M. Particulate matter within the membranous labyrinth: pathologic or normal? Am J Otol. 1994;15(2):173-6.
16. Brandt T, Daroff RB. Physical therapy for benign paroxysmal positional vertigo. Arch Otolaryngol. 1980;106(8):484-5.
17. Semont A, Freyss G, Vitte E. Curing the BPPV with a liberatory maneuver. Adv Otorhinolaryngol. 1988;42:290-3.
18. Epley JM. The canalith repositioning procedure: for treatment of benign paroxysmal positional vertigo. Otolaryngol Head Neck Surg. 1992;107(3):399-404.
19. Epley JM. Positional vertigo related to semicircular canalithiasis. Otolaryngol Head Neck Surg. 1995;112(1):154-61.
20. Hilton M, Pinder D. The Epley (canalith repositioning) manoeuvre for benign paroxysmal positional vertigo. Cochrane Database Syst Rev. 2014;12:CD003162.
21. Glasziou P, Bennett J, Greenberg P, et al. The Epley manoeuvre—for benign paroxysmal positional vertigo. Aust Fam Physician. 2013;42(1-2):36-7.
22. Fife TD, Iverson DJ, Lempert T, et al. Practice parameter: therapies for benign paroxysmal positional vertigo (an evidence-based review): report of the Quality Standards Subcommittee of the American Academy of Neurology. Neurology. 2008;70(22):2067-74.
23. Bhattacharyya N, Baugh RF, Orvidas L, et al. Clinical practice guideline: benign paroxysmal positional vertigo. Otolaryngol Head Neck Surg. 2008;139(5 Suppl 4):S47-81.

24. Tusa RJ, Gore R. Dizziness and vertigo: emergencies and management. Neurol Clin. 2012;30(1):61-74, vii-viii.
25. Ekvall Hansson E, Mansson NO, Hakansson A. Benign paroxysmal positional vertigo among elderly patients in primary health care. Gerontology. 2005;51(6):386-9.
26. Bashir K, Alessai GS, Salem WA, et al. Physical maneuvers: effective but underutilized treatment of benign paroxysmal positional vertigo in the ED. Am J Emerg Med. 2014;32(1):95-6.
27. James AL, Burton MJ. Betahistine for Meniere's disease or syndrome. Cochrane Database Syst Rev. 2001; 1 :CD001873.
28. Dziadziola JK, Laurikainen EL, Rachel JD, et al. Betahistine increases vestibular blood flow. Otolaryngol Head Neck Surg. 1999;120(3):400-5.
29. Soto E, Chávez H, Valli P, et al. Betahistine produces post-synaptic inhibition of the excitability of the primary afferent neurons in the vestibular endorgans. Acta Otolaryngol Suppl. 2001;545:19-24.
30. Gbahou F, Davenas E, Morisset S, et al. Effects of betahistine at histamine H3 receptors: mixed inverse agonism/agonism in vitro and partial inverse agonism in vivo. J Pharmacol Exp Ther. 2010;334(3):945-5.
31. Bertlich M, Ihler F, Sharaf K, et al. Betahistine metabolites, aminoethylpyridine, and hydroxyethylpyridine increase cochlear blood flow in guinea pigs in vivo. Int J Audiol. 2014;53(10):753-9.
32. Hain TC, Yacovino D. Pharmacologic treatment of persons with dizziness. Neurol Clin. 2005;23(3):831-53, vii.
33. McClure JA, Lycett P, Baskerville JC. Diazepam as an anti-motion sickness drug. J Otolaryngol. 1982;11(4):253-9.
34. Brandt T, Zwergal A, Strupp M. Medical treatment of vestibular disorders. Expert Opin Pharmacother. 2009;10(10):1537-48.
35. von Brevern M, Radtke A, Lezius F, et al. Epidemiology of benign paroxysmal positional vertigo: a population based study. J Neurol Neurosurg Psychiatry. 2007;78(7):710-5.
36. van Leeuwen RB, Bruintjes TD. Dizziness in the elderly: diagnosing its causes in a multidisciplinary dizziness unit. Ear Nose Throat J. 2014;93(4-5):162, 164, 166-7.
37. Agus S, Benecke H, Thum C, et al. Clinical and demographic features of vertigo: findings from the REVERT Registry. Front Neurol. 2013;4:48.
38. Kollén L, Frändin K, Möller M, et al. Benign paroxysmal positional vertigo is a common cause of dizziness and unsteadiness in a large population of 75-year-olds. Aging Clin Exp Res. 2012;24(4):317-23.
39. Verhamme KM, Sturkenboom MC, Stricker BH, et al. Drug-induced urinary retention: incidence, management and prevention. Drug Saf. 2008;31(5):373-88.
40. Wetmore SJ, Eibling DE, Goebel JA, et al. Challenges and opportunities in managing the dizzy older adult. Otolaryngol Head Neck Surg. 2011;144(5):651-6.
41. Herdman S J, Tusa RJ. Complications of the canalith repositioning procedure. Arch Otolaryngol Head Neck Surg. 1996;122(3):281-6.
42. Lee NH, Kwon HJ, Ban JH. Analysis of residual symptoms after treatment in benign paroxysmal positional vertigo using questionnaire. Otolaryngol Head Neck Surg. 2009;141(2):232-6.

43. Kim MB, Lee HS, Ban JH. Vestibular suppressants after canalith repositioning in benign paroxysmal positional vertigo. Laryngoscope. 2014;124(10):2400-3.
44. Kim HA, Lee H. Autonomic dysfunction as a possible cause of residual dizziness after successful treatment in benign paroxysmal positional vertigo. Clin Neurophysiol. 2014;125(3):608-14.
45. Deng W, Yang C, Xiong M, et al. Danhong enhances recovery from residual dizziness after successful repositioning treatment in patients with benign paroxysmal positional vertigo. Am J Otolaryngol. 2014;35(6):753-7.
46. Jung HJ, Koo JW, Kim CS, et al. Anxiolytics reduce residual dizziness after successful canalith repositioning maneuvers in benign paroxysmal positional vertigo. Acta Otolaryngol. 2012;132(3):277-84.
47. Kulcu DG, Yanik B, Boynukalin S, et al. Efficacy of a home-based exercise program on benign paroxysmal positional vertigo compared with betahistine. J Otolaryngol Head Neck Surg. 2008;37(3):373-9.
48. Guneri EA, Kustutan O. The effects of betahistine in addition to Epley maneuver in posterior canal benign paroxysmal positional vertigo. Otolaryngol Head Neck Surg. 2012;146(1):104-8.
49. Stambolieva K, Angov G. Effect of treatment with betahistine dihydrochloride on the postural stability in patients with different duration of benign paroxysmal positional vertigo. Int Tinnitus J. 2010;16(1):32-6.
50. Cohen HS, Kimball KT, Stewart MG. Benign paroxysmal positional vertigo and comorbid conditions. ORL J Otorhinolaryngol Relat Spec. 2004;66(1):11-5.
51. Yoda S, Cureoglu S, Yildirim-Baylan M, et al. Association between type 1 diabetes mellitus and deposits in the semicircular canals. Otolaryngol Head Neck Surg. 2011;145(3):458-62.
52. Celikbilek A, Gencer ZK, Saydam L, et al. Serum uric acid levels correlate with benign paroxysmal positional vertigo. Eur J Neurol. 2014;21(1):79-85.
53. Papi G, Guidetti G, Corsello SM, et al. The association between benign paroxysmal positional vertigo and autoimmune chronic thyroiditis is not related to thyroid status. Thyroid. 2010;20(2):237-8.
54. Vibert D, Kompis M, Häusler R. Benign paroxysmal positional vertigo in older women may be related to osteoporosis and osteopenia. Ann Otol Rhinol Laryngol. 2003;112(10):885-9.
55. De Stefano A, Dispenza F, Suarez H, et al. A multicenter observational study on the role of comorbidities in the recurrent episodes of benign paroxysmal positional vertigo. Auris Nasus Larynx. 2014;41(1):31-6.
56. Jang YS, Kang MK. Relationship between bone mineral density and clinical features in women with idiopathic benign paroxysmal positional vertigo. Otol Neurotol. 2009;30(1):95-100.
57. Jeong SH, Choi SH, Kim JY, et al. Osteopenia and osteoporosis in idiopathic benign positional vertigo. Neurology. 2009;72(12):1069-76.
58. Parham K, Leonard G, Feinn RS, et al. Prospective clinical investigation of the relationship between idiopathic benign paroxysmal positional vertigo and bone turnover: a pilot study. Laryngoscope. 2013;123(11):2834-9.
59. Yamanaka T, Shirota S, Sawai Y, et al. Osteoporosis as a risk factor for the recurrence of benign paroxysmal positional vertigo. Laryngoscope. 2013;123(11):2813-6.

60. Mikulec AA, Kowalczyk KA, Pfitzinger ME, et al. Negative association between treated osteoporosis and benign paroxysmal positional vertigo in women. J Laryngol Otol. 2010;124(4):374-6.
61. Jeong SH, Kim JS, Shin JW, et al. Decreased serum vitamin D in idiopathic benign paroxysmal positional vertigo. J Neurol. 2013;260(3):832-8.
62. Talaat HS, Abuhadied G, Talaat AS, et al. Low bone mineral density and vitamin D deficiency in patients with benign positional paroxysmal vertigo. Eur Arch Otorhinolaryngol. 2015;272(9):2249-53.
63. Büki B, Ecker M, Jünger H, et al. Vitamin D deficiency and benign paroxysmal positioning vertigo. Med Hypotheses. 2013;80(2):201-4.

Chapter 14

Surgery for Benign Paroxysmal Positional Vertigo

Gauri Mankekar

INTRODUCTION

Benign paroxysmal positional vertigo (BPPV) is the most common form of positional vertigo, accounting for nearly one half of patients with peripheral vestibular dysfunction. Approximately 18% of patients seen in dizziness clinics[1] and 25% of patients sent for vestibular testing have BPPV.[2] Benign paroxysmal positional vertigo also accounts for ~20% of pediatric referrals.[3]

Majority of the patients with BPPV can be treated successfully with conservative measures such as canal repositioning exercises and vestibular rehabilitation. However, a small percentage of patients are refractory to conservative treatment and may require surgery. Leveque et al.[4] reviewed all articles published from 1972 to 2005 that discussed a specific surgical therapy in BPPV. They reported that singular neurectomy (posterior ampullary nerve transection) and posterior semicircular canal occlusion are the two specific techniques used in intractable BPPV surgery and ~342 and 97 patients, respectively, underwent those two surgeries. They found that the number of surgeries had decreased since the early 1990s due to improvement in symptoms with conservative medical management techniques.

HISTORY

Historically, the first description of positional vertigo has been attributed to Adler[5] in 1897 and subsequently to Barany in 1921.[6] The surgical therapeutic option for benign positional vertigo was described by Gacek[7] in 1974. He described transcanal singular neurectomy in five patients, which abolished their symptoms of BPPV. In 1990, Parnes and McClure[8] introduced posterior semicircular canal occlusion for BPPV, and in 1991, Anthony[9] described partitioning of the labyrinth with laser.

INDICATIONS FOR SURGERY

The surgical procedures for BPPV are difficult and are associated with the risk of hearing loss. Therefore, it is extremely important to identify the ideal candidates for BPPV surgery. First and foremost, one must determine the cause of persistent symptoms despite conservative therapy for BPPV. A concomitant additional vestibular pathology in patients with intractable vertigo must be considered. Patient's history is the most important tool to determine the cause of persistent symptoms despite conservative therapy.[10] Second, one must confirm the diagnosis of BPPV and, finally, confirm the side that is affected.

Surgery is indicated for patients with recurrent and chronic symptoms that are extremely debilitating and warrant an invasive procedure.[10] The patients should also have demonstrated conservative treatment failure, including repeated failures of particle repositioning maneuvers and persistence of symptoms for >1 year.[7] Surgery is contraindicated during acute or subacute episodes of otitis media.[10]

An informed consent with discussion of goals as well as all the potential risks of surgery is essential. This will help the patient to have realistic expectations of the procedure.

SURGICAL PROCEDURES

Singular Neurectomy (Transection of the Posterior Ampullary Nerve)

In 1974, Gacek[7] described amelioration of symptoms in five patients with BPPV who underwent transcanal singular neurectomy. These patients had intractable vertigo despite >1 year of medical as well as physical therapy.

The procedure can be performed under local or general anesthesia. The patient lies down in a supine position with the head turned so that the operating ear is facing upwards towards the surgeon. i.e. toward the surgeon. Gacek[7] recommended a transcanal technique but Silverstein[11] suggested a postauricular approach and Epley[12] suggested a hypotympanotomy approach to reduce the risk of hearing loss. The posterior canal wall flap is elevated after any of the approaches. With the transcanal approach, the posterior external auditory canal wall may require to be curetted in order to expose the round window niche. Using an angled microdrill, the bony overhang is removed so as to visualize the entire round window membrane. The round window can be identified with the round window reflex (movement of the membrane with movement of the ossicles). Occasionally, there may be a mucus membrane covering the round window niche causing confusion. This membrane can be removed with small picks. Once the round window has been completely exposed, the floor of the round window niche inferior to the posterior segment of the round window membrane is drilled to a depth of 1-2 mm. The singular nerve is encountered here in 25-57% of the cases.[11] The singular canal can be identified by the white myelinated nerve bundle that runs at a slight angle to the round window membrane.[10] In some patients, the canal may not be located in this region and may be found superiorly under the attachment of the round window membrane.[10] This region may be visualized drilling and enlarging the existing bony depression to reach the singular canal from the inferior direction. Once the canal is identified, its proximal end is probed with right angle hooks several times. When the procedure is performed under local anesthesia, the patient may feel either pain or vertigo, or both. The distal end of the singular canal is too close to the ampulla of the posterior semicircular canal; hence, it is not advisable to probe it. The area is filled with bone dust to prevent regeneration of the nerve fibers. Gelfoam may be used to fill the bony defect. In case of cerebrospinal fluid leak, a piece of adipose tissue or fascia could be used to plug the leak. At the end of the surgery, the posterior canal wall flap is reposited. The patient may have to stay in hospital postoperatively for 4–5 days depending on the severity of vertigo. Vestibular rehabilitation exercises are commenced as soon as the patient can tolerate head movements.

Nomura et al.[13] have described the use of argon laser for singular neurectomy in a patient with BPPV although they did not identify the nerve prior to section.

Singular neurectomy is a technically challenging procedure and successful outcomes are rare; therefore it has been largely replaced by canal occlusion therefore, it has been largely replaced by canal occlusion.[14]

Posterior Semicircular Canal Occlusion

This procedure was introduced by Parnes and McClure in 1990,[8] and has become the most popular surgical method for the treatment of BPPV. The supposed principle for the surgery is that obstruction of the posterior canal lumen prevents endolymph flow and fixes the cupula rendering it unresponsive to angular acceleration and gravitation.

The surgery is performed under general anesthesia. A cortical mastoidectomy through a postaural approach is performed to gain access to the posterior semicircular canal. Approximately 3–4 mm of the canal is skeletonized and blue-lined through 180° using a diamond burr. Then with a microhook, the endosteal bone is removed to expose the membranous canal (Figs. 14.1 and 14.2). Fibrin glue and bone chips from the cortical mastoidectomy are used to form a plug, which is firmly but gently inserted into the canal to compress the membranous labyrinth. Subsequent secondary fibrosis results further occlusion. In order to avoid a perilymph fistula, a piece of temporal fascia is placed over the semicircular canal and then the wound is closed in layers (Fig. 14.3).

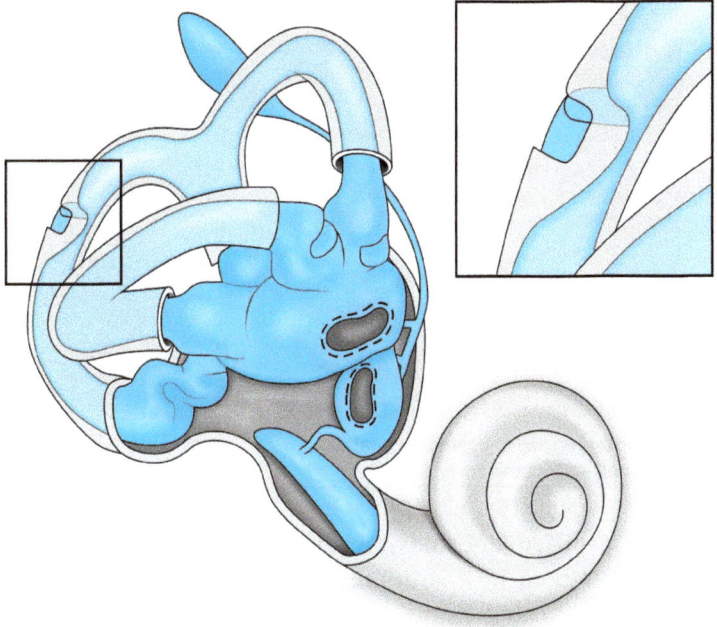

Fig. 14.1: Schematic diagram of posterior canal occlusion surgery.
Courtesy: Northwestern University, Evanston, Illinois, USA

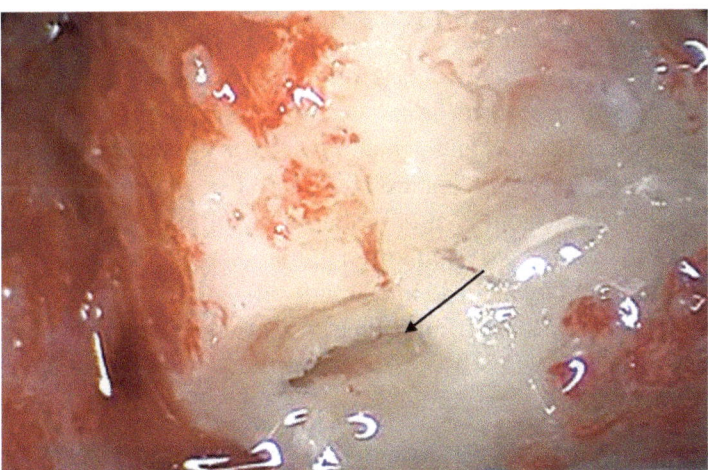

Fig. 14.2: Opening (arrow) created in posterior semicircular canal.
Courtesy: www.dallasear.com.

Some otologists have recommended use of CO_2 laser[15] while others have advocated argon laser[13] to seal the membranous labyrinth prior to occluding the posterior canal. Anthony[9] described the technique of blue-lining the posterior semicircular canal near its ampulla and then vaporizing the blue-lined area. He called it partitioning of the labyrinth

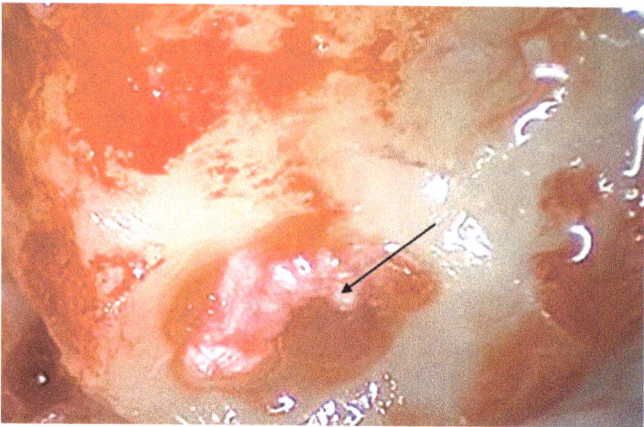

Fig. 14.3: Plugging (arrow) of posterior canal.
Courtesy: www.dallasear.com.

with laser. In a subsequent study,[16] Anthony found that there were histologic changes 24-hour postpartitioning in a guinea pig with creation of bony semicircular canal fistula and constriction of the membranous semicircular canal. The constriction caused decreased endolymphatic flow leading to resolution of BPPV due to long-term obstruction of the membranous canal.

The duration of the hospital stay depends on the severity of postoperative dizziness but use of the CO_2 laser has been associated with a shorter hospital stay as it decreases the incidence of persistent vertigo.[15] The sensation of unsteadiness can last up to several weeks and patients may also experience dizziness when pressure is applied to the postauricular area or ear canal. The vestibular ocular reflex does not fully compensate for almost 15 months after posterior canal occlusion.[10] Therefore, it is imperative to start vestibular rehabilitation exercises as soon as the patient is able to tolerate head movements.

Partitioning of the labyrinth with laser caused resolution of positional vertigo within 7 days in most cases, and within 8 weeks in all uncomplicated cases.[16]

CONCLUSION

Very few patients of BPPV require surgery as the symptoms are known to resolve spontaneously and also with canal repositioning therapies. Prior to surgery, it is essential to rule out other causes of vertigo as patients may have other vestibular lesions causing vertigo, arrive at a confirmed diagnosis of BPPV, and confirm the affected side. Patients as well as surgeons must have realistic expectations of outcomes. An informed consent goes a long way in avoiding misunderstandings.

REFERENCES

1. Nedzelski JM, Barber HO, McIlmoyl L. Diagnoses in a dizziness unit. J Otolaryngol. 1986;15:101.
2. Hughes CA, Proctor L. Benign paroxysmal positional vertigo. Laryngoscope. 1997;107:607.
3. Wiener-Vacher SR. Vestibular disorders in children. Int J Audiol. 2008;47:578.
4. Leveque M, Labrousse M, Seidermann L, et al. Surgical therapy in intractable benign paroxysmal positional vertigo. Otolaryngol Head Neck Surg. 2007;136(5):693-8.
5. Adler D. Ubeden einseitigen Drehschwindel. Dtsch Z Nervenheilkd. 1897;11:358-75.
6. Barany R. Diagnose von Krankheitserscheinungen im bereische des Otolithenapparates. Acta Otolaryngol. 1921;2:434-7.
7. Gacek RR. Transection of the posterior ampullary nerve for the relief of benign paroxysmal positional vertigo. Ann Otol Rhinol Laryngol. 1974;83(5):596-605.
8. Parnes LS, McClure JA. Posterior semicircular canal occlusion for intractable benign paroxysmal positional vertigo. Ann Otol Rhinol Laryngol. 1990;99:330-4.
9. Anthony PF. Partitioning of the labyrinth: application in benign paroxysmal positional vertigo. Am J Otol. 1991;12(5):388-93.
10. Battista RA. Surgery for benign paroxysmal positional vertigo. In: Wiet RJ (Ed.). Ear and temporal bone surgery. Minimizing risks and complications. New York, NY: Thieme Medical Publishers Inc.; 2006. pp. 113-21.
11. Silverstein H. Partial or total eighth nerve section is the treatment of vertigo. Otolaryngology. 1978;86(1):47-60.
12. Epley JM. Singular neurectomy: hypotympanotomy approach. Otolaryngol head Neck surg. 1980;88(3):304-9.
13. Nomura Y, Okuno T, Mizuno M. Treatment of vertigo using laser labyrinthectomy. Acta Otolaryngol. 1993;113(3):261-2.
14. Brandtberg K, Bergenius I. Treatment of anterior benign positional vertigo by canal plugging: a case report. Acta Otolaryngol. 2002;122:281-6.
15. Kartush JM, Sargent EW. Posterior semicircular canal occlusion for BPPV-CO_2 assisted technique. Preliminary results. Laryngoscope. 1995;105(3Pt 1):268-74.
16. Anthony PF. Partitioning the labyrinth for benign paroxysmal positional vertigo: clinical and histologic findings. Am J Otol. 1993;14(4):334-42.

Chapter 15

Atlas of Diagnostic and Repositioning Techniques for BPPV

Gautham Kulamarva, Alessandro De Stefano, Francesco Dispenza, Akhilesh PM

INTRODUCTION

This chapter provides a small picture collection of the most frequent diagnostic tests and therapeutic procedures for benign paroxysmal positional vertigo (BPPV).

The procedures for diagnosing and managing BPPV illustrated in this chapter have been described elsewhere in detail, along with its clinical symptomatology and signs. Please refer to earlier chapters for the detailed explanations.

DIAGNOSTIC TEST

BPPV of the Posterior Canal

Dix-Hallpike Test for Diagnosing Left Posterior Canal BPPV

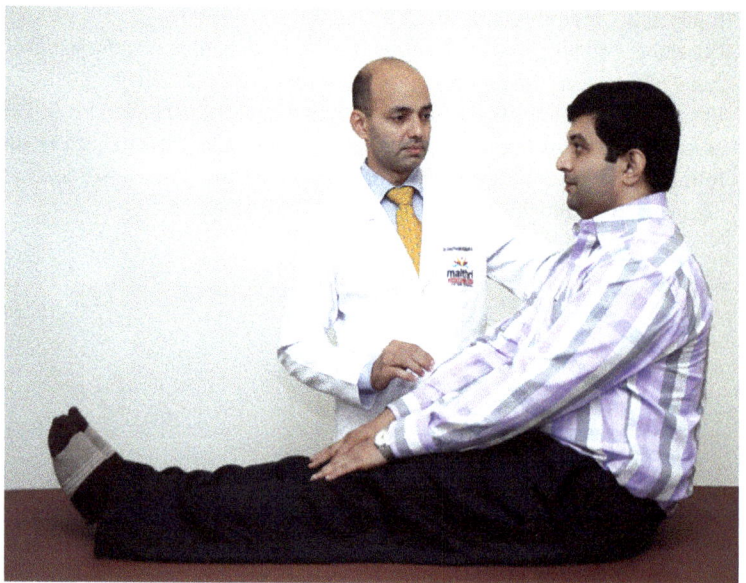

Fig. 15.1: The patient undergoing evaluation is made to sit on a couch with legs extended.

Atlas of Diagnostic and Repositioning Techniques for BPPV | 247

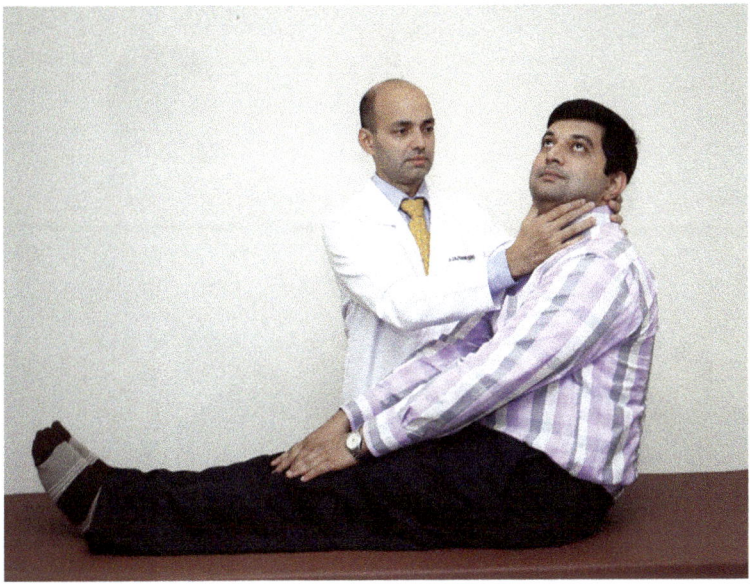

Fig. 15.2: Then the head is turned toward the suspected side (left in this case) of vertigo by 45° and extended by 30°.

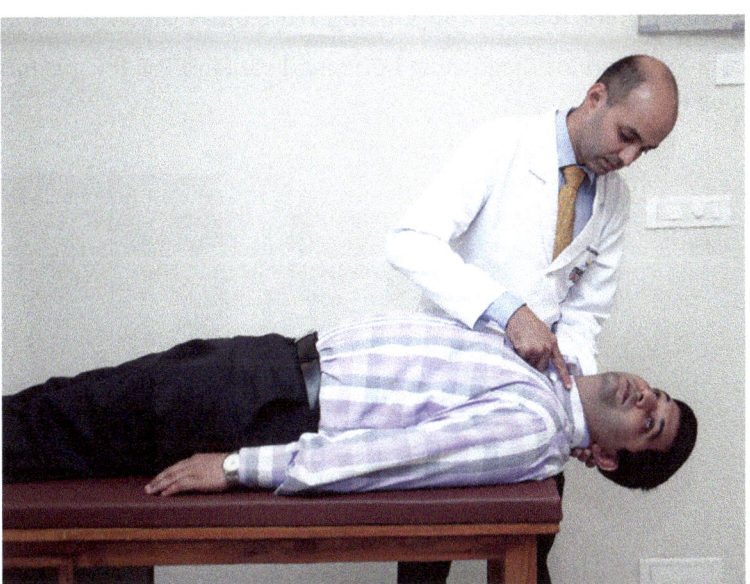

Fig. 15.3: The patient is then made to assume supine position while maintaining the head and trunk positions with the head hanging out of the bed and supported by the examiner. The eyes are observed for the classical nystagmus.

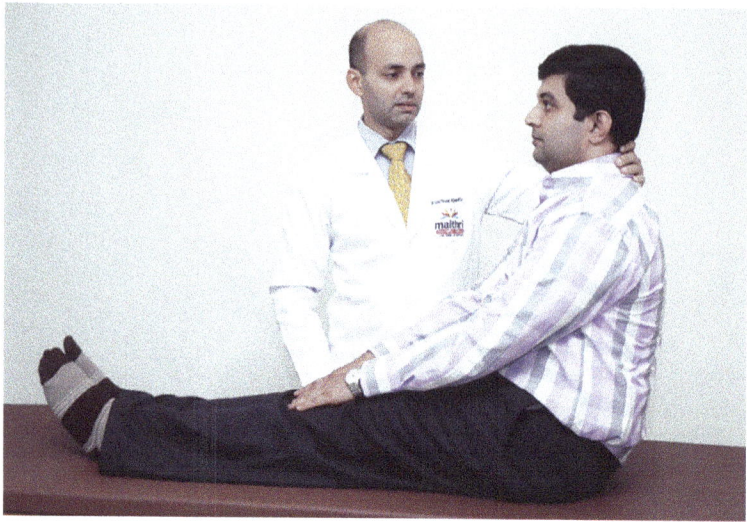

Fig. 15.4: The patient is then brought up back to the sitting position and his eyes are observed again for reversal of nystagmus.

Horizontal Canal BPPV

McClure-Pagnini Test for Diagnosing Horizontal Canal BPPV

This is a test used for diagnosing horizontal canal BPPV. It is performed as follows:

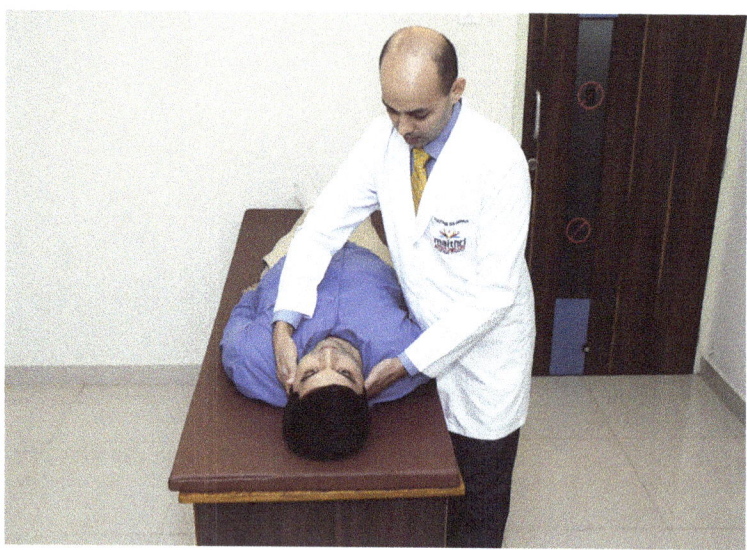

Fig. 15.5: The patient is made to lie down supine with the head in neutral position.

Atlas of Diagnostic and Repositioning Techniques for BPPV | 249

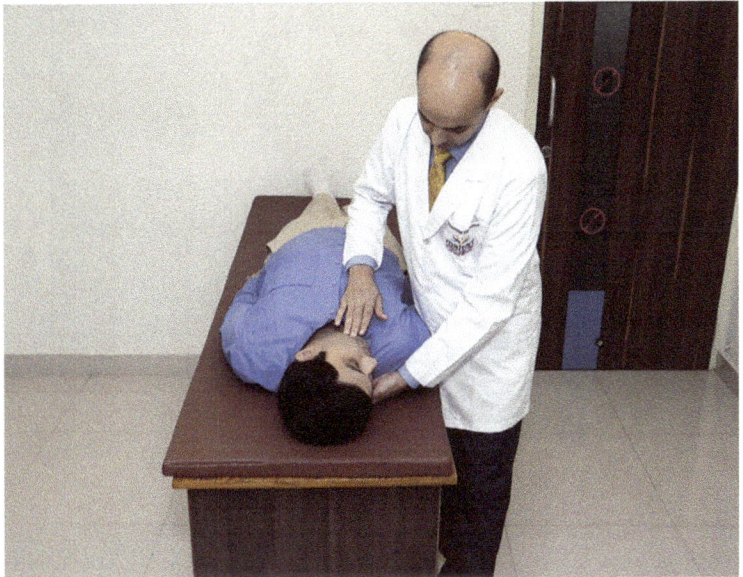

Fig. 15.6: The head of the patient is then turned to right side by 90° and observed for horizontal nystagmus.

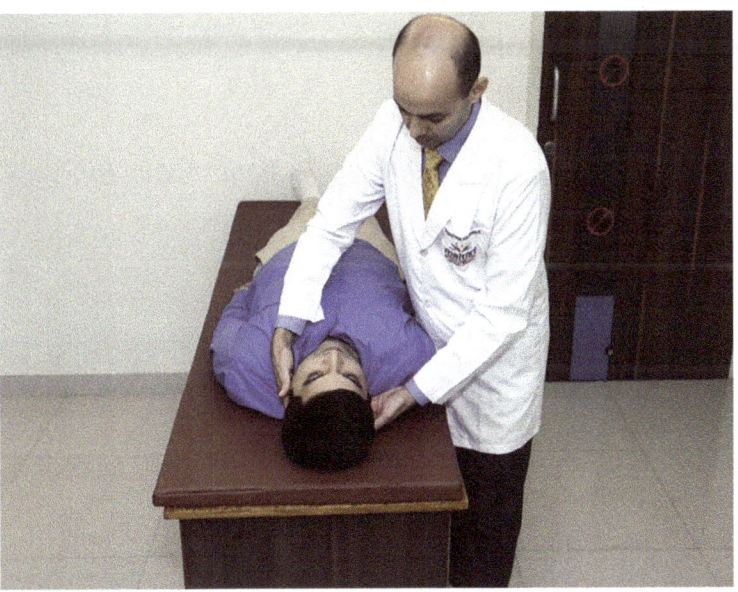

Fig. 15.7: Once the nystagmus stops, the head is returned back to the neutral position in about 10 seconds.

If the nystagmus is beating towards the ground, it is called geotropic type and if the nystagmus is towards the roof it is called apogeotropic type. In the geotropic variant, the affected side demonstrates a stronger

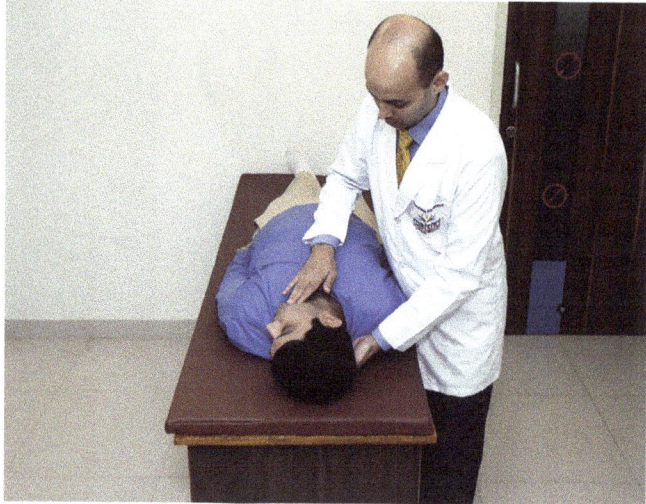

Fig. 15.8: The head is then turned to the left side by 90° and again patient's eyes are observed for nystagmus.

nystagmus whereas in the apogeotropic type the affected side demonstrates a weaker nystagmus. This is in confirmation with Ewald's second law.

THERAPEUTIC TECHNIQUE

Posterior Canal BPPV

Semont Maneuver for Treating Right Posterior Canal BPPV

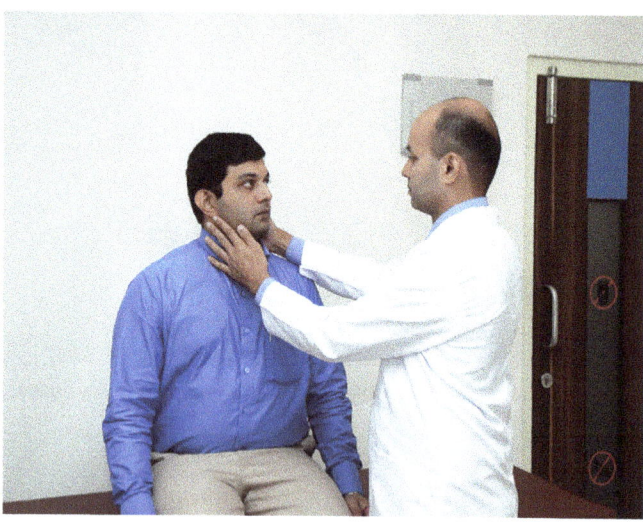

Fig. 15.9: While sitting by the edge of the bed, the patient's head is turned to the uninvolved (left in this case) side by 45°.

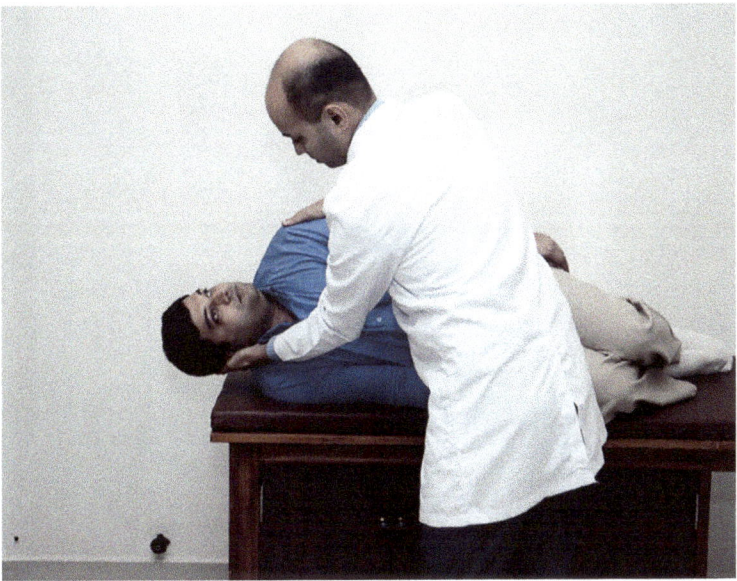

Fig. 15.10: The patient is then quickly made to lie down on his involved side (right in this case) shoulder for 30 seconds.

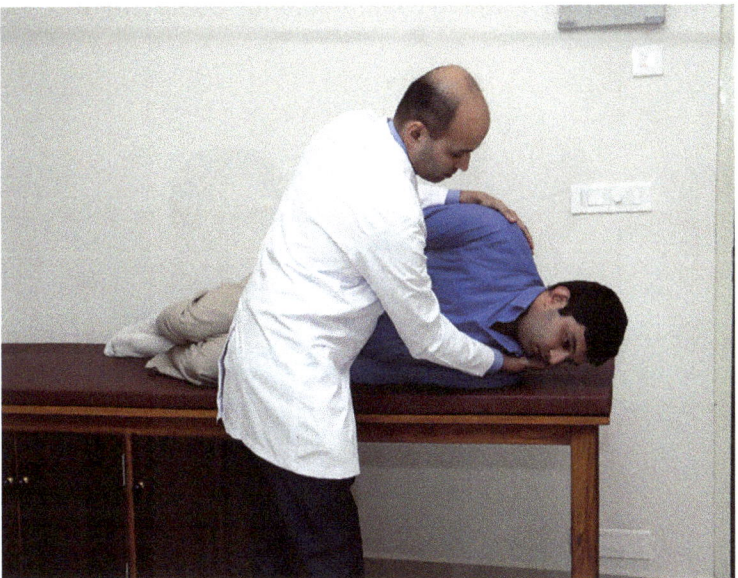

Fig. 15.11: Then, quickly the patient is moved directly to the left side lying-down position, without stopping over in between, while maintaining the positional relation between the head and the rest of the body.

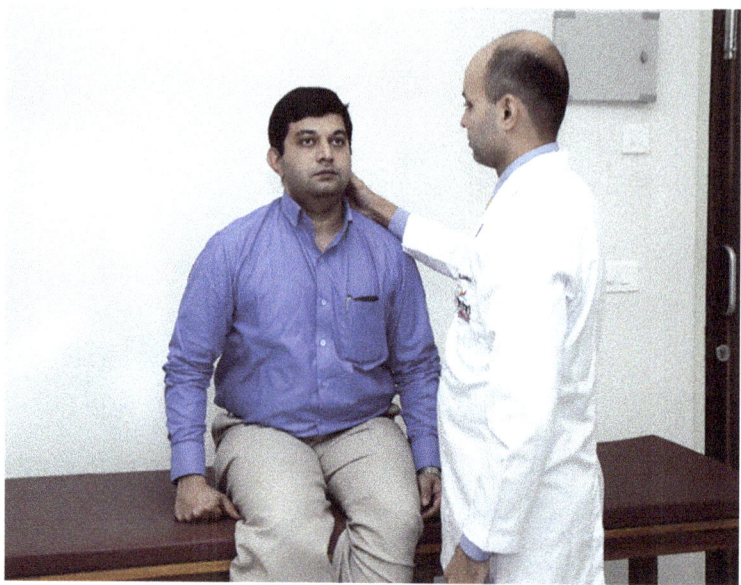

Fig. 15.12: After waiting for another 30 seconds, the patient is returned back to the original sitting position.

Epley Maneuver for Treating Right Posterior Canal BPPV

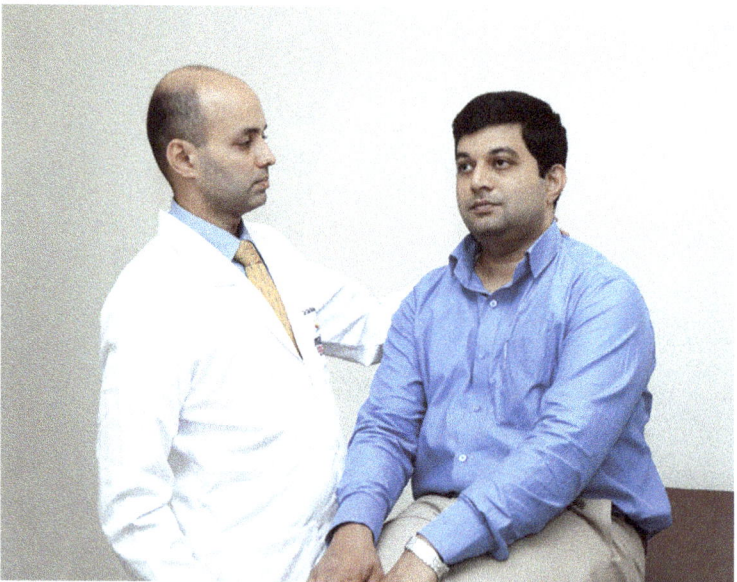

Fig. 15.13: The patient is made to sit on the couch with both legs extended and very close to the edge of the bed toward the side which is to be treated (right in this case).

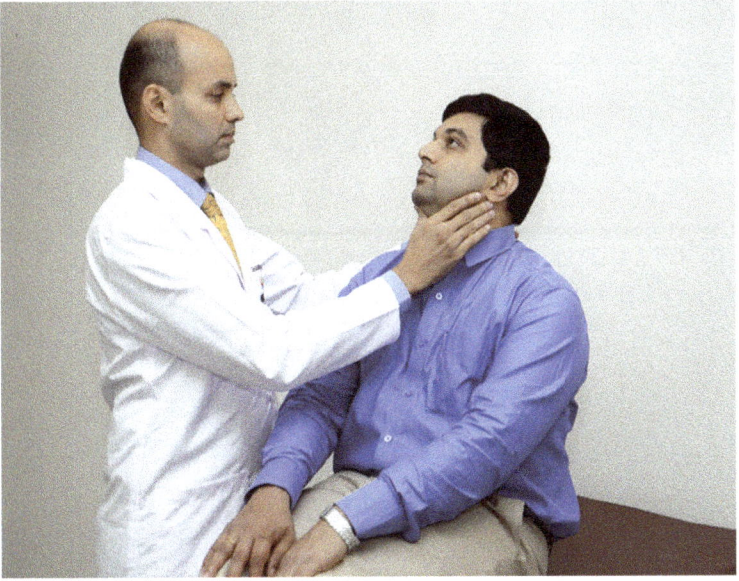

Fig. 15.14: Patient's head is then turned to the affected (right in this case) side by 45° and extended by 30°.

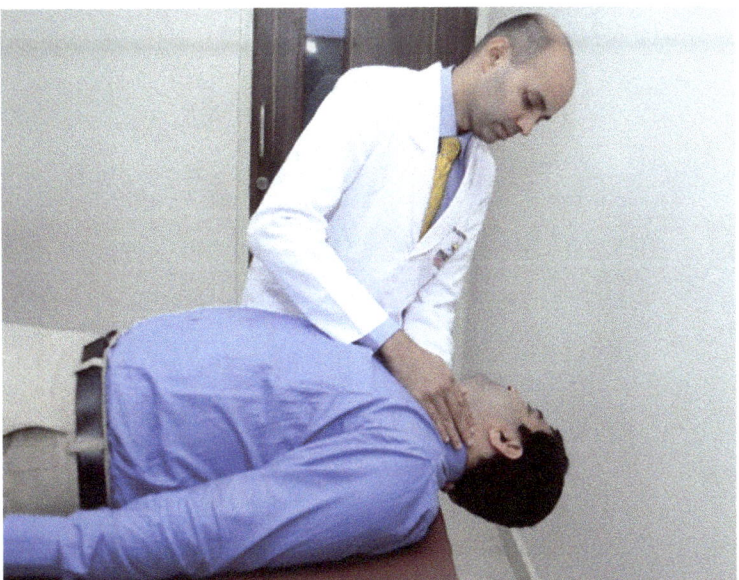

Fig. 15.15A: Patient is then quickly made to lie supine with the head hanging out of the bed, while constantly maintaining the head to trunk positional relation and the head being supported constantly by the therapist.

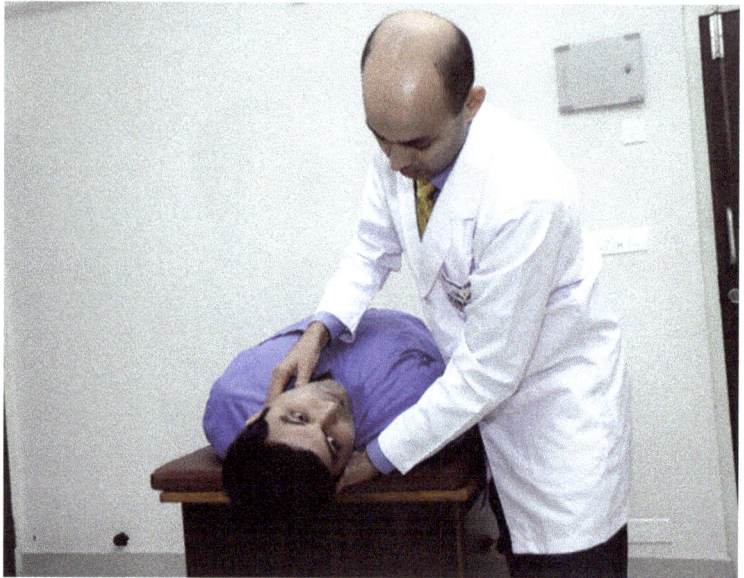

Fig. 15.15B: Patient's eyes are observed for nystagmus and this position is maintained for 1 minute after the disappearance of nystagmus.

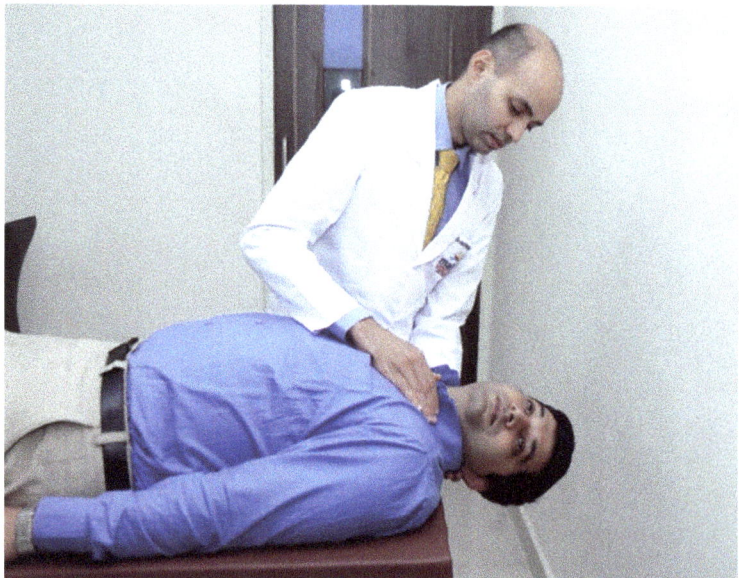

Fig. 15.16A: The head alone is now turned by 90° to the opposite side while still maintaining the extension of the head.

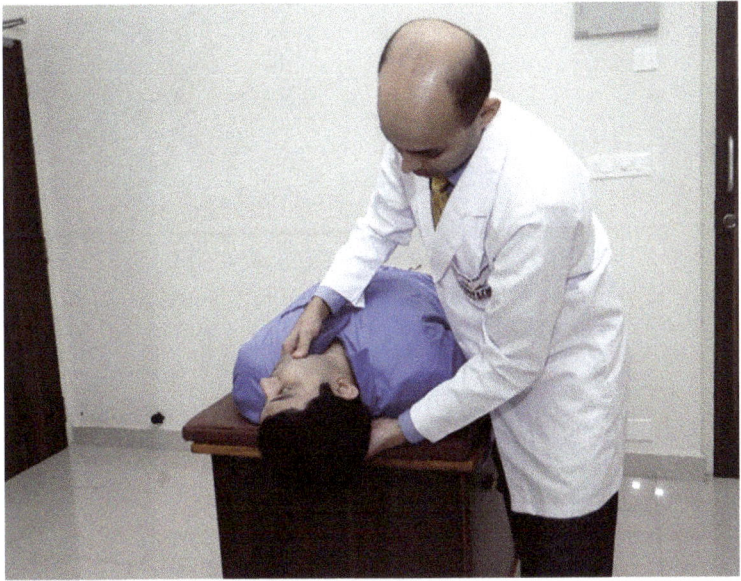

Fig. 15.16B: Again the eyes are observed for nystagmus and the position is maintained for 1 minute after the disappearance of nystagmus.

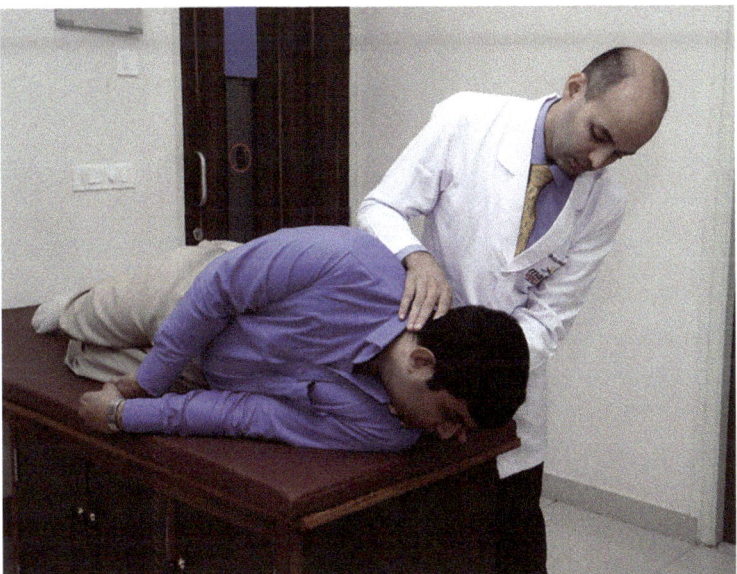

Fig. 15.17: Now the patient is asked to roll over in the bed to the opposite side by another 90° so that he is now facing the floor, while the therapist supports the head and ensures that the head to trunk positional relation is being maintained throughout. Again this position is maintained for 1 minute after the disappearance of nystagmus or vertigo.

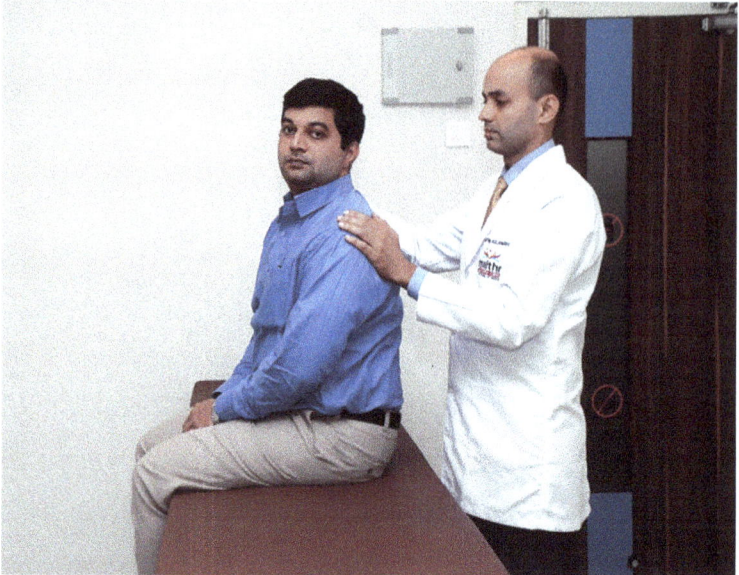

Fig. 15.18: The patient is then made to get up into sitting position with the legs hanging out from the opposite side of the bed from where the treatment started.

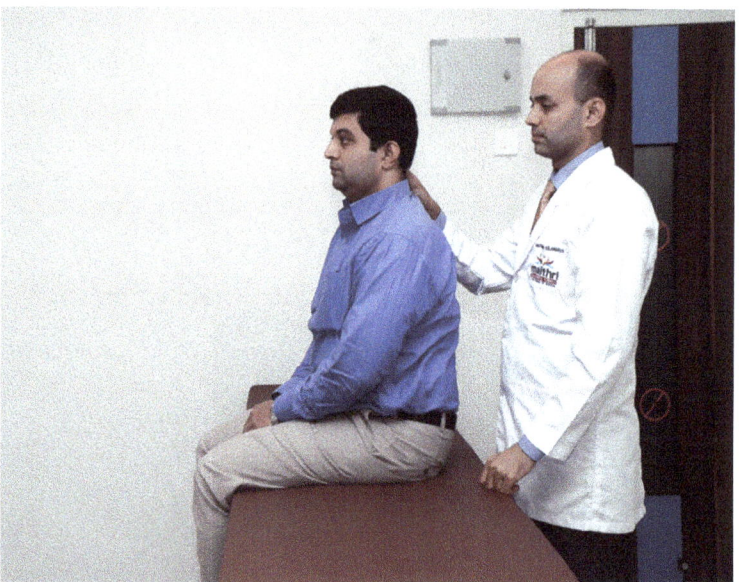

Fig. 15.19: The patient resumes the neutral and natural position of the head.

Gans Maneuver for Treating Right Posterior Canal BPPV

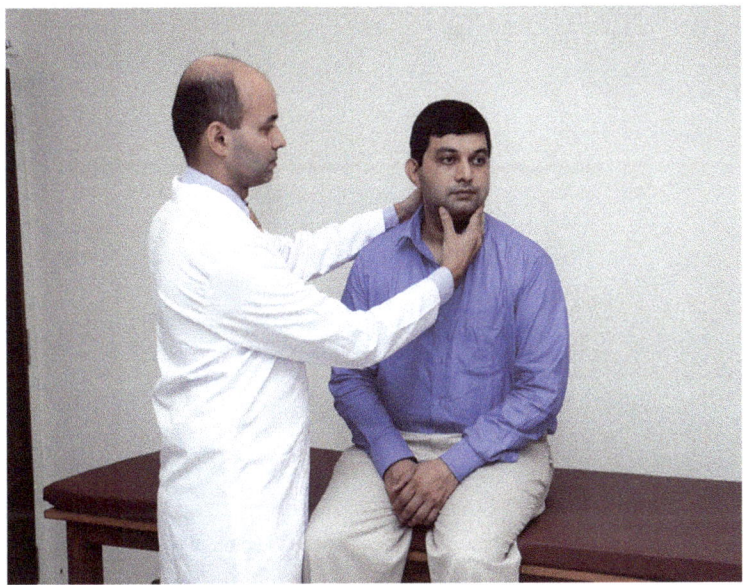

Fig. 15.20: The patient is made to sit by the edge of the bed facing the examiner with legs hanging outside. His head is turned away from the affected side (right in this case) by 45°, without extension of the neck.

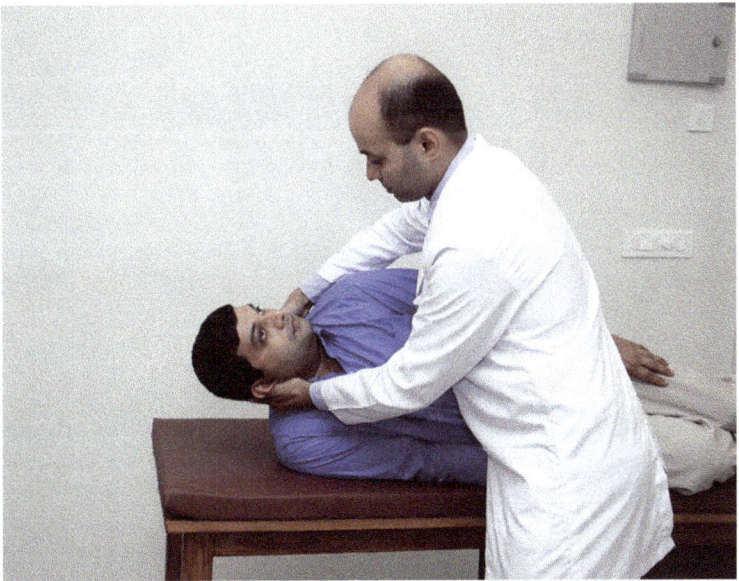

Fig. 15.21: The patient is moved into a side lying position on the involved side (right in this case).

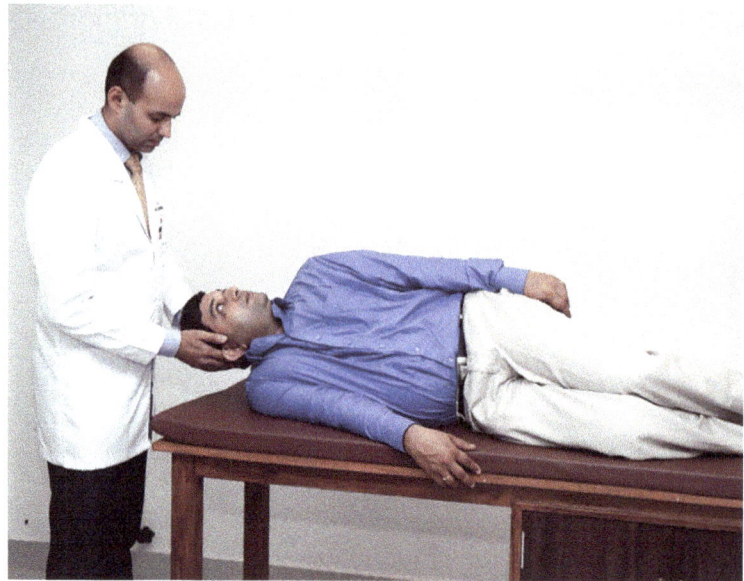

Fig. 15.22: The therapist may move to the head end of the bed for the sake of convenience.

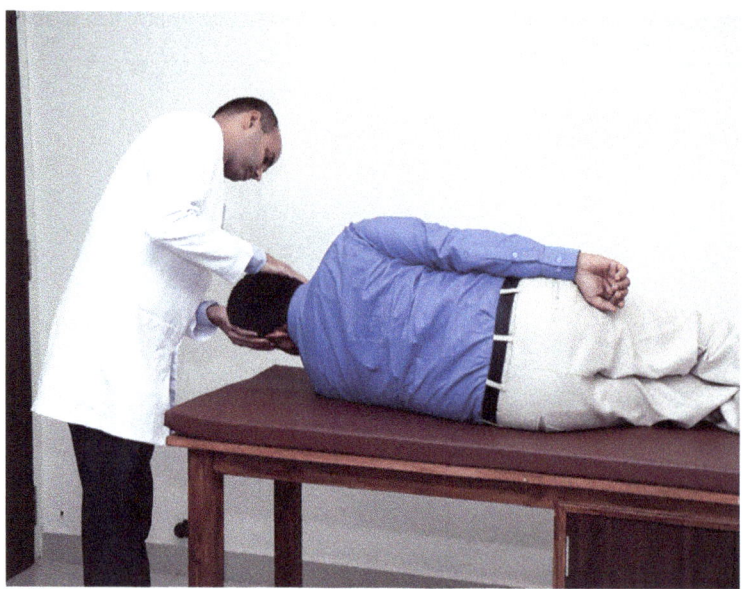

Fig. 15.23: The patient is then rolled over to the opposite side with the head constantly being supported by the examiner in the same positional relation with the trunk.

Atlas of Diagnostic and Repositioning Techniques for BPPV

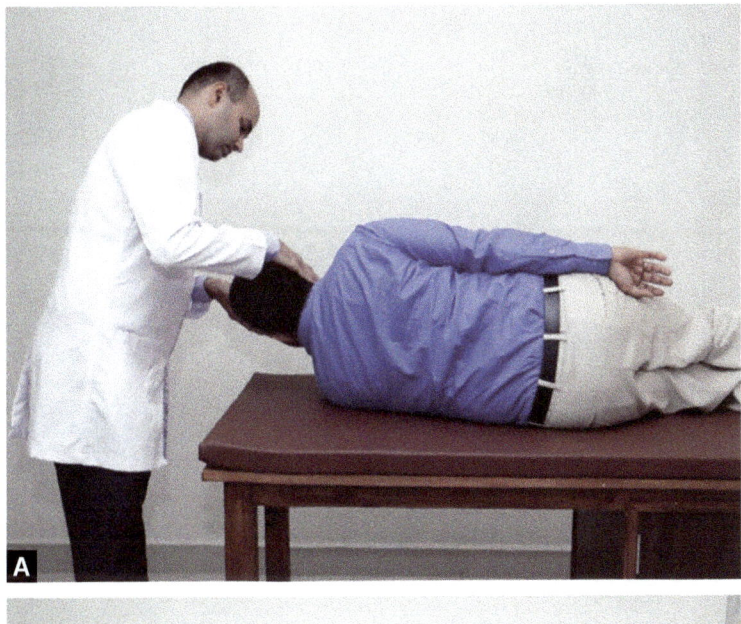

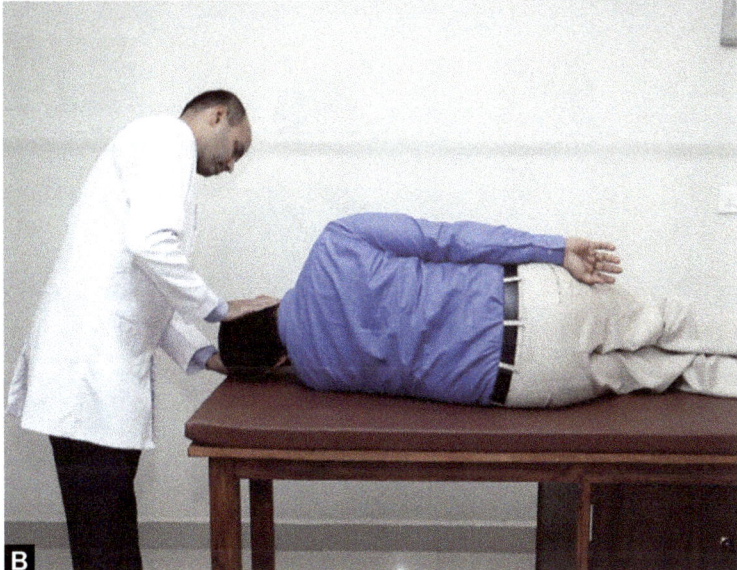

Figs. 15.24A and B: A liberatory head shake is performed by moving the head side to side for 3–4 times so as to move the otoliths through the common crus.

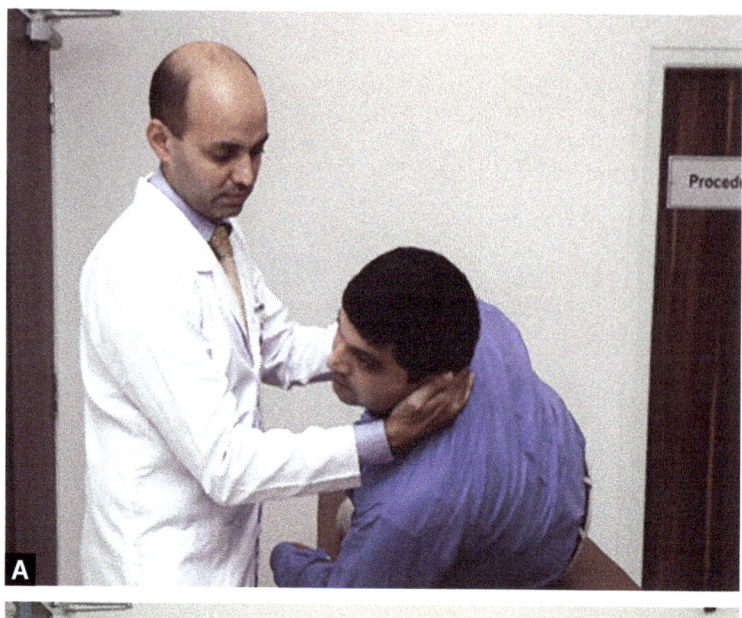
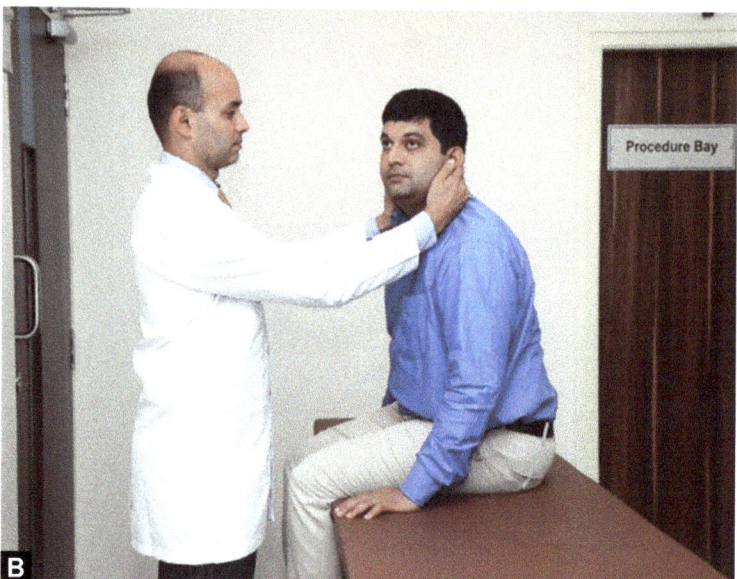

Figs. 15.25A and B: (A) The patient gets up to sitting position (B) while his head is still being supported.

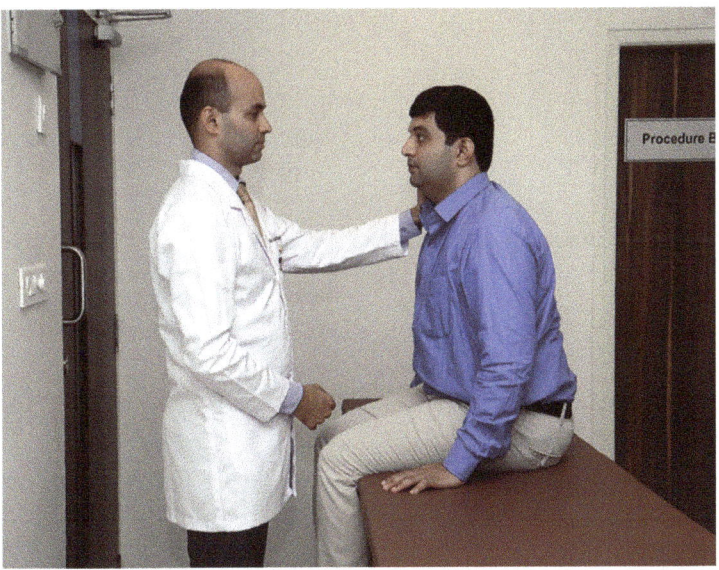

Fig. 15.26: The patient assumes the original neutral position at the end of the therapeutic maneuver.

Horizontal Canal BPPV

Lempert's Barbecue Roll for Left Horizontal Canal BPPV

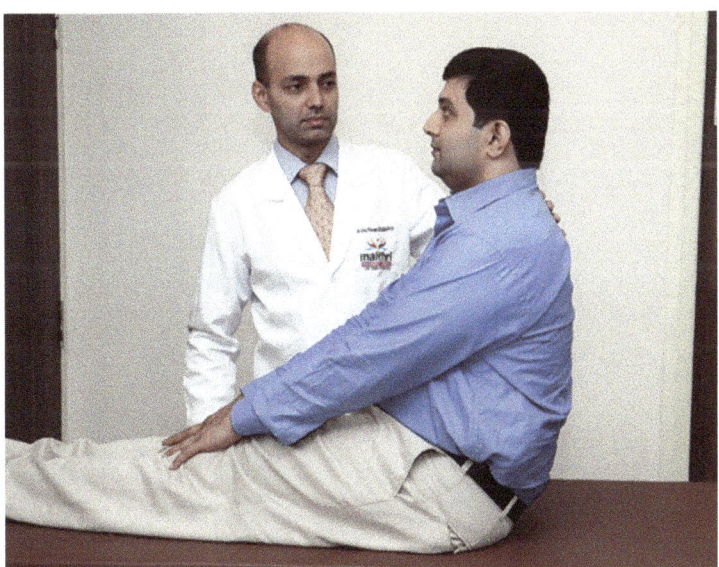

Fig. 15.27: The patient is made to sit on the couch with both legs extended in preparation for the barbecue roll.

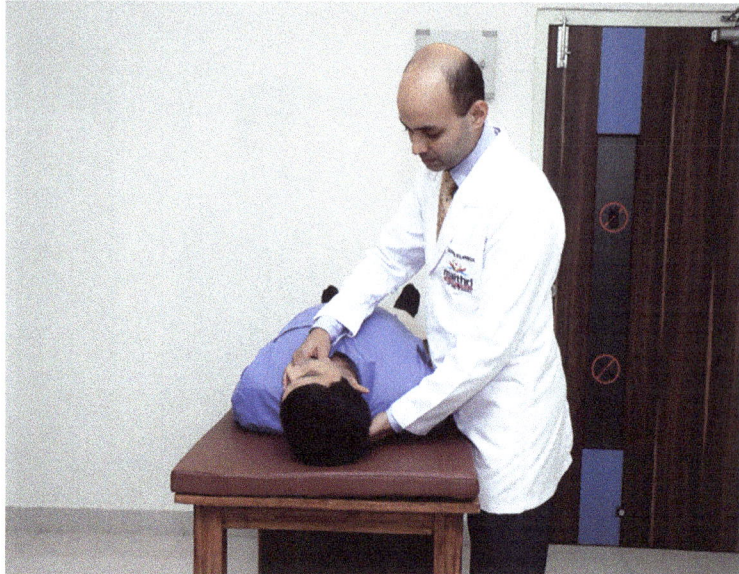

Fig. 15.28: The patient is made to lie down supine with the head turned by 45° to the affected side (left in this case) as the first step of the treatment. Then he is made to hold on for 10–30 seconds in each position before moving on to the next position.

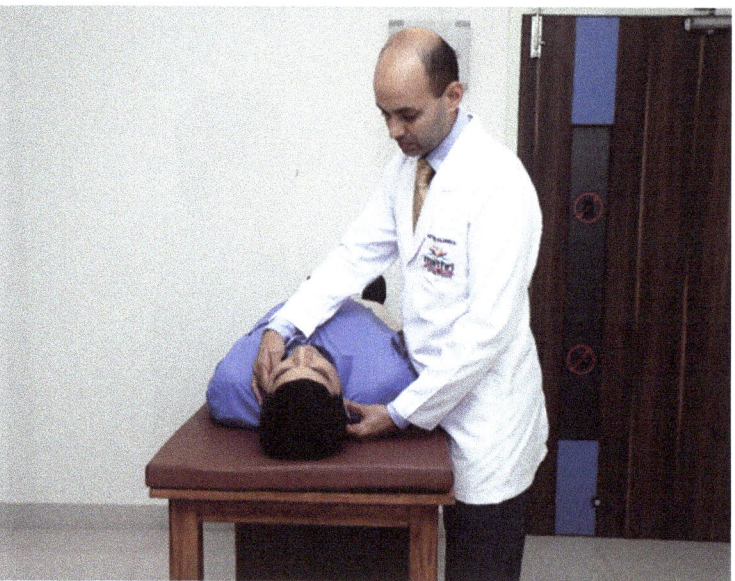

Fig.15.29A

Atlas of Diagnostic and Repositioning Techniques for BPPV | 263

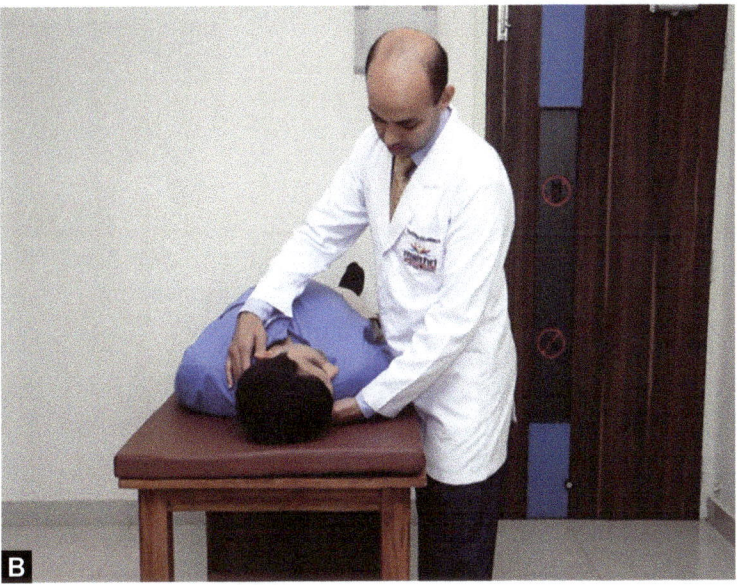

Figs. 15.29A and B: The patients head is then turned towards the unaffected side—(A) first to straight supine then (B) to further 90° to the opposite (unaffected) side.

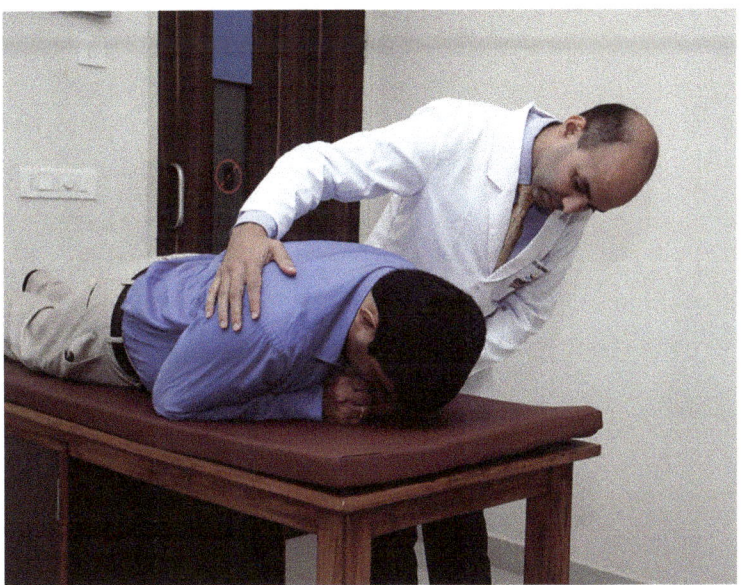

Fig. 15.30: On further turning over both the head and body by 90°, the patient is now lying down on his elbows with head slightly flexed so that the horizontal canal is now vertical.

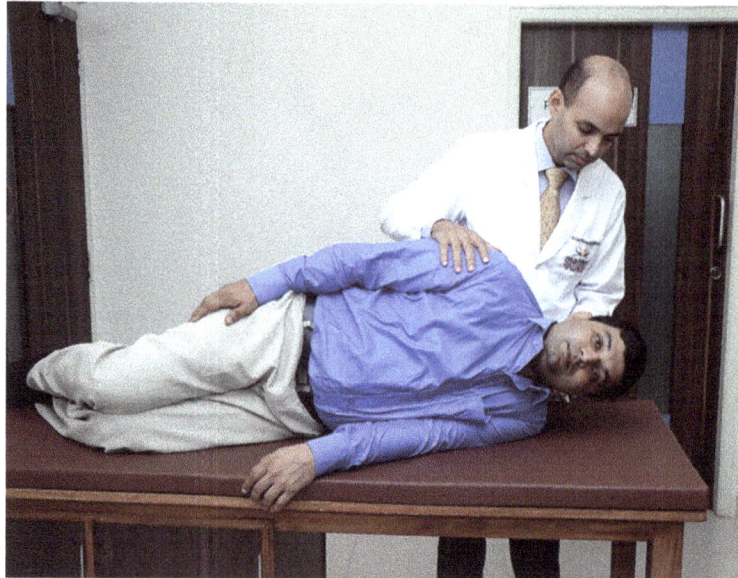

Fig. 15.31: The patient is then rolled over further in the same direction making him lie sideways on his affected side. In this position, the head may need to be supported by the examiner.

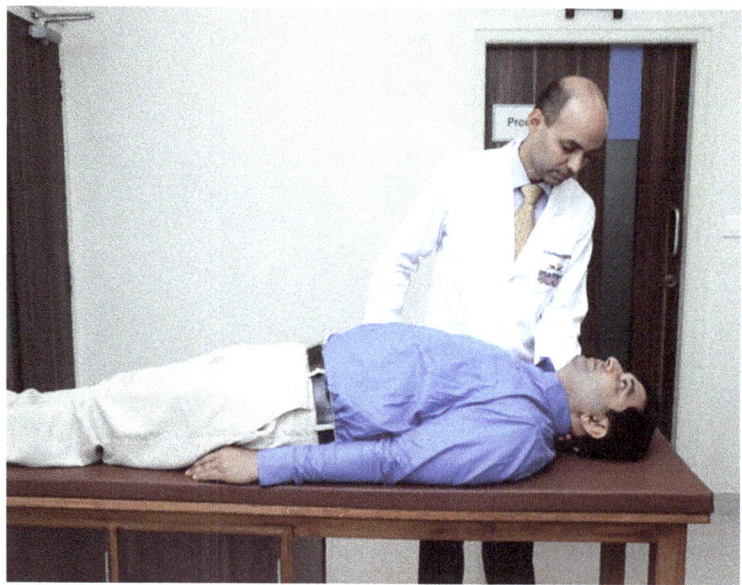

Fig.15.32A

Atlas of Diagnostic and Repositioning Techniques for BPPV | 265

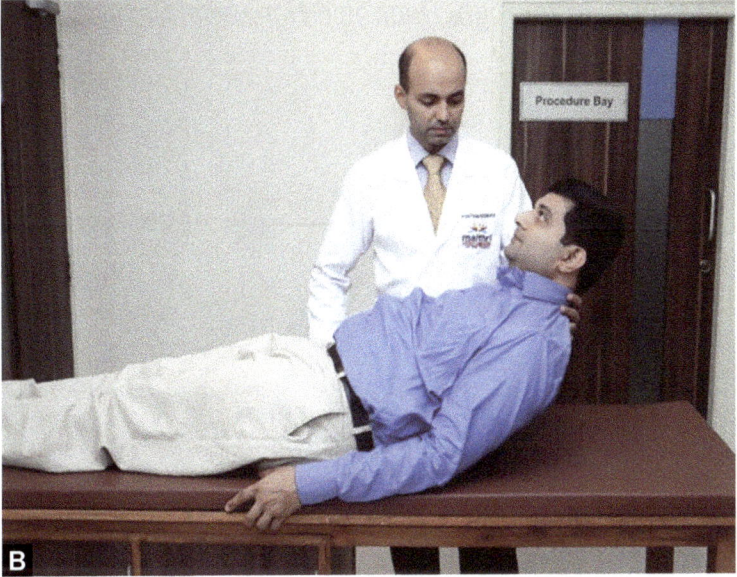

Figs. 15.32A and B: The patient then assumes (A) a straight supine position briefly. (B) while on his way to getting up.

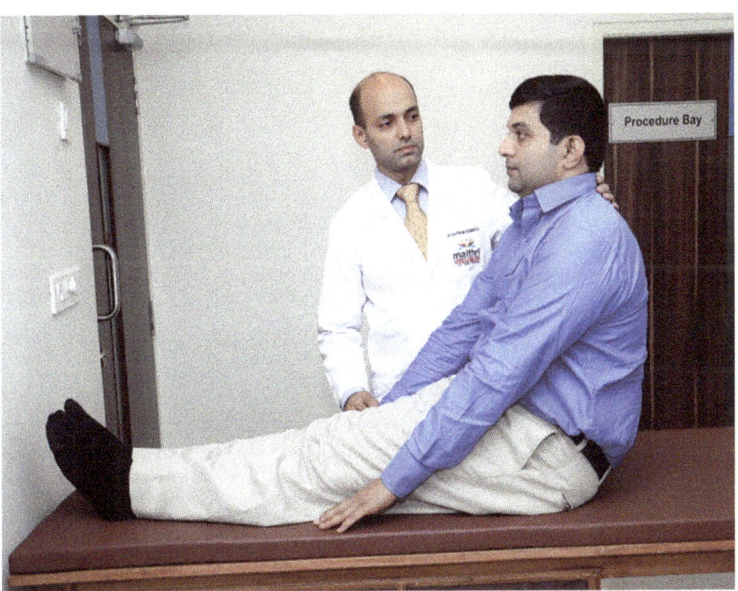

Fig. 15.33: The patient then rapidly assumes the sitting position as an end of the therapy.

Gufoni Maneuver for Right Geotropic Horizontal Canal BPPV

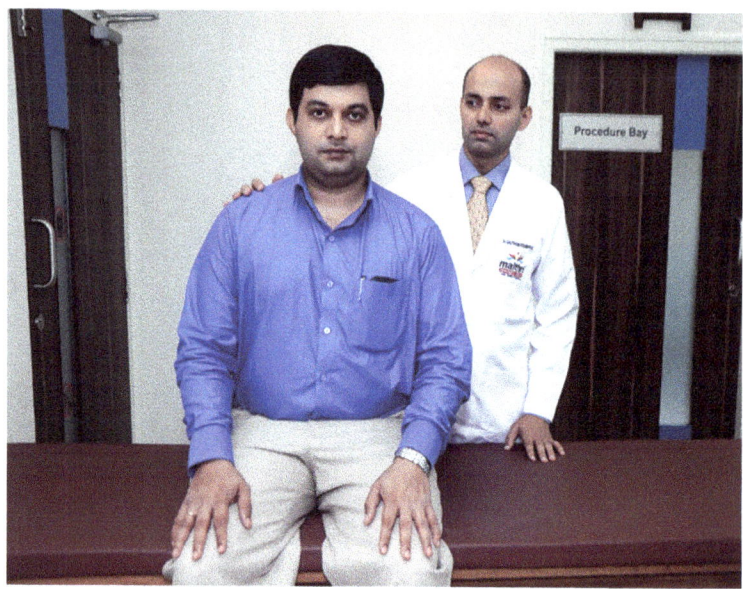

Fig. 15.34: The patient sits by the side of the bed with legs hanging outside.

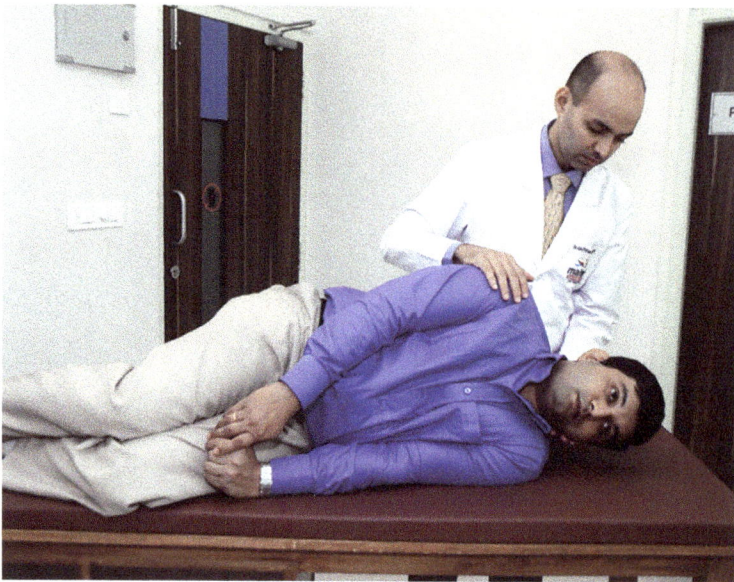

Fig. 15.35: The patient is then made to lie down laterally on the unaffected side (left in this case) for 1 minute.

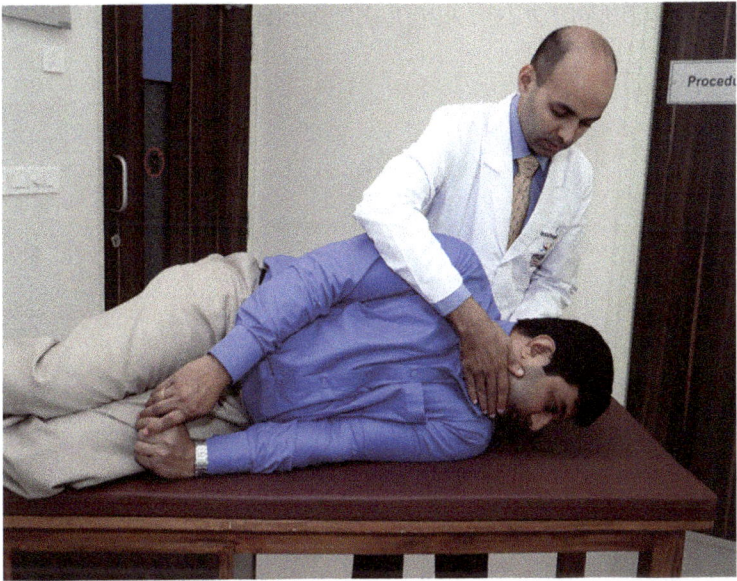

Fig. 15.36: Patient's head is then turned by 45°–60° toward the ground and held in position for 2 minutes.

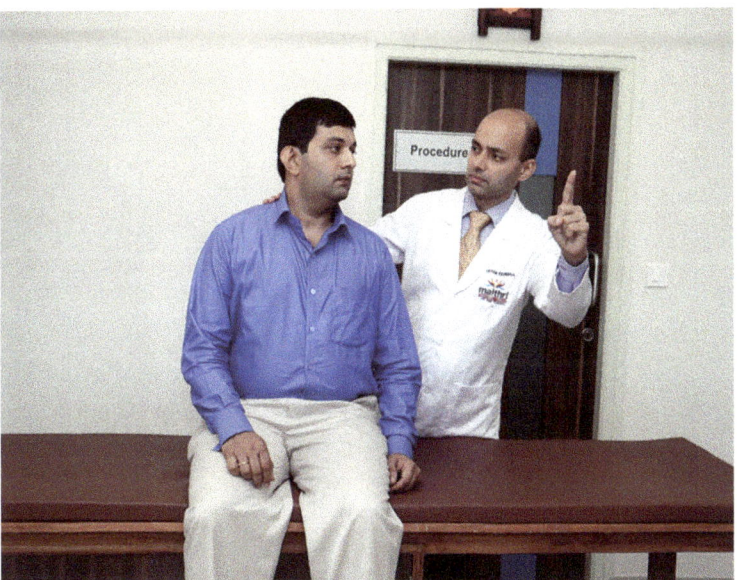

Fig. 15.37: The patient then sits back up with the head in the same position over the unaffected shoulder.

Gufoni Maneuver for Left Apogeotropic Horizontal Canal BPPV

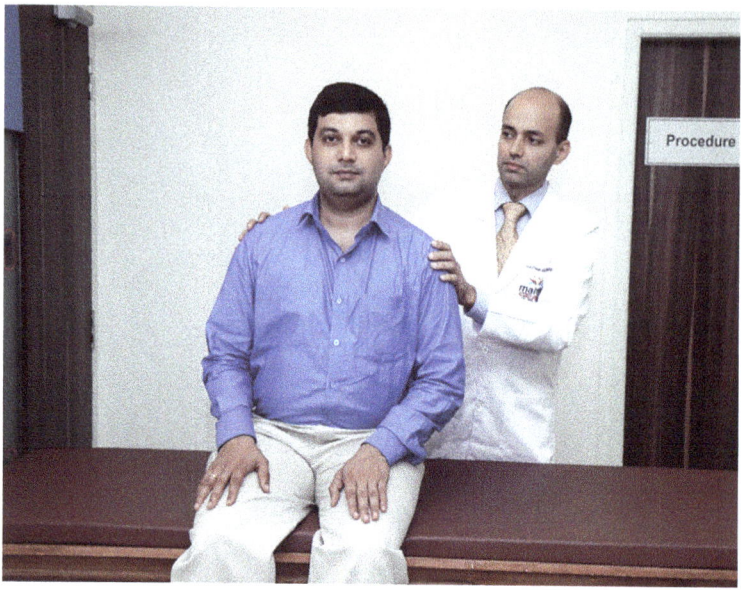

Fig. 15.38: The patient sits with legs hanging outside the bed and head in neutral position.

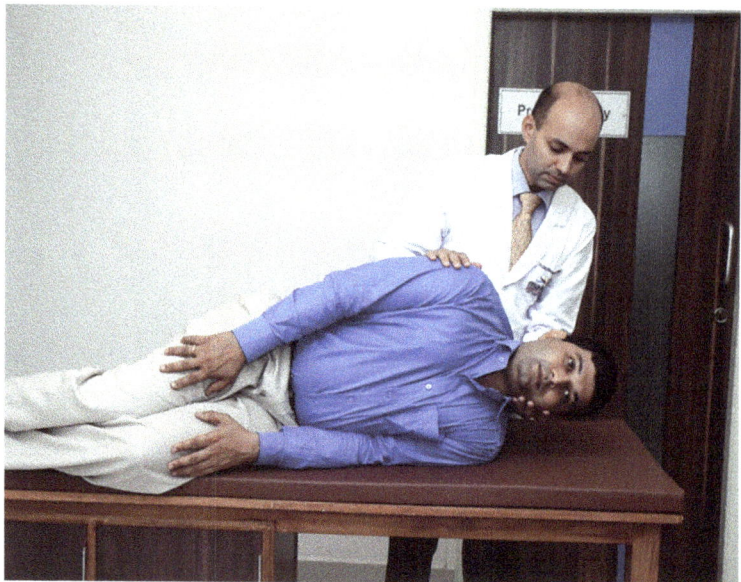

Fig. 15.39: The patient is made to lie down on the affected (left side in this case) lateral position while head is constantly being supported. He is maintained in this position for 2 mins.

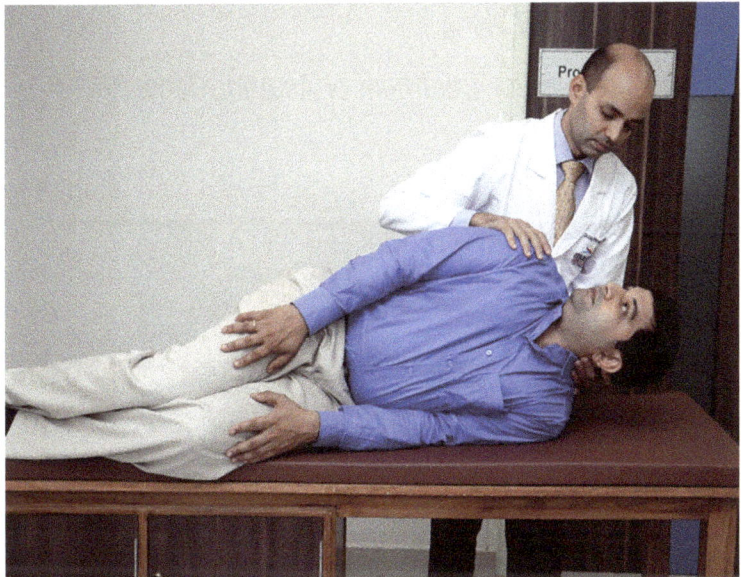

Fig. 15.40: Patient's head is then turned to the opposite side (right in this case) while head is still being supported. This position is maintained again for 2 minutes.

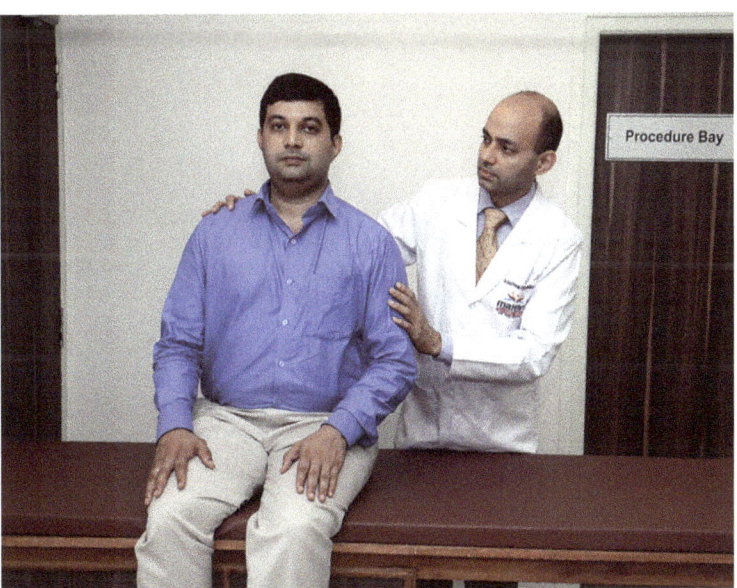

Fig. 15.41: The patient resumes the original sitting position.

Anterior Canal BPPV

Yacovino Maneuver for Treatment of Anterior Canal BPPV

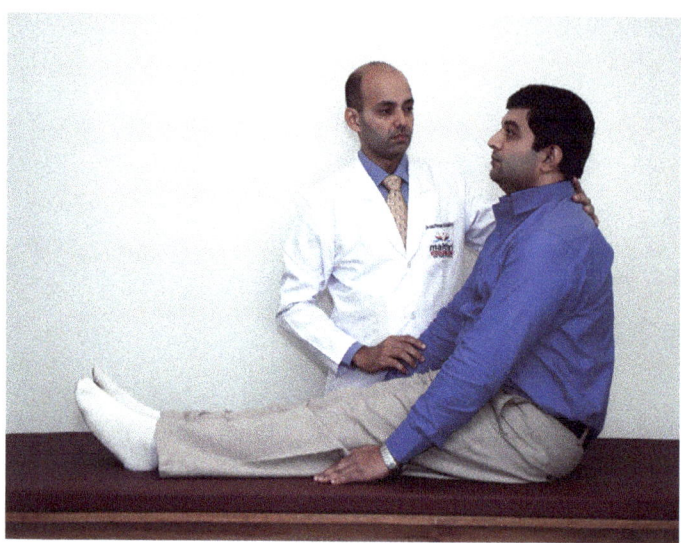

Fig. 15.42: The patient sits in the couch with the legs extended.

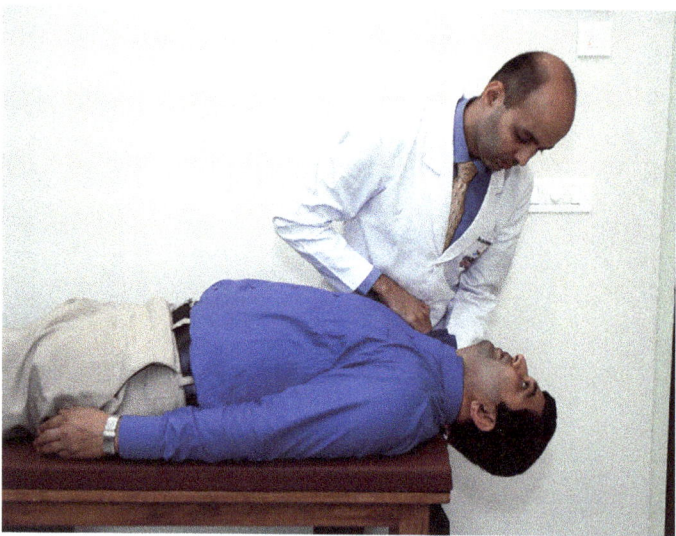

Fig. 15.43: The patient is then quickly made to lie supine with head extended by 30° and hanging outside the bed and supported by the therapist. The position is maintained for 30 seconds.

Atlas of Diagnostic and Repositioning Techniques for BPPV

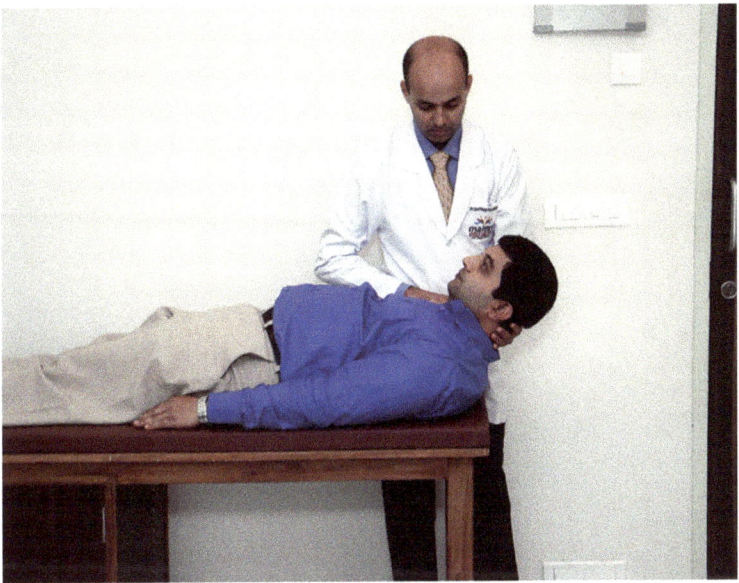

Fig. 15.44: Patient's head is then flexed by 30° for 30 seconds in the same supine position, the head still being supported by the therapist.

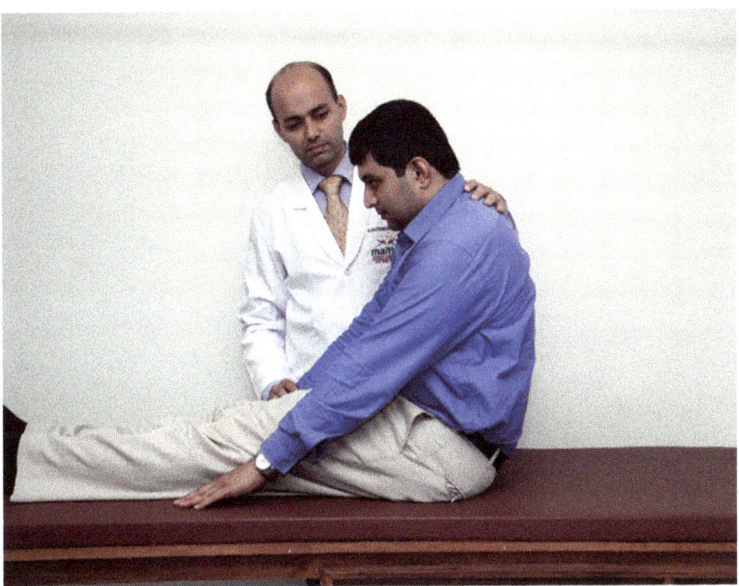

Fig. 15.45: The patient is then brought back to the sitting position with head flexed by 30° for another 30 seconds.

Index

Page numbers followed by f refer to figure and t refer to table.

A

Alprazolam 231
Amitriptyline 217
Ampullary nerve, posterior 241
Analolithiasis, physiological effects
    of 30, 33
Anxiolytic etizolam, low-dose 233
Apogeotropic variant 82
Arnold-Chiari malformation 46, 65,
    66, 114
Asprella maneuver 103, 106
    for right geotropic 107f
Audiological testing 225
Auditory canal, internal 7

B

Balance dysfunction, signs of 138
Barbecue rotation techniques 103
Bed with legs hanging 266f
Benign paroxysmal positional vertigo
    (BPPV) 40, 51f, 94, 95, 98, 99,
    111, 116, 135, 145, 157, 167, 168,
    171, 176, 179, 182, 184, 186, 187,
    193, 212, 214, 215, 216t, 224, 228,
    246, 248
    and migraine, association
        between 213
    anterior 122
        canal 67, 122, 181, 184, 187, 270
        posterior canal 184
    apogeotropic posterior canal 183
        semicircular 183
    bilateral 179
        horizontal canal 186t
    canal 54, 67, 248
        switch 171
    canalolithiasis nystagmus
        features 98t
    classification 95t, 113t
    differential diagnosis of 40
    in childhood 221, 223
    involving multiple canals 176
    medical management of 228
    nystagmus 189t
    of posterior canal 246
    pathophysiology of 30, 40
    patients 37
    phenomenon in 171
    physical therapy for 85
    posterior 184
        canal 67, 187, 250
    pseudovertical multicanal 128
    right geotropic horizontal 106f
    secondary 193
    semicircular canal 99
        function in 36f
    severe 230t
    subjective 157, 168
    surgery for 240
    symptoms of 40
    treating right posterior canal 250
    treatment for 226, 229
        anterior canal 270
        bilateral posterior canal 188
        multicanal 189
        unilateral horizontal canal 186t
        with otologic disease 225
        without nystagmus 44
Benzodiazepines 231
Betahistine 230
Bilateral lithiasis, actual 83
Bone mineral density 138
Brainstem 15, 68
    damage 113
Brandt-Daroff exercises 86f, 141

C

Calcium
    carbonate 12
    crystals 73
    metabolism, disorders of 165
Caloric responses 33
Caloric test 33

Caloric weakness 34
Canal
  cupulolithiasis 147
    posterior 146, 166
  disease
    anterior 188
    posterior 188
  horizontal, lateral 43
  occlusion surgery, posterior 243*f*
  posterior 30, 43, 84
  semicircular 151
  sensitivity axis 21
  switch 108, 171
  vestibulo-ocular reflex 76
Canalith repositioning 229
  maneuvers 123
  procedure 168, 229
Canalolithiasis 74*f*
  mechanism 184
Central nervous system (CNS) 1, 84, 113, 122, 126
  disorders 111
  dysfunction 65
  involvement 46
Central paroxysmal positional vertigo 68, 113, 114
Central positional
  nystagmus 66
  vertigo 64, 69, 111
Central vestibular disorder 126, 139
Cerebellar 113
  artery, anterior-inferior 6
  ataxia 114
  degeneration 66
  disorders 127*f*
  manifestations 147
Cerebellum 68
Cerebrovascular disease 65
Cervical muscles 38
Cervical spondylosis 51
Cervicogenic dizziness 47
Clonazepam 231
Clots 74
Cochlear artery, posterior 201
Cochlear function 225
Craniocervical junction 46
Crista, dysfunction of 203
Cupula, heavy 108

Cupulolithiasis 145, 230
  of lateral semicircular canal 153*t*
  physiological effects of 30, 33

D

Dental care 94
Depression 31, 234
Destroying semicircular canal 193
Diabetes 234
Diazepam 230, 231
Dimenhydrinate 230
Dix-Hallpike examination 204
Dix-Hallpike maneuver 77, 78*f*, 108, 114, 124, 137, 179, 186, 190, 216, 222
Dix-Hallpike position 87, 222
  maneuver 83
Dix-Hallpike test 78, 222*f*
Dizziness 73, 76, 78, 135, 204
  disorders 136, 137
  handicap inventory 159
  problem 141
Domestic injuries 94
Dorsal cerebellar vermis 69
Downbeat nystagmus 65
  causes of 66*t*
Downward facing nonampullary arm 104
Drug toxicity 66
Dysmetria 114

E

Ear 124
  canal 244
  disease 128
    inner 145, 193, 194, 204
  hemorrhage, inner 201
  left 44
  right 44
  surgery 128
Endolymphatic duct 8
Endolymphatic hydrops 194, 200, 203
Endolymphatic sac 8
Episodic vertigo 73
  acute 73
  causes of 73

Epley's Canalith-repositioning
    maneuver 88*f*
Epley's maneuver 147
Epley's original article 135
Erebellar degeneration 65
Eye
    muscles 18
    species 17

F

Female-to-male predominance 214

G

Geo-apogeo conversion 106
Geotropic nystagmus 116
Gufoni liberatory maneuver 103
Gufoni maneuver 106, 106*f*

H

Hair cells 25
Head
    and neck surgery 229
    and rest of body, relation
        between 251*f*
    and trunk positions 247*f*
    extension of 254*f*
    hanging 247*f*
        maneuver 125, 128
    impulse test 35
    pitch test 101
    shaking nystagmus 34
    shaking test 34
    stabilization 3
    thrust test 20
    trauma 197, 202, 207, 223
        postsurgical 197, 202
    yaw test 97, 99*f*, 112
Headache 198
Hydroxyzine 230
Hyperlipidemia 234
Hypertension 234
Hyposthenia 114

I

Imipramine 217

Inner ear
    disease
        chronic 208
        primary 205
    function, loss of 201
International Headache Society 213

L

Labyrinth
    anatomy of posterior 1
    partitioning of 243
    physiology of posterior 1
    vascular supply of 6*f*
Labyrinthine
    disease 21
    function 118
Leukoaraiosis 66
Light cupula 108
Lorazepam 230, 231

M

Macula 12
    dysfunction of 203
Maneuvers performed, common 153*t*
McClure-Pagnini test 97
Meclizine 230
Membranous labyrinth 2*f*
Ménière population 94
Ménière's disease 22, 45, 129, 145,
        194, 195, 200, 206, 225, 231
Metoclopramide 230
Migraine 118, 194, 198, 203, 207, 214
    associated vertigo 212
    positional vertigo 215, 216*t*
Migrainous vertigo 66
Multiple sclerosis 65
Multiple system atrophy 65

N

Nausea 221
Neck hyperextension 53
Neurectomy, singular 241
Neurological signs, abnormal 147
Nonorganic CNS disorder 113
Nortriptyline 217
Nystagmus 78, 98, 204, 216, 250, 254*f*
    direct 115
    direction 98

disappearance of 254*f*
during bowing and leaning 150
fatigue 98
latency 98
of migraine positional vertigo 215
paroxysmal 72
positional 222
quick phase 98

O

Oblique muscle 179
　inferior 17
Ocular
　fixation, increased 164
　tilt reaction 25
Oculomotor signs 147
Ondansetron 230
Osteoarthrosis 234
Otoacoustic emissions 225
Otoconia 12, 32, 164
　debris 221
　large 37
　metabolism of 224
　small 37
Otocyst 1
Otolith 12
　displacement 13*f*
　organs 25
　　fragments of 221
Otolithic dysfunction 89
Otolithic organ 12, 13*f*, 37

P

Paraneoplastic syndromes 66
Patient's eyes 254*f*
Peripheral vestibular
　disease, sign of 69
　disorder 128, 139
Phonophobia 215
Prochlorperazine 230
Promethazine 230
Pseudospontaneous nystagmus 99, 102, 150

R

Rabbits 17
Rectus muscle 179
Residual dizziness 89
Retina 27

S

Saccule 4, 5*f*, 26
Scarpa's ganglion 6
School injuries 94
Scopolamine 230
Segmental amyotrophy 114
Semicircular canal 1, 2*f*, 10, 32, 76
　anterior 49, 74, 95
　involvement 43
　posterior 49, 73, 89*f*, 95, 98, 171, 242, 243*f*
　right posterior 51*f*
　with nystagmus 43*t*
Semont's maneuver 89*f*
Serum levels 73
Spinning dizziness 72
Sports injuries 94
Stroke 234
Sudden sensorineural hearing loss 193, 197, 201, 207
Supine head-hanging 53
Syringomyelia 114

T

Therapeutic maneuver 261*f*
Thyroiditis, chronic 234
Troublesome disorder 90
Trunk 258*f*

U

Unilateral vestibular loss, acute 102
Urinary retention, drug-induced 232
Utricle 4, 5*f*, 25
Utricular function 38
Utricular trauma 198

V

Vannucchi-Asprella maneuver 103, 104, 105*f*
Velocity storage 23
Vertigo 76, 95, 135, 171
　cause of 178
　disorder 136
　duration of 216
　history of 123
　liberatory techniques 103*t*

paroxysmal positional 135, 195
patients 136
right benign positional
  paroxysmal 89*f*
sitting-up 163
symptoms 76
syndrome 73
treatment of central 69
Vestibular evoked myogenic
  potential 38, 225
Vestibular ganglion 6
Vestibular migraine 113-116, 136,
  212, 215, 218
  diagnostic criteria for 213*t*
  treatment of 217
Vestibular nerve 6
  fibers 6
  inferior 199

Vestibular neuritis 102, 129, 194,
  198, 205
Vestibular neuronitis 139
Vestibular nuclei 7
Vestibular organs 221
Vestibulocochlear artery 201
Vestibulo-ocular reflex 9*f*, 42
Videonystagmography 127*f*
Vitamin D 73, 235
  deficiency 235
Vomiting 68, 221

W

White blood cells 74

Y

Yacovino maneuver 270

EU GSPR Authorised Reprsentative
Logos Europe, 9 rue Nicolas Poussin
1700, La Rochelle, France
Phone: +33 (0) 6 67 93 73 78
E-mail: contact@logoseurope.eu